ABC of
Major Trauma

Fourth Edition

ABC series

An outstanding collection of resources for Healthcare Professionals

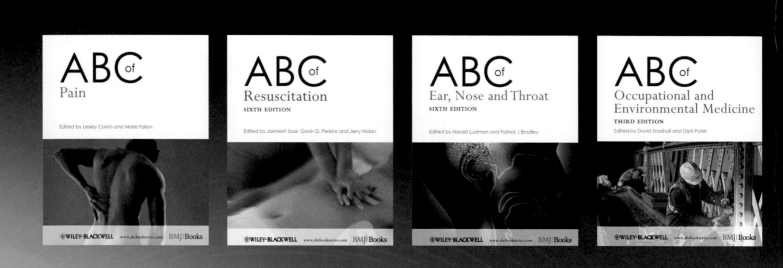

ABC of
Pain

Edited by Lesley Colvin and Marie Fallon

WILEY-BLACKWELL   www.abcbookseries.com   BMJ|Books

ABC of
Resuscitation
SIXTH EDITION

Edited by Jasmeet Soar, Gavin D. Perkins and Jerry Nolan

WILEY-BLACKWELL   www.abcbookseries.com   BMJ|Books

ABC of
Ear, Nose and Throat
SIXTH EDITION

Edited by Harold Ludman and Patrick J Bradley

WILEY-BLACKWELL   www.abcbookseries.com   BMJ|Books

ABC of
Occupational and
Environmental Medicine
THIRD EDITION

Edited by David Snashall and Dipti Patel

WILEY-BLACKWELL   www.abcbookseries.com   BMJ|Books

The *ABC* series contains a wealth of indispensable resources for GPs, GP registrars, junior doctors, doctors in training and specialised Healthcare Professionals

▶ **Highly illustrated, informative and a practical source of knowledge**

▶ **An easy-to-use resource, covering the symptoms, investigations, treatment and management of conditions presenting in day-to-day practice and patient support**

▶ **Full colour photographs and illustrations aid diagnosis and patient understanding of a condition**

For more information on all books in the *ABC* series, including links to further information, references and links to the latest official guidelines, please visit:

www.abcbookseries.com

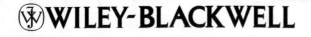

BMJ|Books

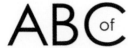

Major Trauma

Fourth Edition

EDITED BY

David V. Skinner
Consultant in Emergency Medicine
John Radcliffe Hospital
Oxford, UK

Peter A. Driscoll
Consultant in Accident and Emergency Medicine
Hope Hospital
Salford, UK

WILEY-BLACKWELL
A John Wiley & Sons, Ltd., Publication

BMJ|Books

This edition first published 2013, © 1991, 1996, 2000, 2013 by Blackwell Publishing Ltd

BMJ Books is an imprint of BMJ Publishing Group Limited, used under licence by Blackwell Publishing which was acquired by John Wiley & Sons in February 2007. Blackwell's publishing programme has been merged with Wiley's global Scientific, Technical and Medical business to form Wiley-Blackwell.

Registered office: John Wiley & Sons Ltd, The Atrium, Southern Gate, Chichester, West Sussex, PO19 8SQ, UK

Editorial offices: 9600 Garsington Road, Oxford, OX4 2DQ, UK

The Atrium, Southern Gate, Chichester, West Sussex, PO19 8SQ, UK

111 River Street, Hoboken, NJ 07030-5774, USA

For details of our global editorial offices, for customer services and for information about how to apply for permission to reuse the copyright material in this book, please see our website at www.wiley.com/wiley-blackwell.

Library of Congress Cataloging-in-Publication Data

ABC of major trauma / edited by David Skinner and Peter Driscoll. – 4th ed.
  p. ; cm.
 Includes bibliographical references and index.
 ISBN 978-0-7279-1859-8 (pbk. : alk. paper)
 I. Skinner, David V. II. Driscoll, P.A. (Peter A.), 1955-
 [DNLM: 1. Wounds and Injuries–therapy. 2. Emergencies. 3. Emergency Medical Services–methods. WO 700]
 617.1′026–dc23

                                                        2011043617

A catalogue record for this book is available from the British Library.

Wiley also publishes its books in a variety of electronic formats. Some content that appears in print may not be available in electronic books.

Cover image: iStock (17389284)
Cover design by Meaden Creative

Set in 9.25/12 Minion by Laserwords Private Limited, Chennai, India

Printed in Singapore by Ho Printing Singapore Pte Ltd

1   2013

Contents

Contents

List of Contributors

Munawar Al-Mudhaffar
Specialist Registrar in Emergency Medicine
Department of Emergency Medicine
John Radcliffe Hospital
Oxford, UK

Orla Austin
Department of Plastic Surgery
Pinderfields Hospital
Wakefield, UK

Dominic Barron
Consultant Radiologist
Leeds General Infirmary
Leeds, UK

John J.M. Black
Medical Director, South Central Ambulance Service;
Consultant in Emergency Medicine
John Radcliffe Hospital
Oxford, UK

Rebecca S. Black
Department of Obstetrics
John Radcliffe Hospital
Oxford, UK

Lizle Blom
Consultant in Emergency Medicine
Royal Berkshire Hospital
Reading, UK

Andrew Blyth
Royal Berkshire Hospital
Reading, UK

Mark Byers
Ministry of Defence
London, UK

Jon Clasper
Defence Professor, Orthopaedics and Trauma
Royal Centre for Defence Medicine
Birmingham, UK

Andre Cromhout
Emergency Physician
Emergency Department
Welllington Hospital
Wellington, New Zealand

Peter R. Davis
Consultant in Emergency Medicine
Defence Medical Services and Honorary Consultant
Southern General Hospital
Glasgow, UK

Martin P. Deahl
Consultant Psychiatrist
South Staffordshire and Shropshire Healthcare NHS Foundation Trust
Stafford, UK

Anthony Deane
Consultant Urologist
William Harvey Hospital
Ashford;
Buckland Hospital
Dover, UK

Peter A. Driscoll
Consultant in Accident and Emergency Medicine
Department of Emergency Medicine
Hope Hospital
Salford, UK

Karen A. Eley
Research Fellow
University of Oxford
Oxford, UK

John Elston
Consultant Ophthalmologist
Oxford Eye Hospital
Oxford University Hospitals NHS Trust
Oxford, UK

Oliver Fenton
Department of Plastic Surgery
Pinderfields Hospital
Wakefield, UK

Andrew Gibson
Consultant Ophthalmologist
The James Cook University Hospital
Middlesbrough, UK

Carl L. Gwinnutt
Consultant Anaesthetist
Hope Hospital
Salford, UK

Deborah J. Harrington
Department of Obstetrics
John Radcliffe Hospital
Oxford, UK

Jill Hill
Senior Sister
Emergency Department
John Radcliffe Hospital
Oxford, UK

Timothy J. Hodgetts
Chief Medical Officer
NATO Allied Rapid Reaction Corps;
Honorary Professor of Emergency Medicine
University of Birmingham
Birmingham, UK

Michael A. Horan
Hope Hospital
Salford, UK

Philip Hormbrey
Consultant in Emergency Medicine
Department of Emergency Medicine
John Radcliffe Hospital
Oxford, UK

Tom Hughes
Consultant in Emergency Medicine
John Radcliffe Hospital, Oxford;
Consultant in Emergency Medicine and Clinical
Director of Emergency Care
Hinchingbrooke Hospital, Huntingdon;
Hon. Senior Lecturer in Emergency Medicine
University of Oxford
Oxford, UK

Bruce Jenner
Trauma Nurse
Royal Air Force
UK

Rohit Kotnis
Specialist Registrar in Trauma and Orthopaedics
John Radcliffe Hospital
Oxford, UK

Peter F. Mahoney
Defence Professor Anaesthetics and Critical Care
Royal Centre for Defence Medicine
Birmingham, UK

Ajith Malalasekera
Department of Urology
Leicester General Hospital
Leicester, UK

Chris A.J. McLauchlan
Consultant in Emergency Medicine
Emergency Department
Royal Devon and Exeter Hospital
Exeter, UK

Lisa E. Munro-Davies
Consultant in Emergency Medicine
University Hospitals Bristol NHS Foundation Trust
Bristol, UK

Virginia Murray
Consultant Medical Toxicologist and Environmental Public Health
Head of Extreme Events and Health Protection
Health Protection Agency
London, UK

David Nicholson
Consultant Radiologist
Department of Emergency Medicine
Hope Hospital
Salford, UK

Jerry P. Nolan
Consultant Anaesthetist
Department of Anaesthesia and Intensive Care Medicine
Royal United Hospital
Bath, UK

Rachael Pery-Johnston
Department of Emergency Medicine
Princess Alexandra Hospital
Brisbane, QLD, Australia

Catherine Peters
Consultant in Critical Care Medicine and Anaesthesia
Department of Intensive Care
Homerton University Hospital
London, UK

Rick Pullinger
Consultant in Emergency Medicine
Department of Emergency Medicine
John Radcliffe Hospital
Oxford, UK

Jaskarn Rai
Department of Urology
Leicester General Hospital
Leicester, UK

James Rankine
Consultant Radiologist
Leeds General Infirmary
Leeds, UK

Colin Robertson
Consultant in Accident and Emergency Medicine
Department of Emergency Medicine
Royal Infirmary of Edinburgh
Edinburgh, UK

Nigel Rossiter
Consultant Trauma and Orthopaedic Surgeon
Basingstoke General Hospital;
Royal Defence Medical College
Basingstoke, UK

Rob Russell
Royal Army Medical Corps Consultant
Emergency Medicine
Royal Centre for Defence Medicine
Birmingham, UK

David V. Skinner
Consultant in Emergency Medicine
John Radcliffe Hospital
Oxford, UK

Andrew Swain
Senior Lecturer and Consultant in Emergency Medicine
University of Otago
Wellington, New Zealand

Timothy Terry
Consultant Urologist
Department of Urology
Leicester General Hospital
Leicester, UK

David Watson
Honorary Professor of Intensive Care Education
Department of Medical Education
Homerton University Hospital
London, UK

Steve R. Watt-Smith
Consultant Maxillofacial Surgeon
Honorary Clinical Senior Lecturer
Oxford University Hospitals NHS Trust
University of Oxford
Oxford, UK

Douglas Wilkinson
Consultant Anaesthetist in Intensive Care
Oxford University Hospitals NHS Trust
Oxford, UK

Keith Willett
Professor of Trauma Surgery
John Radcliffe Hospital
Oxford, UK

Alastair W. Wilson
Consultant in Emergency Medicine
Royal London Hospital
London, UK

Sarah J. Wilson
Consultant in Emergency Medicine
Wexham Park Hospital
Slough, UK

Maralyn Woodford
Executive Director
The Trauma Audit and Research Network
University of Manchester
Manchester, UK

Foreword

As a contributor and user of this book, I am delighted to see a fourth edition published. It represents a most useful core text for those seeking a contemporary practical guide to assess and deliver the best trauma care for those patients who are "candidate major traumas". All counties and healthcare systems are different and some changing, but the core principles of management are common. This text, through its breadth of expert contributors, succinctly describes these. Reading each chapter feels like you've just had a really good tutorial on the subject and represents a very efficient method of acquiring knowledge. I would certainly recommend you keep a copy of this publication close by whether preparing for your on-call day or a teaching session.

Keith Willett
Professor of Trauma Surgery
John Radcliffe Hospital
Oxford, UK

Preface

This edition of the *ABC of Major Trauma* has had a long gestation, being 12 years since the third edition.

Trauma care continues to evolve and improve both in the 'front line' and nationally with the development of Trauma Centres and supporting networks. Prevention is also playing its part, with deaths on the roads continuing to fall.

There is, however, no room for complacency and we hope this fourth edition will remind our readership of the crucial importance of a thorough, stepwise assessment of the trauma patient and that attention to detail, not least in spinal care, can avoid the devastating consequences of the 'second' injury.

This edition sees extensive revision of all its chapters and the addition of further material. At the time of publishing all information is current.

The book is aimed at all clinicians involved in front line trauma care, paramedics, hospital doctors and nurses as well as those members of the 'team', crucial to optimal management, including radiographers, radiologists and laboratory staff.

Chapter 29 reminds us of the excellent facilities available to us in UK practice. However, this chapter also shows us that simple manoeuvres can be life saving in the Third World environment.

The continuing conflicts around the world involving UK armed forces has resulted in improved trauma management in these conflict zones. Lessons learnt and techniques developed have been shared with civilian clinicians to the benefit of patients. Many authors in this edition have put themselves in 'harms way' to manage victims of conflict. This edition is dedicated to them.

David V. Skinner

Acknowledgements

I would like to acknowledge the help and guidance afforded to me by all at Wiley-Blackwell during the course of the production of this fourth edition of the *ABC of Major Trauma*.

I would like in particular to thank Adam Gilbert, Vicki Donald, Ilaria Meliconi, Laura Quigley, Kate Newell, Cathryn Gates and Helen Harvey whose support, encouragement, good humour and pure professionalism have seen this task to completion.

David V. Skinner

List of Abbreviations

5-HT	5-hydroxytryptamine		FRC	functional residual capacity
ABC	airway, breathing, circulation		GCS	Glasgow Coma Scale
ACE	angiotensin-converting enzyme inhibitor		GDP	Gross Domestic Product
AIC	ambulance incident commander		GP	general practitioner
AIS	Abbreviated Injury Scale		HART	hazardous area response team
AP	anteroposterior		HBOC	haemoglobin-based oxygen carrier
APLS	Advanced Paediatric Life Support		HCT	hospital co-ordination team
ARDS	acute respiratory distress syndrome		HCVR	hypercapnic ventilatory response
ASD	acute stress disorders		HPA	Health Protection
ATLS	Advanced Trauma Life Support			Agency/hypothalamo-pituitary-adrenal
ATP	adenosine triphosphate		HR	heart rate
BATLS	Battlefield Advanced Trauma Life Support		HVR	hypoxic ventilatory response
BP	blood pressure		ICP	intracranial pressure
BVM	bag-valve-mask		ICU	intensive care unit
CAT	computed axial tomography		I/E	inspiratory/expiratory
CBF	cerebral blood flow		IED	improvised explosive device
CBT	cognitive-behavioural therapy		IO	intraosseous
CCS	casualty clearing station		IPE	individual protective equipment
CHaPD	Chemical Hazards and Poisons Division		ISS	Injury Severity Score
COPD	chronic obstructive pulmonary disease		ITU	intensive therapy unit
CPB	cardiopulmonary bypass		IV	intravenous
CPP	cerebral perfusion pressure		MAP	mean arterial pressure
CPR	cardiopulmonary resuscitation		MERIT	medical emergency incident response team
CRT	capillary refill time		MIC	medical incident commander
CSF	cerebrospinal fluid		MODS	multiorgan dysfunction syndrome
CT	computed tomography		MRI	magnetic resonance imaging
CXR	chest X-ray		NAI	non-accidental injury
DCLHb	diaspirin cross-linked haemoglobin solution		NGT	nasogastric tube
DIC	disseminated intravascular coagulation		NICE	National Institute for Health and Clinical Excellence
DPL	diagnostic peritoneal lavage		NPIS	National Poisons Information Service
DVT	deep venous thrombosis		NSAID	non-steroidal anti-inflammatory drug
ECG	electrocardiogram		PEEP	positive end-expiratory pressure
ECMO	extracorporeal membranous oxygenation		PPE	personal protective equipment
ED	emergency department		PPH	postpartum haemorrhage
EEG	electroencephalogram		PTA	post-traumatic amnesia
ET	endotracheal		PTC	Primary Trauma Care
ETA	expected time of arrival		PTSD	post-traumatic stress disorder
ETCO$_2$	end-tidal carbon dioxide concentration		RSI	rapid-sequence induction
FAST	focused assessment with sonography in trauma		RTA	road traffic accident
FBC	full blood count		RTC	road traffic crash
FFP	fresh frozen plasma		RTS	Revised Trauma Score
FiO$_2$	fraction of inspired oxygen		SaO$_2$	oxygen saturation

SCIWORA	spinal cord injury without radiological abnormality	TNF	tumour necrosis factor
SHO	senior house officer	US	ultrasound
SIGN	Scottish Intercollegiate Guidelines Network	USAR	urban search and rescue
SIRS	systemic inflammatory response syndrome	WHO	World Health Organization
SXR	plain radiograph of the skull	ZPP	zone of partial preservation
TARN	Trauma Audit and Research Network		

CHAPTER 1

Initial Assessment and Management: Primary Survey and Resuscitation

David V. Skinner[1] and Peter A. Driscoll[2]

[1]John Radcliffe Hospital, Oxford, UK
[2]Hope Hospital, Salford, UK

OVERVIEW

- Initial management of trauma victims requires a team approach in which each member carries out a specific task. Collectively, the team should aim to treat all the immediately life-threatening conditions and identify the need for surgery early.

- The ABC (airway, breathing, circulation) approach provides an optimal system whereby urgent, potentially life-threatening conditions are dealt with first.

- The critically injured patient requires a calm rapid response to his/her injuries, in the field, resuscitation room and operating theatre. If prehospital personnel, the resuscitation room team and its leader, as well as the appropriate surgeons can deliver this, then lives will be saved and unnecessary deaths avoided. Any deaths that do occur will have been unavoidable. The team should also be aware of this and suitably debriefed.

Morbidity and mortality in seriously injured patients, managed in UK hospitals, remain higher than necessary. Recognition of this problem over the last 25 years has seen a variety of initiatives designed to improve the situation, including the introduction of Advanced Trauma Life Support (ATLS) to clinical practice, the widespread use of the auditing tool TARN (Trauma Audit and Research Network), and the deployment of multidisciplinary trauma teams to manage trauma victims in emergency department (ED) resuscitation rooms. Increasingly, consultant-delivered services, where available, will further enhance care.

For each individual patient, however, survival and reduction of long-term disability depend on the rapid deployment of skilled prehospital clinicians (paramedics and/or doctors), the skills and experience of the receiving clinicians (trauma team) and the human and other resources available round the clock to deal with patient injuries in a timely and effective fashion.

Most seriously injured patients seen in UK EDs have suffered blunt trauma. This, by its very nature, presents its own unique set of difficulties for the clinician, not least because serious life-threatening injuries may be initially covert, especially in the young. Prehospital clinicians may not recognise potential problems; this may be further compounded by a failure of recognition by the receiving hospital, leading to inappropriate triage. Lone junior doctors may then find themselves assessing a deteriorating trauma patient in an unmonitored area of the ED, leading to potential catastrophe.

All ED doctors should therefore be ATLS trained and encouraged to have a very low threshold for 'upgrading' such patients without delay to the resuscitation room for a team response. Such upgrade should include not only the deteriorating patient, but also those in whom the mechanism of injury suggests the possibility of serious problems. In the authors' experience, most problems arise from a failure to understand, or take note of, the mechanism's injurious potential, rather than poor management of an overtly seriously injured patient.

Comprehensive management protocols (usually ATLS) must be followed to the letter. Short cuts expose patients to risk which will lead some into difficulty. The 'experienced' clinician's personal opinion must be outweighed every time by the multitude of experienced clinicians who devised the protocol. Such protocols are frequently driven by the need to avoid the errors of the past.

The introduction of trauma centres will hopefully produce a further improvement in trauma care but in the end, individual clinicians, either working alone or as trauma team leaders, bear the responsibility for ensuring optimum care.

Effective ED care depends on the following.

- Safe, accurate receipt of prehospital information regarding the trauma victim or victims.
- Assembly of a competent trauma team, competently led, and dressed in protective clothing.
- The team's ability to identify immediately life-threatening problems and begin their correction.
- Limiting investigations and interventions to those crucial to addressing life-threatening problems.
- Ready availability of all investigation modalities, and a suitably urgent response by labs, radiology, intensive therapy units (ITU) and theatres.
- The additional ability to sensibly allocate resources when a multivictim response is needed.

Trauma centre 'feeder units' will not have the resources and manpower to provide a full trauma team response 24 hours a day,

7 days a week. In spite of this and given the difficulty of complete triage accuracy in the prehospital field, seriously injured patients will continue to arrive at such feeder centres. It is crucial therefore that such patients are managed in a logical way, based on ATLS, before possible onward transfer to a trauma centre. The main difference will be that the resuscitation phase will take longer given the reduced numbers in the trauma team.

Where a trauma team can be made available round the clock then it is in the patient's interests that it should be deployed. The following text suggests one way in which such a team should be developed and deployed. Individual centres will decide on the exact composition of such teams and comparative national data will identify the optimum team size and composition.

The trauma team

Personnel

The trauma team (Figure 1.1) should initially comprise four doctors, five nurses and a radiographer. The medical team consists of a team leader, an 'airway' doctor and two 'circulation' doctors. The nursing team comprises a team leader, an 'airway' nurse, two 'circulation' nurses and a 'relatives' nurse.

Team members' roles

Examples of paired roles and tasks are given below but assignments may vary among units depending on the resources available. To avoid chaos, no more than six people should be touching the patient. The other team members must keep well back. The objectives of the trauma team are shown in Box 1.1.

> Box 1.1 **Objectives of the trauma team**
>
> - Identify and correct life-threatening injuries.
> - Commence resuscitation.
> - Determine the nature and extent of other injuries.
> - Prioritise investigation/treatment needs.
> - Prepare and transport the patient to a place of continuing care.

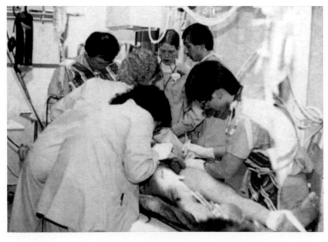

Figure 1.1 Trauma team in action.

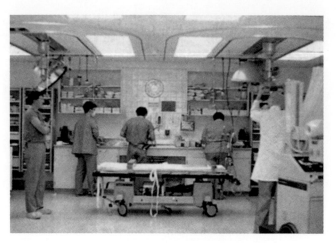

Figure 1.2 The resuscitation room: preparing for the patient's arrival.

Before the patient arrives

All EDs should be warned by the ambulance service of the impending arrival of a seriously injured patient. This communication system can also provide the trauma team with helpful information about the patient's condition and the paramedics' prehospital interventions.

After the warning, the team should assemble in the resuscitation room (Figure 1.2) and put on protective clothing. A safe minimum would be rubber latex gloves, plastic aprons and eye protection because all blood and body fluids should be assumed to carry HIV and hepatitis viruses. Ideally, full protective clothing should be worn by each member of the team, and all must have been immunised against tetanus and the hepatitis B virus. Trauma patients often have sharp objects such as glass and other debris in their clothing and hair and on their skin, and therefore suitable precautions must be taken by all team members.

While protective clothing is being put on, the team leader should brief the team, allocating roles and responsibilities. A final check of the equipment by the appropriate team members can then be made. As the resuscitation room must be kept fully stocked and ready for use at any time, only minimum preparation should be necessary.

Roles of trauma team members

Medical and other staff
Team leader

- Co-ordinates the activities of the whole team.
- Performs a rapid initial primary survey to identify any immediately life-threatening problems.
- Ensures that airway and circulation team members are managing their roles rapidly.
- Allocates a suitably skilled team member to any task necessary, e.g. chest drain.
- Constantly prioritises patient's needs and team's activities.
- Ensures all information from prehospital team is noted.

- Ensures that other specialist clinicians are urgently alerted as soon as their need is identified.

Airway doctor

- Clears and secures the airway while taking appropriate cervical spine precautions.
- Inserts central and arterial lines if required.

Circulation doctors

- Assist in the removal of the patient's clothes.
- Establish peripheral intravenous infusions and take blood samples for investigations.
- Carry out other procedures depending on their skill level.

Radiographer

- Takes three standard X-ray films on all patients subjected to blunt trauma: chest, pelvis and lateral cervical spine.

Nursing staff
Team leader

- Co-ordinates the nursing team and liaises with the medical team leader.
- Records clinical findings, laboratory results, intravenous fluid and drug infusion, and the vital signs as called out by the circulation nurse.
- Prepares sterile packs for procedures.
- Assists the circulation nurses and brings extra equipment as necessary.

Airway nurse

- Assists in securing the airway and the cervical spine.
- Establishes a rapport with the patient in the resuscitation room. Ideally all information should be fed through this nurse to the patient.

Circulation nurses

- Assist in the removal of the patient's clothes.
- Assist with starting intravenous infusions, blood bottle labelling and other tasks allocated to the circulation doctor.
- Measure the vital signs and connect the patient to the monitors.

Relatives' nurse

- Cares for the patient's relatives.

Reception and transfer

The team leader should meet the patient and prehospital team in the ambulance bay and accompany them to the resuscitation room. The essential prehospital information required by the trauma team is shown in Box 1.2. The nursing team leader should start the stop clock so that accurate times can be recorded.

Box 1.2 **Essential prehospital information**

- Nature of the incident.
- Number, age and sex of the casualties.
- The patient's complaints, priorities and injuries.
- Airway, ventilatory and circulatory status.
- The conscious level and spinal status.
- Estimated time of arrival.

The transfer of the patient from stretcher to trolley must be co-ordinated to avoid rotation of the spinal column or exacerbation of pre-existing injuries (see Chapter 8). Team members should also check that lines and leads are free so that they do not become disconnected or snagged.

Primary survey and resuscitation

The objectives of this phase are to identify and treat any immediately life-threatening condition (Box 1.3). Each patient should be assessed in the same way, and the appropriate tasks performed automatically and simultaneously by the team. It is vital that problems are anticipated and prepared for, rather than reacted to. If the patient deteriorates at any stage, the medical team leader must reassess the patient, beginning again with the airway.

Box 1.3 **Objectives**

- **Primary survey and resuscitation**
  Airway and cervical spine control
  Breathing
  Circulation and haemorrhage control
  Dysfunction of the central nervous system
  Exposure and environmental control
- **Secondary survey**
- **Definitive care**

As previously suggested, the team leader should perform a rapid primary survey to identify immediately life-threatening conditions. This should take no longer than 1–2 min. The management of individual problems identified in this rapid primary survey is detailed below. The tasks are allocated to team members and take place concurrently rather than in a stepwise approach as laid out below.

Airway management, with cervical spine protection

Assume that the cervical spine has been damaged if there is a history of a high-speed impact, head injury, neck pain or any positive neurology. If the ambulance service have immobilised then assume a C-spine injury until proven otherwise. The doctor dealing with the airway should talk to the patient with the neck immobile and if the patient replies appropriately with a normal voice, then the airway is patent and the brain is being perfused adequately with oxygenated blood. If there is no reply, the patient's airway should be checked, cleared and managed appropriately. This is the first and pre-eminent priority.

The complications of alcohol ingestion and possible injuries to the chest and abdomen increase the chance of regurgitation. If the patient does vomit and is on a spinal board, the trolley should be tipped head down by 20° and the vomit sucked away with a rigid sucker as it appears in the mouth. If not on a spinal board then log roll the patient and suck out.

Progressively interventionist manoeuvres should be employed as necessary including chin lift/jaw thrust, Guedel airway (Figure 1.3) insertion (although these can precipitate vomiting) and deployment of a nasopharyngeal airway (Figure 1.4) which is preferred (less likely to cause vomiting) provided that there is no evidence of a base of skull fracture.

Apnoeic patients require ventilation with a bag-valve-mask device initially but this may lead to gastric distension with air and can induce vomiting, so early intubation should be considered. Orotracheal intubation with in-line stabilisation of the neck is

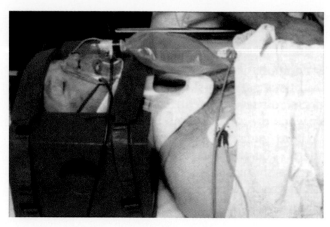

Figure 1.5 Patient with rigid collar in place.

recommended, rather than nasotracheal intubation. If this proves impossible (rarely) then a surgical airway must be provided.

Once the airway has been cleared and secured, every patient should receive 100% oxygen at a flow rate of 15 L/min. The neck must then be examined for wounds, tracheal position, venous distension, surgical emphysema and laryngeal crepitus. Confirmation of the security of the cervical spine, using a semi-rigid collar, sand bags and tape, is crucial. The only exception is the restless and thrashing patient. Here the cervical spine can be damaged by immobilising the head and neck while allowing the rest of the body to move. Suboptimal immobilisation with just a semi-rigid collar is therefore accepted (Figure 1.5).

Breathing

Listed in Box 1.4 are five immediately life-threatening thoracic conditions that must be urgently identified and treated during the primary survey and resuscitation phase (see Chapter 4).

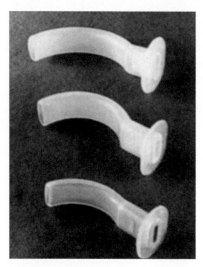

Figure 1.3 Guedel airway.

> Box 1.4 **Immediately life-threatening thoracic conditions**
>
> - Tension pneumothorax.
> - Cardiac tamponade.
> - Open chest wound.
> - Massive haemothorax.
> - Flail chest.

All clothes covering the front and sides of the chest must be removed. The respiratory rate, effort and symmetry must be noted. These are sensitive indicators of underlying pulmonary contusion, haemothorax, pneumothorax and fractured ribs. The team leader must examine both sides of the chest for bruising, abrasions, open wounds and evidence of penetrating trauma. Cardiac tamponade after trauma is usually associated with a penetrating injury. The team leader should also remember that because of intercostal muscle spasm, paradoxical breathing is seen with a flail chest only if the segment is large or central, or when the patient's muscles become fatigued. The patient with a flail

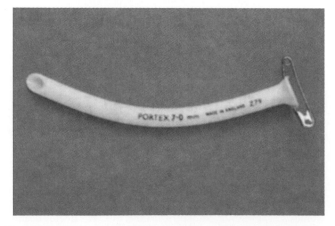

Figure 1.4 Nasopharyngeal airway.

chest usually has a rapid, shallow, symmetrical respiratory pattern initially.

After inspection, the chest should be auscultated and percussed to assess symmetry of ventilation and resonance. As listening over the anterior chest detects mainly air movement in the large airways, it is recommended that the medical team leader also listens over the axillae to gain a more accurate assessment of pulmonary ventilation. A tension pneumothorax or massive haemothorax can thus be identified. Early chest X-ray (CXR) is crucial: clinical examination in the context of major trauma is unreliable. Pneumothorax or haemothorax should be treated by inserting a chest drain with a gauge of >28 in the fifth intercostal space just anterior to the midaxillary line. This enables air and fluid to be drained but should always be preceded by intravenous lines. During examination of the chest, the patient should be attached to a pulse oximeter. Common causes of inadequate ventilation are shown in Box 1.5.

Box 1.5 Common causes of inadequate ventilation

- Bilateral
  - Obstruction of the upper respiratory tract
  - Leak between the face and mask
- Unilateral
  - Pneumothorax
  - Haemothorax
  - Intubation of the right main bronchus
  - Foreign body in a main bronchus, significant lung contusion

---

Circulation and haemorrhage control

The medical team leader will look for clinical signs of shock (see Chapter 5), apparent with tachycardia, poor capillary refill and peripheral perfusion. It is important to remember that up to 30% loss of blood volume produces tachycardia and reduces the pulse pressure, but the blood pressure may stay within normal limits (particularly in the young).

There is a consistent fall in the systolic blood pressure only when more than 30% of the blood volume has been lost.

The circulation doctor must control any major external haemorrhage by direct pressure. Tourniquets are usually only used when the affected limb is deemed unsalvageable.

A pelvic splint should be used when there is a suspected pelvic fracture and this may already have been applied by the prehospital team.

Concurrently with the above, two wide-bore (14–16 gauge) peripheral lines must be inserted, preferably in the antecubital fossae. If this is impossible, venous access should be gained by a venous cutdown or by inserting a short, wide-bore central line into the femoral or subclavian vein. If a subclavian approach is used and a chest drain is already in place, the central line must be inserted on the same side. As central vein cannulation can cause serious injury, it should be carried out only by experienced personnel.

Once the first cannula is in position, 20 mL of blood should be drawn for group, type or full cross-match, full blood count, and measurement of urea and electrolyte concentrations. An arterial sample should also be taken for blood gas and pH analysis, but this can wait until the end of the primary survey. While venous access is being gained, a circulation nurse must measure the blood pressure and record the rate, volume and regularity of the pulse. An automatic blood pressure recorder and electrocardiogram (ECG) monitor should also be attached to the patient. In seriously ill patients, palpating femoral and carotid pulses is a quick and reliable method of establishing whether there is some cardiac output when no blood pressure can be recorded, either automatically or otherwise.

In the UK, the type of fluid initially given to injured patients to maintain fluid balance depends on departmental policy. Some start with colloid while others use crystalloid such as physiological saline. It is therefore important for team leaders to know the local policy. The aim of fluid management in a hypotensive resuscitation should be to restore critical organ perfusion until haemorrhage that is amenable to surgery is stemmed. Therefore the initial approach in a standard adult trauma victim is to give 1 L of warm colloid (or 2 L of crystalloid) and then reassess the patient. Remember that the best colloid is blood and, where necessary, this should be given as soon as possible. This underlines the importance of early cross-match and an effective chain between the resuscitation room, labs and back again!

When there is a limited response to the fluid bolus, or after a major injury, blood is urgently required. To reduce the incidence of hypothermia, all fluids must be warmed before use.

In reassessing the circulatory state one of three responses will be seen (Figure 1.6).

- The vital signs return to normal after infusion of less than 1 L of colloid solution (or 2 L of physiological saline). Such patients have lost less than 20% of their blood volume and are probably not actively bleeding.
- The vital signs initially improve with the infusion but then deteriorate. These patients are actively bleeding and have usually lost more than 20% of their blood volume. They require transfusion with typed blood and the source of the bleeding must be controlled. This often requires surgery.
- The vital signs do not improve at all. This suggests either that the shock has not been caused by hypovolaemia or that the patient is bleeding faster than blood is being infused. History, mechanism of injury and physical findings will help to distinguish between these possibilities.

Measurement of the central venous pressure and, in particular, its change after a fluid bolus may assist in diagnosis. There are a limited number of anatomical sites of bleeding: external, into the chest or abdomen, or around a fractured pelvis or long bones. Skilled FAST (focused assessment with sonography in trauma) ultrasound will confirm intra-abdominal blood and clinical examination and CXR will identify the others.

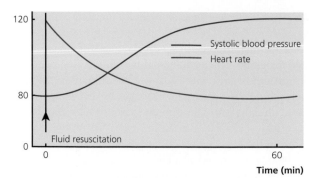

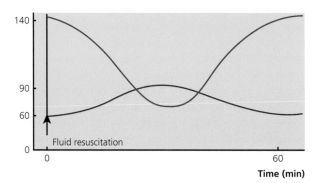

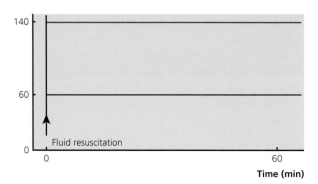

Figure 1.6 The three responses to fluid resuscitation.

Patients with hypovolaemia whose vital signs do not improve at all have lost more than 40% of their blood and usually require immediate operation (Box 1.6). It is crucially important that the likely 'operators', usually the general surgeons, have been fast-bleeped to the resuscitation room as soon as this possibility has been entertained by the team leader. They can then be involved in the diagnostic process and this results in earlier surgery.

Box 1.6 Circulation and haemorrhage control

- Patients with hypovolaemia whose vital signs do not improve at all when fluid is administered have lost more than 40% of their blood volume.
- The source of the bleeding is usually in the thorax, abdomen or pelvis (and/or long bones), and requires immediate operation.

Dysfunction of the central nervous system

A rapid assessment of brain and spinal cord function is made by assessing the pupillary reflexes and by asking patients to 'put out your tongue', 'wiggle your toes' and 'squeeze my fingers'. The patient must also be assessed on the AVPU scale (Box 1.7). Remember, however, that these quick manoeuvres will detect only gross neurological damage. A more detailed assessment, including assessment of the Glasgow Coma Scale, can be used if there is time, but is often delayed until the secondary survey.

Early recognition of spinal injury mandates continuing close attention to spinal protection and early involvement of spinal surgeons and relevant investigations. Head injuries are obvious but spinal injuries less so. One of the trauma team's principal roles is to 'do no further harm'. Inadvertent movement of a trauma patient with an unstable spinal column injury may damage a thus far uninjured cord. Such 'second' injuries are irreversible and life-long.

Box 1.7 Conscious level can be assessed by the ATLS system of AVPU

A = Alert
V = Responds to voice
P = Responds to pain
U = Unconscious

Exposure and environment

By this stage, all clothing impeding the primary survey should have been cut away with minimal patient movement, using large, sharp scissors. Remaining clothing should now be removed. To prevent patients subsequently becoming cold, they should be covered with warm blankets (and/or a Bair Hugger) when not being examined and the resuscitation room kept warm.

By the end of the primary survey and the team's interventions, the medical team leader must make sure that all the allocated tasks have been completed. The vital signs should continue to be recorded every 5 min, to detect the patient's progress or deterioration. Only when all ventilatory and circulatory problems have been corrected (which may mean surgery) can the team continue with the more detailed secondary survey (in the resuscitation room or later after surgery).

While the primary survey and resuscitation phase is under way, the relatives' nurse should greet any of the patient's friends or relatives who arrive. He or she can then take them to a private room that has all necessary facilities and stay there with them, providing support and information. Relatives should not be prevented from seeing the patient in the resuscitation room. However, they must be accompanied by the relatives' nurse so that they can be fully informed (see Chapter 16).

Team leader co-ordination

As well as the direction of the above, the team leader has a vital role in ensuring appropriate and timely ongoing care. Those patients who are critically ill cannot be satisfactorily 'stabilised' in the resuscitation room. For example, intra-abdominal or continuing intrathoracic bleeding can only be corrected in the operating theatre. Those patients with intracranial haemorrhage require accurate definition of their pathology by computed tomography (CT) scan and potentially neurosurgery to achieve stability and survival. Such cases mandate the early appearance of a senior neurosurgeon.

These sorts of interventions are time critical and life saving. They are therefore properly part of the primary survey and the team leader is crucially responsible for ensuring that the patient is 'in the right place with the right surgeon' in a timely fashion. This means prioritising the patient's injuries, and therefore requirements, and avoiding delay. This often requires tact and varying degrees of 'assertiveness'.

Whilst an arterial line (15 min) and central line (15 min) could be advocated (and frequently are), they must not take precedence over the operating theatre for the ruptured spleen in the shocked patient. Similarly unnecessary investigations must not delay the head-injured patient's transfer for essential neurosurgery. Such theatre or scanning interventions frequently follow on directly from the resuscitation room episode and the team leader is pivotal in ensuring that they occur, and quickly.

Further reading

American College of Surgeons Committee on Trauma. (1997) *Advanced Trauma Lift Support Course for Physicians.* Chicago: American College of Surgeons.

Bickles W, Wait M, Pepe P, *et al.* (1994) A comparison of immediate versus delayed fluid resuscitation for hypotensive patients with penetrating torso injury. N Engl J Med 331: 1105–9.

Driscoll P, Vincent C. (1992) Variation in trauma resuscitation and its effects on outcome. Injury 23: 111–15.

Driscoll P, Vincent C. (1992) Organising an efficient trauma team. Injury 23: 107–10.

CHAPTER 2

Initial Assessment and Management: Secondary Survey

Rachael Pery-Johnston[1] *and David V. Skinner*[2]

[1]Princess Alexandra Hospital, Brisbane, QLD, Australia
[2]John Radcliffe Hospital, Oxford, UK

OVERVIEW

The secondary survey of the trauma patient involves the following.

- History
  - AMPLE history, interview ambulance staff and witnesses
  - Give analgesia
  - Universal precautions, wear lead gowns
- Head-to-toe
  - Log roll: five persons
  - Systematic head-to-toe examination
  - Splint fractures, photograph and dress wounds
  - Tetanus and antibiotic prophylaxis
  - Discover injuries missed in primary survey
  - Regular reassessment of vital signs
- Investigations
  - Radiography including CT or ultrasound
  - Blood tests, ECG and arterial blood gas sampling
  - Urine dip including pregnancy test
- Management plan
  - Interventions as appropriate to manage the patient, e.g. urinary catheter, chest drain
  - Documentation of all findings and investigations with time and signature
  - Specialist consultations with detailed handover if transferring care
  - Operating theatre or interhospital transfer to closest centre with appropriate facilities
  - Liaison with police for blood samples, collection of clothing for evidence

---

Objectives

The secondary survey of the trauma patient is co-ordinated by the trauma team leader and comprises:

- taking a focused **history**
- performing a systematic and thorough **head-to-toe assessment**
- interpreting results of **investigations** (radiological, laboratory, etc.) in light of clinical findings

---

ABC of Major Trauma, Fourth Edition. Edited by David V. Skinner and Peter A. Driscoll.
© 2013 Blackwell Publishing Ltd. Published 2013 by Blackwell Publishing Ltd.

- formulating a **management plan** for the patient and documenting all findings.

The secondary survey is undertaken ONLY after the primary survey is complete and the patient is responding to resuscitation. The goal is to identify and plan treatment for every single injury the patient has sustained. This may include life-threatening conditions which have not yet been appreciated. Injuries missed during the secondary survey may have implications for the patient's immediate well-being or long-term functional status. Regular re-evaluation of vital signs should take place during the secondary survey and if the patient appears to deteriorate, the primary survey must be repeated immediately. Universal precautions should be continued during the secondary survey and lead gowns worn. The patient needs to remain nil by mouth until non-surgical definitive care is confirmed.

History

AMPLE is a well-recognised mnemonic.

> **A**– Allergies/antitetanus status
> **M**– Medications currently taken
> **P**– Past medical history/pregnancy
> **L**– Last ate when?
> **E**– Exact events/environment resulting in injury

Information should be gathered from the ambulance officers or any witnesses to the event regarding the **mechanism of injury**. They may have a photograph of the damage to the patient's vehicle or be able to estimate the height the patient has fallen. This is useful because certain injury patterns occur predictably based on the amount of force involved and the part of the body affected (Box 2.1). Co-morbid conditions and medications need to be considered, as up to 38% of trauma victims in the UK have co-existing medical problems. These may have a significant influence on how a patient will respond to injury and therapy.

In the case of road traffic accidents, it is important to know whether the patient was wearing a seatbelt or child restraint and the approximate speed involved. This information can alert the clinician to injury patterns expected and the higher risk patient who was not restrained by a seatbelt. Airbags save lives but recent data show that they are responsible for a significant rise in forearm and shoulder injuries in car crash victims. If the patient was ejected from the vehicle or there were fatalities in the same accident, that patient has clearly been subject to considerable violence and a vigilant search for injuries must be undertaken.

Box 2.1 **Mechanism of injury and related suspected injury patterns**

Mechanism of Injury	Suspected Injury Patterns
Frontal impact	
• Bent steering wheel	• Cervical spine fracture
• Knee imprint, dashboard	• Anterior flail chest
• Bull's-eye fracture, windscreen	• Myocardial contusion
	• Pneumothorax
	• Traumatic aortic disruption
	• Fractured spleen or liver
	• Posterior fracture/dislocation of hip, knee
Side impact automobile	• Contralateral neck sprain
	• Cervical spine fracture
	• Lateral flail chest
	• Pneumothorax
	• Traumatic aortic disruption
	• Diaphragmatic rupture
	• Fractured spleen/liver, kidney depending on side of impact
	• Fractured pelvis or acetabulum
Rear impact, automobile collision	• Cervical spine injury
	• Soft-tissue injury to neck
Ejection, vehicle	• Ejection from the vehicle precludes meaningful prediction of injury patterns, but places patient at greater risk from virtually all injury mechanisms
Motor vehicle impact with pedestrian	• Head injury
	• Traumatic aortic disruption
	• Abdominal visceral injuries
	• Fractured lower extremities/pelvis

If the patient's injuries may be the result of criminal activity, it is necessary to collect all clothing and belongings in a bag for evidence. Police personnel can legally request permission to take a blood sample from a patient if they suspect him or her of driving whilst intoxicated.

Analgesia

If the patient is conscious they can indicate where they have pain and how severe it is. Scoring pain on a scale of 1 (minimal pain) to 10 (very severe pain) has been validated as a reliable way to assess severity and can be used to monitor response to analgesics. Pain relief should also be administered to the unconscious patient.

Morphine should be given intravenously and the dose titrated to effect. Intramuscular injections have no place in treating pain from trauma: absorption rates are unpredictable. Oral analgesia can be given after contraindications have been ruled out during the secondary survey.

Head-to-toe assessment

Log roll

The patient should be taken off the spinal board as soon as possible after the primary survey and resuscitation has commenced. Delay can result in pressure sores and the board decreases the quality of radiological imaging.

The log roll is a manoeuvre involving five people who carefully roll the patient onto his side, maintaining head and body in alignment to prevent exacerbation of any spinal injury that must be assumed to be present (Figure 2.1). The spinal board can then be removed and the assessing doctor must thoroughly examine the patient's back from head to toe. The back of the scalp can be inspected and palpated for bruising and fractures and the scapulae and every individual vertebral spinous process examined for tenderness and crepitus. The buttocks must be separated to check for wounds and to assess saddle sensation. A rectal exam is done to assess anal tone, confirm the normal location of the prostate and detect bleeding of the mucosa occasionally found with pelvic fractures. Clothes and windscreen glass can be removed from the patient's mattress.

Head
Brain

A brief neurological examination should be performed including formal documentation of the Glasgow Coma Scale (GCS). Pupillary findings and the presence of any lateralising signs should be noted, and comparison made with findings during the primary survey. This examination should be repeated frequently if head injury is a concern and any deterioration should prompt a return to the primary survey and elucidation of a cause. Early consultation with neurosurgery is required if serious head or spinal injuries are present. Prevention of secondary brain injury can be achieved

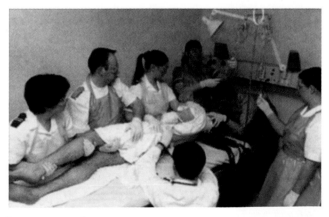

Figure 2.1 Log roll.

by maintaining a normal temperature, blood pressure and blood glucose, and avoiding hypoxia or hypercarbia.

Scalp

The rest of the scalp should be palpated systematically (having checked the back of the head during the log roll). Scalp bleeding can be torrential and wounds may need to be dealt with promptly using a pressure bandage or a couple of well-placed large sutures. If possible, staples should be avoided as the metal creates artifact on computer tomography (CT) images. Wounds which need exploration and suturing later should be documented.

Face

The face needs to be inspected and palpated to detect fractures. The skull base tends to fracture along a line from the mastoid process to the orbit and this can result in the characteristic pattern of bruising seen with 'raccoon eyes' and Battle's sign (Figures 2.2 and 2.3).

The maxilla may become disconnected from the other bones. If the maxilla is grasped above the upper incisors and gently

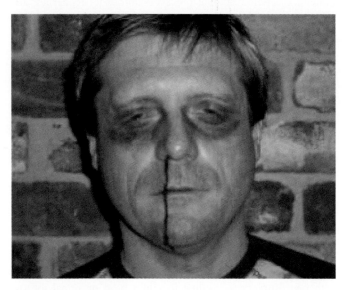

Figure 2.2 Raccoon eyes.

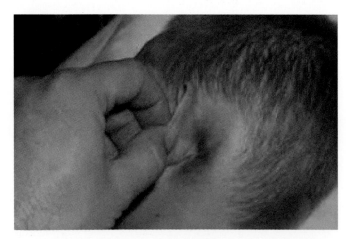

Figure 2.3 Battle's sign.

pulled forwards, abnormal mobility will be found when it has fractured. In some circumstances this midface fracture can create airway problems due to haemorrhage or the fragment collapsing backwards into the pharynx; if this occurs, it must be pulled forwards and the airway secured. Nasal airways and nasogastric tubes are contraindicated when there are significant facial injuries as there is a risk of insertion into the brain.

The mandible and each temporomandibular joint should be examined. A mandibular fracture may cause the tongue to loll backwards into the pharynx; the tongue can be pulled forward with a suture with the ends taped firmly to the neck. Conscious patients can be asked to open and close their mouth: they will be able to feel if their teeth are maloccluding.

The inside of the mouth should be inspected; jaw fractures may be open injuries at risk of infection. Any missing or loose teeth should be noted; they are occasionally seen on the chest radiograph!

Eyes

An early inspection is a good idea as periorbital swelling (Figure 2.4) can make examination difficult.

Pupil size and reactivity need to be documented and each eye inspected with the ophthalmoscope looking for any penetrating injury, haemorrhages, corneal abrasions or contact lenses (which should be removed). If indicated, eyelid eversion should be performed to find and remove debris. The patient can be asked to read small print on a label with each eye to assess satisfactory visual acuity. If the eyes are injured, the retina should be inspected for obvious haemorrhage or retinal detachment. It is important to examine eye movements as some facial fractures can cause ocular muscle entrapment.

Ears

Whilst a member of staff manually stabilises the head, the C-spine collar can be undone at the front and the ears inspected for lacerations or an auricular haematoma. Clear or bloody fluid draining from the ear (or nose) may be cerebrospinal fluid (CSF). Both tympanic membranes should be examined for rupture or haemotympanum (which may be the only sign of a basal skull fracture). Hearing can be assessed as grossly intact with simple bedside tests. Earrings obscure detail on a C-spine film and must be removed.

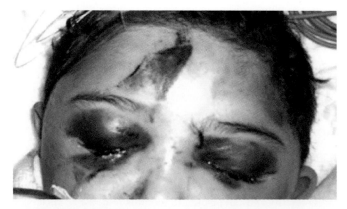

Figure 2.4 Massive periorbital swelling/bruising.

Neck

A cervical spine injury must be assumed to be present in a trauma patient, until this can be specifically excluded radiologically and/or clinically. While the C-spine collar has been released briefly (see above paragraph), the front of the neck can be inspected for wounds or bruising. Any wound penetrating the platysma needs exploration in the operating theatre. A careful examination should be made for crepitus or surgical emphysema and the opportunity taken to check that the trachea is midline. A bruit may alert the clinician to carotid or subclavian artery injury. The bony midline of the cervical spine needs to be palpated for crepitus and deformity, and tenderness if the patient is conscious. Every multiply injured patient requires a C-spine series of radiographs. This includes a lateral film showing the junction between C7 and T1, anteroposterior and peg views.

Chest

Chest injuries can be life threatening. A patient with a significant chest injury may have pain, hypoxia or an abnormal respiratory rate. If there are signs of a tension pneumothorax or cardiac tamponade (i.e. distended neck veins, tachycardia or hypotension), these must be decompressed as soon as they are discovered. A small open pneumothorax or a flail segment may have been overlooked during the primary survey, but these are serious injuries requiring immediate attention.

A thorough visual inspection of the entire chest wall should identify wounds, bruising and unequal thoracic movements. The seatbelt can fracture a clavicle or sternum and leave bruises across the chest and abdomen as a clue to underlying injury (e.g. to the aorta, pancreas or small bowel). The patient may have been thrown against the steering wheel, causing a sternal fracture or cardiac contusion. An electrocardiograph may show ST segment abnormalities (injury pattern) consistent with this. Systematic palpation of the chest should detect subcutaneous emphysema and rib or sternal fractures. There are case reports of airbag inflation causing rib fractures and even aortic transection. It is important to listen for breath sounds at the posterior axillae (decreased in haemothorax) and anterior chest (decreased in pneumothorax).

If not already performed, a chest radiograph needs to be arranged (erect if the patient's condition allows). It is possible to see a haemothorax or pneumothorax on this film, as well as widening of the mediastinum which suggests major vessel injury. Maintaining a high index of suspicion is essential, as it is easy to miss subtle diagnoses such as diaphragmatic or oesophageal rupture. Lung contusions may not be visible on early radiographs. Children have a pliable ribcage which will allow substantial damage to underlying structures without rib fractures. Further evaluation of chest injuries can be made with CT scanning if necessary, once the patient is stable. An arterial blood gas sample (from the radial or femoral artery) is useful to assess adequacy of oxygenation and gas exchange and to assess end-organ perfusion, as the lactate level will rise in patients with inadequate blood supply to the tissues.

Abdomen and pelvis

The secondary survey includes a thorough re-evaluation of the abdomen and vital signs, ideally by the same doctor each time.

The decision to be made is whether the patient needs an urgent laparotomy. Examining the abdomen in an unconscious or intoxicated patient can be unreliable. Serious intra-abdominal injury is suggested by a patient with a distended, tender or rigid abdomen or simply persistent tachycardia or hypotension with no alternative cause identified. Bruising from a seatbelt or a penetrating injury may be present. Exposed bowel should be covered with moist gauze and any wounds dressed and referred to the surgical team to explore formally in the operating theatre. A recent randomized, controlled trial supports the use of focused assessment with sonography in trauma (FAST) to detect free fluid in the abdomen, as an alternative to CT scan or diagnostic peritoneal lavage. CT scan is the current gold standard for detection of intra-abdominal injuries for haemodynamically stable patients. If there are any concerns whatsoever, general surgical consultation is necessary. See also Chapter 9, Abdominal Trauma.

Pelvic fractures can be suspected from the mechanism of injury and may result in exsanguinating haemorrhage. Both sides of the patient's pelvis should be pressed simultaneously only ONCE to elicit instability and then stabilised in a bedsheet firmly tied around the patient. There are also proprietary devices which achieve the same effect. Any patient with blunt trauma to the pelvis requires an anteroposterior pelvic radiograph. (Along with the chest and C-spine films, this completes the 'trauma series'.) If catastrophic internal bleeding is suspected, there are interventional radiological as well as surgical techniques which can address this and save the patient's life. Early referral is critical.

The perineum, vagina and urethral meatus should all be inspected for bleeding and wounds. If urethral bleeding is present, a retrograde urethrogram study needs to be done before insertion of a urinary catheter. One of the most sensitive markers of adequate end-organ perfusion is the production of urine, so monitoring of urine output is mandatory in patients with any significant degree of injury. A urinary pregnancy test can be performed at this time, and urine sent for toxicology or microbiology if required. If the urine has blood in it, this should raise the suspicion of a renal injury, and appropriate contrast investigation of this may be arranged with radiology.

Neurological system

Weakness, paralysis or loss of sensation suggests a serious injury to the spinal cord or peripheral nervous system. Findings must be accurately documented when discovered and spinal precautions used when moving the patient to protect them from further injury. Spinal shock presents as hypotension without tachycardia due to loss of sympathetic tone causing peripheral vasodilation. This may be less profound if the cord injury is lower as major sympathetic outflow is in the cervical region. It is important initially to use intravenous fluid to correct low blood pressure in the setting of trauma, as hypovolaemia is a more common cause of hypotension than spinal injury.

Musculoskeletal system

The mechanism of injury is a useful guide to the extremity examination. For instance, landing upright from a height puts the patient at risk for calcaneal, spinal and wrist fractures. Knee and acetabular fractures may result when a car occupant is thrown forward against the dashboard.

Systematic inspection and palpation of every limb are crucial. This begins with the clavicles for the upper limb. At each joint, range of movement should be assessed and note made of peripheral nerve function and vascular supply at extremities. Every digit must be individually assessed for swelling, deformity, tenderness and decreased range of movement as missed injuries of the hands may lead to long-term functional deficits for the patient. During this assessment, the clinician should remain aware that other more painful injuries may distract the patient from acknowledging the degree of pain from examined structures (distracting injuries).

Prompt reduction of deformity and splinting of fractures are important, to improve the vascular and neurological outcome and reduce pain and haemorrhage. Careful note should be made of any ischaemic-looking skin or wounds overlying a fracture and iodine-soaked dressings applied. It is best to photograph the wound to avoid further exposure to infection from repeated inspections. Antitetanus and antibiotic prophylaxis are also necessary.

Any injured limb needs to be considered at risk of a compartment syndrome. Muscle swelling after limb injury causes compression of blood vessels and nerves, leading to muscle ischaemia within fascial compartments. The affected area will feel tense to palpation and be excruciatingly painful. The limb is at risk if the high pressure is not relieved quickly and therefore a compartment syndrome is a surgical emergency.

Further reading

American College of Surgeons Committee on Trauma. (2004) *ATLS, Advanced Trauma Life Support Program for Doctors*, 7th edn. Chicago, IL: American College of Surgeons.

Melniker LA, Leibner E, McKenney MG, Lopez P, Briggs WM, Mancuso CA. (2006) Randomized controlled clinical trial of point-of-care, limited ultrasonography for trauma in the emergency department: the first sonography outcomes assessment program trial. Ann Emerg Med 48(3): 227–35.

Miller MT, Pasquale MD, Bromberg WJ, Wasser TE, Cox J. (2003) Not so FAST. J Trauma 54(1): 52–9; discussion 59–60.

Stengel D, Bauwens K, Sehouli J, *et al.* (2005) Emergency ultrasound-based algorithms for diagnosing blunt abdominal trauma. Cochrane Database Syst Rev 2: CD004446.

Wallis LA, Greaves I. (2002) Injuries associated with airbag deployment. Emerg Med J 19(6):490–3.

Wardle TD. (1999) Co-morbid factors in trauma patients. Br Med Bull 55(4): 744–56.

CHAPTER 3

The Upper Airway

David Watson and Catherine Peters

Homerton University Hospital, London, UK

OVERVIEW

- Airway management is vital in the resuscitation of a trauma patient.
- Provision of oxygen via a managed airway is integral to successful resuscitation.
- Ventilatory support may be necessary.

First vital minutes

All severely injured patients experience hypoxaemia to some degree. As soon as medical help arrives, the priority must be to ensure that the patient's airway is clear and ventilation is unimpaired. Immediate administration of supplementary oxygen to the unobstructed airway is of paramount importance.

Remember that the cervical spine of any patient with trauma should be considered broken until proved otherwise. The neck must be kept stabilised without traction (for example, by using a spinal board, sand bags, tape and a semi-rigid collar) at all times until the possibility of neck injury is excluded.

In an unconscious patient any obstruction to the airway must be removed under direct vision. For the signs and symptoms of upper airway obstruction, see Box 3.1. The laryngeal and pharyngeal reflexes should then be assessed and respiratory performance examined. If protective reflexes are adequate (for example, the patient is coughing), retracting the tongue forward by employing the chin lift or jaw thrust manoeuvre or inserting an anaesthetic type airway or nasopharyngeal airway may suffice. If the reflexes are depressed or absent (that is, there is no gag reflex when oropharyngeal suction is attempted in an unconscious patient), the airway must be secured at the earliest opportunity by intubation with an appropriately sized endotracheal tube with a low-pressure cuff. A laryngeal mask airway is not a substitute for a cuffed tube in the trachea, and its role in the resuscitation of the injured patient has not yet been fully defined. When a trauma patient has a laryngeal mask airway in place on arrival in the emergency department, the patient must be reassessed and a decision made whether the laryngeal airway should be removed and replaced with a cuffed endotracheal tube (Box 3.2).

Box 3.1 **Signs and symptoms of upper airway obstruction**

- Hoarse voice, noisy breathing.
- Increased effort of breathing: increased use of accessory muscles, tracheal tugging; intercostal recession; abdominal see-saw movement.
- Inability to lie flat.
- Cyanosis (late).
- Apnoea (late).

Box 3.2 **Indications for securing an airway with an endotracheal tube**

- Apnoea.
- Obstruction of upper airway.
- Protection of lower airway from soiling with blood or vomitus.
- Respiratory insufficiency.
- Impending or potential compromise of airway, for example, after facial burns.
- Altered consciousness, continuous seizures.
- Uncooperative patient requiring further assessment (for example, CT scanning).
- Raised intracranial pressure requiring controlled ventilation.

Ventilation and intubation

Patients with hypoxia or apnoea must be ventilated and oxygenated before intubation is attempted. Ventilation can be achieved with a mouth-to-mouth mask or bag-valve-face mask (Figure 3.1). Studies suggest that ventilation techniques with a bag-valve-face mask are less effective when performed by one person rather than two people, when one of the pair can use both hands to ensure a good seal. When only one person is present to provide ventilation, the method employing the mouth-to-mouth mask is preferred. During such manoeuvres the neck must be kept immobilised.

ABC of Major Trauma, Fourth Edition. Edited by David V. Skinner and Peter A. Driscoll.
© 2013 Blackwell Publishing Ltd. Published 2013 by Blackwell Publishing Ltd.

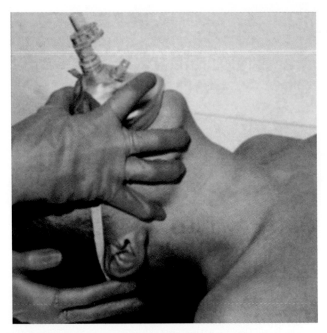

Figure 3.1 Mouth-to-mouth mask, preferred to a bag-valve-face mask when only one person is available to provide ventilation.

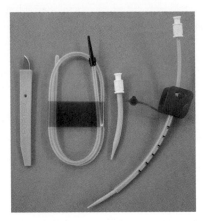

Figure 3.2 Apparatus for emergency cricothyroidotomy. Scalpel, guidewire, dilator and uncuffed endotracheal tube.

If intubation is performed, a large-bore gastric tube should also be passed. Nasal passage of a gastric tube is contraindicated in patients with suspected basal skull fractures or injury to the cribriform plate.

Tracheostomy is rarely necessary as an emergency procedure. Severe distorting injury to the structures above or at the level of the larynx can render endotracheal intubation impossible, but cricothyroidotomy (Figure 3.2) is preferred to emergency tracheostomy in such circumstances.

In patients with fractured ribs with or without a pneumothorax, chest drainage on the side of the fractures should be considered before artificial ventilation is undertaken. A tension pneumothorax should always be suspected when a patient with a recent crush injury has obvious respiratory distress or cyanosis. In patients with a chest injury complicated by pneumothorax, an apical chest drain should be inserted through the space between the fifth and sixth

ribs, just anterior to the midaxillary line. If there is blood in the pleural cavity an additional basal drain may be required.

An open pneumothorax should be managed initially by inserting a chest tube to release any accumulated air and prevent the development of a tension pneumothorax. The opening can then be closed temporarily with a petroleum jelly gauze or other non-porous dressing.

Indications for oxygenation and ventilation

Once the airway is secured, the adequacy of respiratory gas exchange must be evaluated (Box 3.3). The respiratory rate can be recounted and respiratory effort reassessed. Measurements of blood gas tensions should be undertaken as soon as is practicable.

Box 3.3 **Indications for oxygenation and ventilation.**

- Ventilatory assistance is required when there is excessive respiratory work or obvious ventilatory insufficiency.
- Failure of adequate oxygenation (PaO_2 <9 kPa) when the patient is breathing a high inspired oxygen concentration (10 L/min O_2 by facemask) demands consideration of endotracheal intubation and assisted positive pressure ventilation.

Artificial ventilation in patients without respiratory failure must also be considered when there is coincidental head injury, agitation or recurrent seizures. Hypercapnia and hypoxaemia from asphyxia or inadequate ventilation with fluctuations in arterial blood pressure can cause considerable deterioration in cerebral function. This is probably secondary to alterations in cerebral blood flow that adversely affect intracranial pressure.

Hospital management

An anaesthetist experienced in caring for victims of trauma should be available to examine the patient's airway immediately on arrival at hospital. Evaluation of the patient's airway must proceed simultaneously with treatment. If the airway is satisfactory, treatment may consist simply of increased oxygen delivery. If the airway is compromised or the patient needs ventilatory support, a secure endotracheal airway, if not already in place, is required. Patients with hypoxia or apnoea must be ventilated and oxygenated before intubation is attempted.

The route of choice for securing the airway depends on several factors (Box 3.4). Blunt trauma of the head and face is associated with an incidence of cervical spine fractures of 5–10%. Patients with trauma should be assumed to have a cervical fracture until proved otherwise; manipulation of the neck is strictly contraindicated. Doctors in the United Kingdom generally accept that laryngoscopy and orotracheal intubation after induction of anaesthesia and muscle paralysis can be performed by a competent operator with minimal changes in the position of the cervical vertebrae while an assistant holds the patient's head.

Although optimum exposure of the larynx is not achievable under such conditions, experienced anaesthetists can intubate patients without clearly visualising the vocal cords. This may require aids such as gum elastic bougie (Figure 3.3) or alternative laryngoscopes. Pressure on the cricoid must be provided by another skilled assistant in an attempt to protect the patient from aspirating gastric contents. The stomach may already have been emptied as much as possible by the passage of a gastric tube with the neck immobilised. Alternatively, if the patient's condition permits, fibreoptic endoscopy may facilitate difficult orotracheal or nasotracheal intubation.

Surgical cricothyroidotomy (Figure 3.4) may be necessary for patients who cannot be intubated nasally or orally. Often these patients have massive facial trauma. Although surgical cricothyroidotomy can be performed through a small midline incision in the cricothyroid membrane, life-saving oxygenation can also be provided by cannula cricothyroidotomy with a cannula connected to wall oxygen at 15 L/min with a Y-connector or a sidehole in the tubing attached between the oxygen source and the cannula. Spontaneous respiration after cannula cricothyroidotomy, however, can be extremely difficult, requiring large pressure changes in the airway and considerable ventilatory effort. Intermittent insufflation (for which sedation and muscle paralysis are necessary) can be achieved by occluding the open end of the Y-connector or the sidehole of the oxygen tubing. The patient can be ventilated by this technique for only 30–45 min; this limits its usefulness, particularly in those with head injuries. Jet insufflation must also be used with caution when obstruction by a foreign body is suspected in the glottic area.

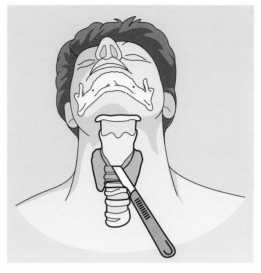

Figure 3.4 Cricothyroidotomy with scalpel.

Anaesthetic considerations

Anaesthetists caring for patients who are critically ill give reduced doses of all anaesthetic agents because hypovolaemia and hypotension alter the distribution and pharmacokinetics of drugs, thereby exaggerating their clinical effects. Intravenous opiates (morphine, fentanyl or alfentanil) and anaesthetic induction agents (thiopentone, etomidate or propofol) are therefore given in smaller doses to avoid cardiovascular depression. Ketamine (1–2 mg/kg) is useful in trauma that is complicated by haemorrhagic shock. Ketamine and halogenated hydrocarbons such as enflurane may raise intracranial pressure and are therefore contraindicated in head trauma. Muscle relaxants given to facilitate and maintain intubation include suxamethonium (1–2 mg/kg), rocuronium (0.6–0.9 mg/kg), pancuronium (0.1–0.2 mg/kg), vecuronium (0.1–0.2 mg/kg) or atracurium (0.4 mg/kg). Drugs contraindicated in trauma are shown in Box 3.5.

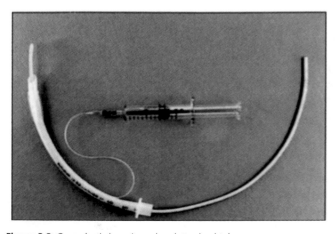

Figure 3.3 Gum elastic bougie and endotracheal tube.

Rapid-sequence intubation with anaesthetic agents, neuromuscular blocking drugs and oesophageal occlusion by cricoid pressure should be performed only by those trained in their use, knowledgeable of their inherent complications and skilled in the techniques of airway maintenance, endotracheal intubation and assisted ventilation. In the UK this usually means anaesthetists.

Patients may have taken drugs such as opiates, cocaine and marijuana before suffering trauma. These may interact with anaesthetic agents. Ethanol enhances the effect of anaesthetics and sedatives and reduces the minimum alveolar concentration of volatile general anaesthetics required.

Before embarking on intubation, an anaesthetist will check the equipment, including the suction and oxygen delivery apparatus. Anaesthetic agents should be ready in labelled syringes, and duplicate ampoules should be easily accessible. Vasoactive drugs such as atropine should also be ready in syringes in case untoward bradycardia complicates extended laryngoscopy. A skilled assistant must be at hand to apply pressure on the cricoid. The neck must also be kept stabilised. Secure venous access is mandatory. A pulse oximeter should be attached to the patient's earlobe or finger to give a continuous display of the arterial haemoglobin oxygen saturation.

Anaesthesia is induced with the best possible monitoring available and only after administration of oxygen. Pressure on the cricoid is maintained by the assistant. Neuromuscular blockade is produced by suxamethonium, and intubation proceeds with the onset of paralysis and relaxation of the jaw.

Patients with responsive airway reflexes require induction of anaesthesia and muscle paralysis for the airway to be secured by an oral or a nasotracheal route. Deeply unconscious patients with head and brain injury should not be intubated without prior administration of a cerebral sedative and muscle relaxant, hence avoiding dangerous increases in cerebral blood volume and intracranial pressure during laryngoscopy. Nasotracheal intubation should not be undertaken if fractures of the base of the skull or of the cribriform plate are suspected.

Intubation technique

The procedure for endotracheal intubation is shown in Box 3.6. The anaesthetist takes the laryngoscope in his or her left hand and inserts it into the right-hand side of the patient's mouth, thereby moving the tongue to the left. While carefully observing the back of the tongue, he or she advances the curved blade of the laryngoscope until the epiglottis comes into view (Figures 3.5, 3.6).

Box 3.6 **Rapid-sequence induction endotracheal intubation**

- All equipment and drugs checked.
- Patient monitoring established.
- Patient preoxygenated with 100% oxygen.
- Intravenous anaesthetic agents administered followed by suxamethonium (unless contraindicated).
- Cricoid pressure applied.
- Laryngoscopy and endotracheal intubation performed.
- Inflation of endotracheal tube cuff.
- Confirmation of tracheal placement.
- Release of cricoid pressure.

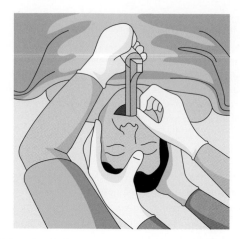

Figure 3.5 Inserting the laryngoscope.

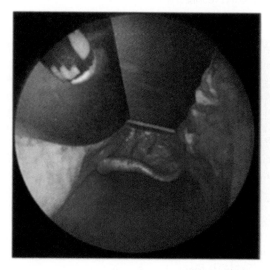

Figure 3.6 Lifting the root of the tongue.

The tip of the blade is moved anterior to the epiglottis and the whole lower jaw lifted upwards, taking care not to move the neck. This should expose the arytenoid cartilages and vocal cords (Figure 3.7). The tracheal rings should be visible beyond. Under direct vision, the anaesthetist advances a gum elastic bougie or the endotracheal tube, aiming for the left vocal cord. If a gum elastic bougie is used, a cut cuffed endotracheal tube of the appropriate size is subsequently 'rail roaded' into the trachea. A size 8 tube is usually suitable for women and a size 9 for men. The cuff of the endotracheal tube is then inflated with air from a syringe until an airtight seal is secured.

The chest should be auscultated in both axillae to exclude intubation of the right main bronchus or oesophagus (Figure 3.8). An end-tidal carbon dioxide monitor attached to the endotracheal tube between the adaptor and the ventilator device will rapidly confirm that the endotracheal tube is in the trachea. Pressure on the cricoid can only now be released and the tube secured with tapes.

After intubation, oxygen-enriched ventilation should proceed with a tidal volume of about 10 mL/kg at a rate of about 10 breaths/min. To facilitate ongoing respiratory support, sedation and

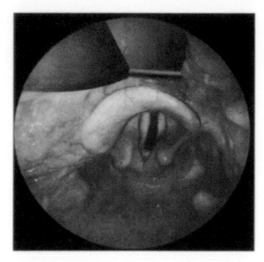

Figure 3.7 Direct visualisation of the glottis.

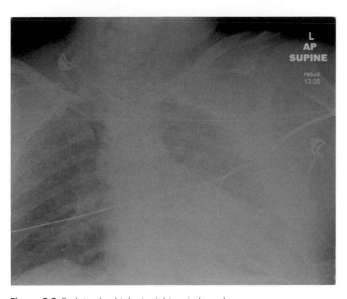

Figure 3.8 Endotracheal tube in right main bronchus.

analgesia may need to be maintained by intravenous administration of benzodiazepines (e.g. midazolam) or anaesthetic induction agents (e.g. propofol) and opiates (e.g. morphine, fentanyl or alfentanil) together with neuromuscular blocking drugs (e.g. atracurium, vecuronium, rocuronium or pancuronium) for muscle paralysis. Although capnography and pulse oximetry may provide immediate non-invasive assessment of oxygenation and the adequacy of ventilation, the arterial blood gas tensions should be analysed at the first opportunity. Radiography of the chest should also be performed routinely after endotracheal intubation to check the position of the endotracheal tube in the bronchial tree and gastric tube in the stomach.

Summary

In conclusion, providing oxygen and ventilatory support as early as possible is a prerequisite for successful resuscitation in victims of major trauma. Otherwise, as Haldane observed, hypoxia not only stops the machine but wrecks the machinery.

Acknowledgement

Illustrations of the technique of intubation (Figures 3.6 and 3.7) are reproduced from *A Systematic Guide to Intubation* (by P. Lotz, F.W. Annefeld and W.K. Hirlinger), Atelier Flad, Eckental, Germany.

Further reading

Morris CG, McCoy W, Lavery GG. (2004) Spinal immobilization for unconscious patients with multiple injuries. BMJ 329: 495–9.

Scott RPF. (1998) Onset times and intubating conditions. Br J Anaesth 80: 417–19.

Sellick BA. (1961) Cricoid pressure to control regurgitation of stomach contents during induction of anaesthesia. Lancet ii: 404.

CHAPTER 4

Thoracic Trauma

Andrew Blyth

Royal Berkshire Hospital, Reading, UK

OVERVIEW

Thoracic trauma leads to:

- respiratory and cardiovascular inplications
- hypoxia
- hypovolaemia
- reduced cardiac output.

Untreated, it will be fatal.

Trauma in the United Kingdom annually results in 720,000 admissions and over 6 million attendances to emergency departments. There are over 17,000 trauma deaths, with nearly 25% of these directly attributable to thoracic injuries. Many of these patients will die at the scene of the injury, with patients reaching hospital already a self-selected group who have a good chance of survival with early appropriate management. Evidence suggests that a significant proportion of in-hospital deaths from thoracic trauma are preventable, with injuries either not being recognised or being inadequately treated.

Only 10–15% of patients with blunt trauma and 15–30% of those with penetrating trauma ultimately require surgery. The remainder can be treated successfully in the emergency department through the application of fundamental principles of initial trauma management as well as through direct interventions within the scope of practice of emergency physicians. These management principles are especially important as thoracic trauma impacts directly on the heart and lungs, the two organs most integral to the provision of oxygenation and perfusion.

Successful management of thoracic trauma depends ultimately on effective prioritisation of resuscitation through the ABC principles with rapid detection and treatment of life-threatening injuries.

Mechanisms and patterns of chest injury

Chest injuries can be broadly classified as penetrating or blunt, the latter encompassing direct blunt trauma as well as crush, acceleration or deceleration injuries and blast injuries. An understanding of the specific mechanisms involved in individual trauma patients is important as patterns of injury are produced with significant differences in pathophysiology and clinical course (Table 4.1). Life-threatening injuries without obvious external signs can be missed as attention is paid to more visible but clinically less serious injuries. Diagnosis therefore often depends on maintaining a high index of suspicion of specific injuries which are associated with the underlying mechanism of trauma and tailoring the clinical assessment and investigation to look for and exclude those injuries. Predictors of thoracic injury include head and abdominal injuries, evidence of major haemorrhage in the absence of abdominal swelling or major bony injury, wounds, bruising or seatbelt marks on the chest wall and any degree of respiratory distress.

Penetrating injuries frequently cause pneumothorax or haemothorax and blood loss with cardiac or vascular injuries may be catastrophic. Patients often deteriorate rapidly but with appropriate management, have the potential to improve rapidly. Surgical intervention is frequently necessary, but special investigations are less commonly required than in blunt trauma.

Blunt trauma typically causes organ damage by compression, acceleration or deceleration and shear forces. In contrast to penetrating trauma, the majority of blunt injuries are managed non-operatively, responding to emergency department interventions such as intubation and ventilation or intercostal drainage.

Table 4.1 Patterns of chest injury

Mechanism	Common injuries
Penetrating	Laceration of heart, great vessels, intercostal vessels, lung parenchyma, airways, oesophagus and diaphragm
Blunt	
Direct blunt trauma	Cardiac contusion, pulmonary contusion, rib fractures with or without flail segment, thoracic spine fractures
Crush	Ruptured bronchus, ruptured oesophagus, cardiac and pulmonary contusion, bilateral rib fractures with or without flail segment
Deceleration	Aortic disruption, major airway injury, diaphragmatic rupture
Blast	Disruption of any intrathoracic organ, pulmonary contusion

ABC of Major Trauma, Fourth Edition. Edited by David V. Skinner and Peter A. Driscoll.
© 2013 Blackwell Publishing Ltd. Published 2013 by Blackwell Publishing Ltd.

Blunt injuries are typically more difficult to diagnose and additional investigations such as computed tomography (CT) scanning are frequently required. Injuries such as pulmonary contusion may only manifest some time after the initial trauma and anticipation of the potential to develop such problems may allow the emergency physician to tailor management in an effort to reduce the risk of avoidable complications.

Regardless of mechanism, the main consequences of thoracic trauma are the combined effects on both respiratory and cardiovascular function, leading to hypoxia, hypovolaemia and reduced cardiac output, which not only impact directly on the thoracic organs but compound the effects of injuries to other organ systems.

Hypoxia and impairment of gas exchange

Hypoxia is the most common pathophysiological manifestation of moderate to severe chest injury. It may be the direct result of impairment of gas exchange at a pulmonary level or occur at a tissue level through inadequate perfusion despite normal or near-normal pulmonary gas exchange.

Patients with lung injury may experience significant impairment of gas exchange as a result of diffuse interstitial and alveolar haemorrhage, as seen in pulmonary contusion, which is a significant cause of delayed morbidity and mortality associated with chest trauma. Experimental and clinical studies have shown that the condition is progressive. Initial haemorrhage and oedema are followed by interstitial fluid accumulation and decreased alveolar membrane diffusion. These changes produce relative hypoxaemia, increased pulmonary vascular resistance, decreased pulmonary vascular flow and reduced lung compliance.

In patients with impaired respiratory function because of pulmonary injury, the associated mediastinal shift secondary to haemothorax, pneumothorax or both may result in compression of the non-injured lung, further compromising ventilation. This ventilation–perfusion mismatch can lead to an intrapulmonary shunt of more than 30% that contributes significantly to hypoxaemia, especially in the period soon after injury. Later, this hypoxia-induced pulmonary vasoconstriction will divert the blood away from the non-ventilated alveoli, thus reducing the intrapulmonary shunt to about 5%.

Hypovolaemia

All mechanisms of chest injury have the potential to cause major haemorrhage, leading to profound hypovolaemia. It is most often seen with aortic transection, great vessel rupture or laceration, pulmonary hilar injury or penetrating cardiac injuries not producing tamponade. The resulting decrease in cardiac output compounds the effects of hypoxia at a tissue level through reduced perfusion and worsens the outcome for other injuries, both thoracic and elsewhere.

Reduced cardiac output

Reduction in cardiac output in the setting of thoracic trauma may result from poor diastolic filling due to hypovolaemia, or from the secondary effects of hypoxia and reduced coronary perfusion on myocardial function, or may be caused by direct cardiac injuries. Such injuries include myocardial contusion in blunt trauma, transection of coronary arteries, blunt or penetrating heart valve injury and cardiac tamponade.

Blunt myocardial injury can reduce cardiac contractility and compliance of the ventricles, resulting in a low cardiac output state. Injury to coronary arteries or smaller vessels, either through direct penetrating trauma or within contused areas, can cause tissue necrosis and infarction leading to heart failure or cardiogenic shock. This is exacerbated by the reduction in coronary perfusion that results from hypovolaemia and hypoxaemia due to multiorgan trauma, and which further compromises global myocardial function.

Traumatic injury to the heart valves may result in acute volume overload of the ventricles, and severe regurgitation may cause acute congestive cardiac failure and death. Acute insufficiency of any valve may go unnoticed in the presence of more obvious injuries, with the result that valve lesions are not often detected during the initial post-trauma survey and resuscitation phase. Their recognition requires a high index of suspicion and further investigation (such as echocardiography).

The ultimate goal of treatment of thoracic trauma is therefore to restore and maintain both oxygenation and tissue perfusion, aiming to restore ventilation to all viable lung tissue and optimise cardiac output, through rapidly identifying and treating those injuries which compromise respiratory and cardiac function.

Primary survey and resuscitation

The primary survey is a rapid, focused assessment following the **ABC** principles (see Chapter 1).

During the course of resuscitation, major life-threatening thoracic injuries will be uncovered during the primary survey (and immediately addressed) whilst other potentially serious thoracic problems will be identified in the secondary survey. The following adjuncts are crucial to the identification of thoracic injuries.

Diagnostic adjuncts to the primary survey

The chest X-ray

The plain anteroposterior (AP) chest radiograph done in the resuscitation area of the emergency department remains the most important standard initial image in chest trauma. It should be performed within 10 min of the patient's arrival in the emergency department. Clinical signs in thoracic trauma are often subtle or misleading and the chest radiograph is a valuable tool which helps to identify important problems which require intervention as well as guiding decision making on further investigations such as CT scanning.

In blunt trauma, with the risk of spinal injury, the X-rays are performed in the supine position and should be sufficiently penetrated to allow some visualisation of the thoracic spine as well as the outline of the aorta. In penetrating trauma, where possible, the chest X-ray is done with the patient sitting upright to increase its sensitivity in detecting small haemothoraces or pneumothoraces as well as diaphragmatic injuries. It requires 400–500 mL of blood or fluid to obliterate the costophrenic angle on the erect chest X-ray. Widening and shift of the mediastinum and rib fractures may be evident (Figures 4.1–4.5).

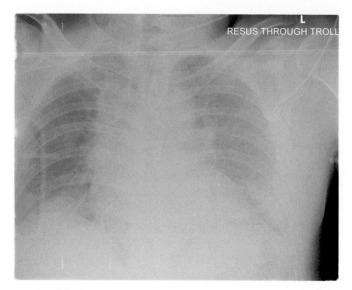

Figure 4.1 Widened mediastinum needing urgent further investigation.

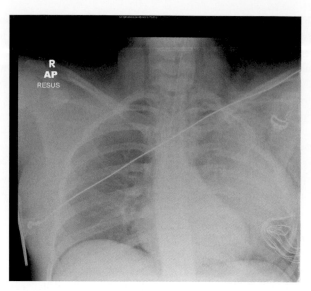

Figure 4.3 Multiple rib fractures with signs of haemothorax and surgical emphysema.

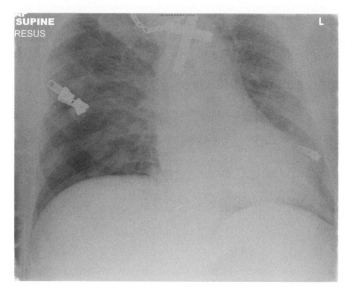

Figure 4.2 Subtle right pneumothorax.

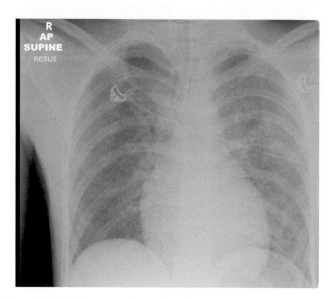

Figure 4.4 Right lung contusion on chest X-ray.

The arterial blood gas

Arterial blood gas analyses should be performed on all patients with significant thoracic trauma, in particular those patients who are intubated and ventilated. This will not only give specific measures of oxygen and carbon dioxide, but also indicate acid–base status via pH, base excess and bicarbonate. Many blood gas machines will also provide haemoglobin estimation as well as lactate measurement which is a useful indicator of tissue perfusion and oxygenation.

Focused assessment with sonography for trauma examination

Focused assessment with sonography for trauma (FAST) is a rapid ultrasound assessment tool used in haemodynamically unstable patients with blunt trauma. It is performed in the resuscitation area

of the emergency department and, aside from its role in abdominal trauma, may be useful in identifying the presence of pericardial blood or haemothorax, though the latter may only be detectable when >200 mL. It may be similarly useful in certain cases of penetrating thoracic trauma. It requires an operator specifically trained in FAST.

Immediate life-threatening injuries

Six specific thoracic injuries identified on the primary survey may be rapidly fatal if not recognised and treated promptly (Box 4.1): airway obstruction or rupture (see Chapter 1), tension pneumothorax, open pneumothorax, flail chest, massive haemothorax and cardiac tamponade. During the primary survey, the signs that will aid

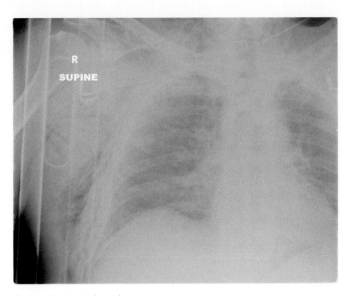

Figure 4.5 Surgical emphysema.

in diagnosis should be actively sought and treatment should be initiated as the problems are identified (Table 4.2).

Box 4.1 Life-threatening injuries: primary survey

- Airway obstruction or airway rupture.
- Tension pneumothorax.
- Open pneumothorax.
- Flail chest.
- Massive haemothorax.
- Cardiac tamponade.

Tension pneumothorax

A traumatic tension pneumothorax is the progressive build-up of air within the pleural space, caused by a one-way leak from lacerations to lung, airway or chest wall. Air enters the pleural space on inspiration but cannot escape during expiration due to the effective formation of a one-way flap valve. The result is progressive accumulation of air with initial collapse of the ipsilateral lung, causing hypoxia, followed by shift of the mediastinum to the opposite side, compressing the contralateral lung and decreasing venous return to the heart. The resulting combination of worsening hypoxia, impaired ventilation and reduced cardiac output leads to traumatic arrest unless the tension is decompressed.

Tension pneumothorax can complicate either blunt or penetrating trauma or be iatrogenically caused through the insertion of central venous lines or the incorrect application of occlusive dressings to penetrating chest wall wounds. It is most commonly seen in patients with a simple pneumothorax or visceral pleural injury who are put on positive pressure ventilation. Such patients may deteriorate rapidly after initiation of ventilation or may present insidiously hours later. Awareness of this potential for deterioration and early recognition and treatment are the key to management. It is a clinical diagnosis and delays in decompression while radiological evidence is obtained may have fatal consequences.

The clinical presentation of tension pneumothorax is that of progressive respiratory distress, chest pain and air hunger. The presentation may mimic airway obstruction as effective ventilation decreases. The classic signs are of tracheal deviation away from the side of the tension, hyperinflation, reduced chest movement with hyper-resonance to percussion and reduced breath sounds on the affected side, elevated jugular venous pressure, tachycardia and hypotension. Untreated, this process will progress to full circulatory collapse and cardiac arrest with pulseless electrical activity.

However, classic signs are often absent, with tachycardia and tachypnoea being the only overt signs. Percussion note and breath sounds are often difficult to hear in the noisy trauma environment, while elevation of venous pressure may not occur with hypovolaemia. In rare cases, tension pneumothorax may be bilateral.

Treatment is the immediate decompression of the affected side, converting tension pneumothorax into simple pneumothorax. This is achieved by the insertion of a large-calibre cannula, around 16 gauge, into the second intercostal space (just above the third rib) in the midclavicular line. The corresponding hiss of air confirms decompression and the cannula should be left open. The chest should be re-examined and an intercostal drain inserted on the same side without delay (see 'Procedures associated with the primary survey' below). as needle thoracostomies can easily become kinked or displaced, allowing the tension to recur. It is possible for drains to become blocked and the patient to re-tension, so any deterioration in the patient's condition should be followed by immediate reassessment. In the ventilated patient, open thoracostomy is an effective technique to treat tension and prevent recurrence. Formal drains can be inserted later.

Because of the potential for developing tension pneumothorax, all patients on positive pressure ventilation who have any evidence of pneumothoraces or have multiple rib fractures should be considered for intercostal drain insertion, particularly if they require transfer.

Open pneumothorax

An open pneumothorax is a pneumothorax which communicates with the exterior via a chest wall defect. The thickness of chest wall is much less than the length of the trachea with the result that any chest

---

Table 4.2 Interpretation of chest examination findings. Both the position of the patient and the severity of the injury will affect the findings on examination

Injury	Tracheal deviation	Expansion	Percussion	Breath sounds
Tension pneumothorax	Away	Decreased	Hyper-resonant	Reduced
Simple pneumothorax	Central	Decreased	Usually normal	Reduced
Massive haemothorax	Central	Decreased	Dull	Reduced
Lung collapse	Towards	Decreased	Normal	Slightly reduced

wall defect more than 75% of the size of the trachea provides less resistance to air flow. During inspiration, which generates negative intrathoracic pressure, air is preferentially sucked through the chest wall defect and into the pleural space, rather than down the trachea. This reduces the effectiveness of ventilation and compromises oxygenation. If a flap valve effect is created either by the chest wound itself or dressings applied to it, tension pneumothorax can result.

The diagnostic clinical signs are of a chest wound that appears to be sucking air on inspiration and bubbling on expiration. The patient is typically tachypnoeic with a shallow breathing pattern. Breath sounds on the affected side are reduced with resonance on percussion. However, other than the wound itself, signs may easily be overlooked.

Initial management consists of applying a sterile occlusive dressing taped down on three sides, providing a flutter valve effect which prevents air ingress during inspiration, but lifts on the untaped side during expiration, allowing egress of both air and blood. This may be difficult to apply on large wounds. A commercial dressing, the Asherman chest seal, has a one-way valve that achieves the same objective. Definitive management involves wound closure with insertion of an intercostal drain.

Massive haemothorax

Haemothorax is an accumulation of blood in the pleural space following blunt or penetrating trauma and is typically caused by rib fractures, lung parenchymal injuries or vascular injuries. The majority of haemothoraces are small and self-limiting, but following penetrating injuries to heart, great vessels and hilar structures or less commonly following blunt trauma, bleeding into the pleural space may be severe.

A massive haemothorax is defined as loss of more than 1500 mL of blood or more than one-third of blood volume into either the pleural space or out via an intercostal drain. Examination may reveal evidence of a penetrating wound or bruising to the chest wall with crepitus from rib fractures.

The cardinal signs of massive haemothorax are of hypovolaemic shock with dullness to percussion and reduced or absent breath sounds on the affected side. Neck veins are typically collapsed secondary to hypovolaemia, but may be distended if there is associated tension pneumothorax or cardiac tamponade. It is unusual for the haemothorax itself to shift the mediastinum sufficiently to cause visible distension of neck veins.

The key to management of massive haemothorax is the restoration of circulating blood volume together with drainage of the haemothorax via a wide-bore intercostal chest tube (28 French or larger) inserted in the fourth or fifth intercostal space just anterior to the midaxillary line. (See Procedures associated with the primary survey, below.) If decompression of the haemothorax takes place before venous access is obtained and volume resuscitation commenced, haemodynamic decompensation can rapidly occur, particularly if the source of bleeding is uncontrolled. Volume resuscitation is initially with crystalloid, but the need for blood should be recognised early and transfusion commenced with type-specific blood until fully cross-matched blood becomes available. If there is significant drainage of blood via an intercostal drain, autotransfusion can be considered.

During resuscitation, systemic blood pressure should not be allowed to rise uncontrollably through overvigorous fluid administration if cardiac or vascular injury is suspected as this may precipitate further bleeding (permissive hypotension). In addition, the initiation of positive pressure ventilation during resuscitation can also dramatically increase bleeding from pulmonary vessels through mechanical clot displacement. The potential for sudden haemodynamic deterioration following intubation and ventilation should therefore be anticipated and recognised by the emergency physician, though this does not change the indications for ventilation in trauma patients.

Thoracotomy in theatre is likely to be required if initial drainage of blood is more than 1500 mL or ongoing drainage exceeds 200 mL/h for 2 or more hours. Initial volume drained is typically less important than ongoing drainage and the need is based on the patient's clinical status as well as ongoing requirement for blood transfusion. Early cardiothoracic opinion should therefore be obtained.

Flail chest

Injuries to the chest wall are extremely common following blunt trauma and vary from minor bruising to severe bilateral crush injuries with multiple rib fractures which compromise ventilation. Rib fractures may be associated with pulmonary contusion and fractures of the first rib should raise the suspicion of underlying vascular injury.

When a segment of chest wall loses bony continuity with the thoracic cage, it becomes flail and will move paradoxically on respiration, reducing tidal volume and compromising ventilation. In addition, rib fractures may be accompanied by significant blood loss. The principal cause of hypoxia after flail chest is the development of severe pulmonary contusion.

Diagnosis is usually clinical, by observation of abnormal chest wall movement and the palpation of crepitus, although splinting of the chest wall may initially make it difficult to detect. The chest radiograph will not always reveal rib fractures or costochondral separation, although arterial blood gas analysis may reveal hypoxia and/or hypercapnia.

Treatment is initiated with high-flow oxygen and lung expansion must be restored by intermittent positive pressure ventilation if required and any haemopneumothoraces must be drained. Intercostal chest drains are almost always required, particularly if positive pressure ventilation is needed. The aim of further management is to preserve respiratory function.

Pain reduces the tidal volume and inadequate ventilation of the basal lung segments results in atelectasis. Pain also inhibits coughing, allowing secretions to obstruct bronchi and cause acute respiratory failure. Effective pain relief is required so that regular physiotherapy can be carried out with the patient's full co-operation. Epidural anaesthesia may be extremely effective in the management of patients with flail chest.

Careful fluid management is essential because the injured lung, with its increased capillary leakage, is sensitive both to inadequate perfusion and also to fluid overload.

A flail segment in itself does not justify mechanical ventilation, although elective intubation and ventilation are often appropriate.

The degree of respiratory distress and hypoxia determines the need for ventilation (Box 4.2) and it is important to be aware that pulmonary contusion may develop insidiously over hours to days. Functional, not physical, integrity of the ribcage is required and adequate analgesia and careful fluid management are essential. Operative stabilisation of fractures is rarely indicated.

Box 4.2 **Indications for ventilation in flail chest**

- Significant impedance to ventilation due to the flail segment.
- Large pulmonary contusion.
- Unco-operative patient, e.g. head injuries.
- Development of respiratory failure: hypoxia/hypercapnia.
- General anaesthesia for another indication.

Cardiac tamponade

Bleeding into the pericardium is usually the result of penetrating trauma to the heart or great vessels, although blunt trauma may also damage these structures. Many patients with lacerations to the heart will exsanguinate quickly but in cases that are not rapidly fatal, bleeding may be contained within the pericardium. In the acute setting, the pericardial space has a fixed volume and only a small amount of blood accumulating is sufficient to exert pressure that restricts cardiac filling and compromises cardiac output.

Many of the signs of cardiac tamponade overlap with tension pneumothorax and this should first be excluded. The classic Beck's triad of elevated central venous pressure, hypotension and muffled heart sounds is not commonly seen in the emergency department. Neck veins may not be distended if there is significant hypovolaemia and heart sounds can be difficult to assess in a noisy environment. Other signs of tamponade include Kussmaul's sign of paradoxical elevation of central venous pressure during inspiration and exaggeration of the physiological phenomenon of pulsus paradoxus. Systolic blood pressure decreases during spontaneous (rather than assisted) inspiration and a systolic drop of >10 mmHg is considered abnormal. Both Kussmaul's sign and pulsus paradoxus may be difficult to detect in the trauma setting.

The diagnosis of tamponade should be suspected in any patient with penetrating injury and shock, or with blunt trauma and shock that does not respond to fluid resuscitation and in whom tension pneumothorax has been ruled out. X-rays are typically normal, although access to FAST may aid in the diagnosis.

Immediate pericardiocentesis is indicated in patients with suspected cardiac tamponade who have failed to respond to initial resuscitative measures. (See 'Procedures associated with the primary survey', below.) Removing as little as 10–20 mL of blood from the pericardial space can considerably improve the condition of the patient with cardiac tamponade. Although pericardiocentesis may be life saving in certain circumstances, it has also caused death through cardiac laceration and should be performed with caution. In 25% of cases the blood within the pericardium has clotted and aspiration will not be possible. A fine balance between internal and external cardiac pressures may prevent exsanguination in cardiac tamponade, and aspiration of blood from the pericardium may contribute to fatal haemorrhage by reducing the external cardiac pressure and allowing a rise in intracardiac pressures.

In the arrested patient, pericardiocentesis should not be allowed to delay immediate thoracotomy. Patients with a positive pericardiocentesis should always undergo formal surgical exploration in the operating theatre.

Procedures associated with the primary survey

Intercostal drain insertion

Drainage of typically air or blood from the pleural space via intercostal drain insertion is the most common intervention in thoracic trauma. Despite being a simple procedure within the skills of the emergency physician, it has a complication rate of up to 10%. Adherence to proper technique will prevent many of the serious complications. Indications for intercostal drain insertion are shown in Box 4.3.

Box 4.3 **Indications for intercostal drain insertion**

- Pneumothorax: simple, open or tension (decompress first).
- Haemothorax.
- Traumatic arrest: typically bilateral drain insertion.
- Rib fractures in patients requiring positive pressure ventilation (relative indication).

Drains are typically inserted after plain chest radiographs are taken, but in certain circumstances such as the arrested patient or patients who have had tension pneumothoraces decompressed, it may be appropriate to insert an intercostal drain without first obtaining a chest X-ray. The technique for inserting an intercostal drain is shown in Box 4.4. Acute and chronic complications of this procedure are shown in Boxes 4.5 and 4.6 respectively.

Box 4.4 **Inserting an intercostal drain: technique**

1 Approach is typically in the fourth or fifth intercostal space just anterior to the midaxillary line, over the rib below the chosen space. In practical terms, this is usually the highest space in the axilla that can be easily accessed.
2 The area is cleaned and draped appropriately.
3 In the conscious patient, 10–20 mL of 1% lidocaine should be infiltrated into the skin and periosteum as well as down to the pleura, with the needle passing above the rib to avoid the neurovascular bundle. Aspiration of air will confirm position.
4 The skin is incised down to the rib. The track is then established above the rib by blunt dissection down to and through the pleura. Trocars should NOT be used.
5 Once the pleura is punctured, a gloved finger is inserted into the pleural cavity and a finger sweep performed to clear pleura or clots and to prevent damage to lung and other organs when the drain is inserted.
6 A large-bore (>28) drain is then introduced along the track with a surgical forceps. It should slide easily into position through

(continued)

---

the track. It is essential that the drain is inserted far enough for all sideports to lie within the chest cavity, but not so far as to abut the mediastinum.

7 The tube is connected to an underwater drain system which should always be positioned below the level of the patient. Bubbling or swinging of the drain helps to confirm placement.

8 Once positioned, the drain should be secured with 0 gauge sutures. Purse-string sutures are no longer advised.

9 The chest must be re-examined and position and efficacy of the drain confirmed on X-ray.

10 The tube should not be clamped after insertion.

Box 4.5 Acute complications (usually related to poor technique)

- Laceration of intercostal vessels (cause – approach under the rib instead of over).
- Penetration of diaphragm or abdominal cavity (cause – drain placed too low).
- Laceration of lung (cause – pleural adhesions not cleared).
- Injury to stomach or bowel (cause – failure to identify diaphragmatic hernia).
- Subcutaneous tube placement.
- Tube in too far, causing pain.
- Tube displacement (cause – not adequately secured).

Box 4.6 Chronic complications

- Infection or empyaema.
- Clotted haemothorax.
- Blocked tube (usually due to clot).

Pericardiocentesis

Pericardiocentesis is indicated in suspected or confirmed cardiac tamponade. The diagnosis should be suspected in patients with penetrating injury and shock, or with blunt trauma and shock that does not respond to fluid resuscitation. The aspiration of as little as 10 mL of blood may improve blood pressure. The technique for pericardiocentesis is described in Box 4.7. The complications of this technique are shown in Box 4.8.

Box 4.7 Pericardiocentesis: technique

1 Patient's vital signs and ECG must be monitored throughout and following the procedure.
2 The skin is prepared and landmarks identified.
3 In conscious patients, the puncture site should be anaesthetised with 1% lidocaine.

---

4 A 16–18 gauge over-the-needle catheter at least 15 cm in length attached to a 50 mL syringe is required. Consider a three-way tap on the syringe.
5 The skin is punctured 1–2 cm inferior to the left xiphochondral junction with the needle at 45° to the skin, aimed at the tip of the left scapula.
6 As the needle is advanced, aspirate until the syringe fills with blood, while observing the monitor for ECG changes. Aspirate as much blood as possible.
7 Electrocardiogram changes such as widening/enlarging of the QRS complex, marked ST changes or frequent ectopics suggest that the needle is too far advanced and must be withdrawn until the changes resolve. ECG changes may also occur during aspiration as the pericardial sac is drained. Again, slight withdrawal of the needle is indicated.
8 After aspiration is complete, remove the needle, leaving the catheter in place, attached to a three-way tap.
9 Secure the catheter in place.
10 Aspiration via the catheter can be repeated if the signs of tamponade recur.
11 Surgical exploration is usually required following positive pericardiocentesis.

Box 4.8 Complications of pericardiocentesis

- Aspiration of ventricular blood.
- Laceration of myocardium.
- Coronary vessel injury: may cause new haemopericardium and tamponade.
- Arrhythmias, typically ventricular fibrillation.
- Pneumothorax.
- Infection.

Emergency department thoracotomy

This remains a controversial topic and is a procedure that carries a high mortality. By no means can indiscriminate emergency room thoracotomy by the untrained be advocated, in particular when the potential exists for the procedure to be done by an experienced surgeon in the more controlled environment of an operating theatre. However, knowledge of the indications and principles of thoracotomy is important for any doctor dealing with major trauma and in a select group of patients, it can be a life-saving procedure. The exact criteria defining that selection remain controversial. With a recent increase in the number of patients presenting to many emergency departments with penetrating chest trauma, in particular stab wounds, this knowledge may become increasingly relevant.

Overall survival rates for patients undergoing emergency department (ED) thoracotomy are 4–33% across numerous studies, with mechanism and location of injury as well as the presence or absence of vital signs being the most important determinants of survival. Stab wounds have a better prognosis than gunshot wounds and survival may approach 70% in isolated stab wounds with cardiac tamponade. Outcome in blunt trauma is dismal, with studies showing survival rates of 0–2.5%. However, the patient with blunt trauma who is exsanguinating via an intercostal drain due to a ruptured pulmonary vessel may be salvageable with thoracotomy and immediate cross-clamping of the bleeding vessel. Survival rates in both blunt and penetrating trauma patients who have not exhibited signs of life at any point are extremely poor.

Box 4.9 shows the indications for ED thoracotomy. Contraindications are shown in Box 4.10.

Box 4.9 Indications for ED thoracotomy

Penetrating thoracic injury

- Traumatic arrest with previously witnessed cardiac activity (prehospital or in-hospital).
- Hypotension unresponsive to treatment (BP <70 mmHg).
- Rapid exsanguination from intercostal drain or into airways.

Blunt thoracic injury

- Unresponsive hypotension (BP <70 mmHg).
- Rapid exsanguination from intercostal drain or into airways.

Box 4.10 Contraindications to ED thoracotomy

- Blunt thoracic injuries with no witnessed cardiac activity.
- Multiple blunt trauma.

It is outside the scope of this text to provide details of the specific surgical techniques of emergency thoracotomy, but its aims mirror its indications (Box 4.11).

Box 4.11 Aims of ED thoracotomy

- Relief of cardiac tamponade.
- Control of haemorrhage.
- Access for internal cardiac massage.

A left lateral thoracotomy approach can also occasionally be used to provide access for aortic cross-clamping in uncontrolled exsanguinating haemorrhage distal to the thoracic aorta. Following initial stabilisation, the patient should be immediately transferred to an operating theatre for definitive management.

Whatever the indication, if the opportunity exists, thoracotomy should always take place in an operating theatre in the hands of an experienced trauma surgeon. Survival rates are hugely improved when thoracotomy takes place in the theatre environment.

Secondary survey

Once immediately life-threatening conditions have been excluded or diagnosed and treated, the patient can be more thoroughly assessed. This assessment includes a detailed history, full examination, an upright chest radiograph if clinically possible, measurement of arterial blood gases, ECG and other diagnostic tests relevant to the clinical setting.

Several potentially life-threatening injuries may not be identified on the primary survey and require more detailed examination and investigation to diagnose (Box 4.12). A high index of suspicion based on the mechanism of injury and knowledge of common injuries associated with certain mechanisms (see Table 4.1) may aid considerably in reaching a diagnosis. Identification of certain injuries should prompt a thorough search for other associated injuries, for example great vessel injuries associated with first rib or scapular fractures. Missed injuries contribute to significantly increased mortality in the post-traumatic period. As in the primary survey, a structured, organised approach is required.

Box 4.12 Potentially life-threatening injuries identified on the secondary survey

- Tracheobronchial injury.
- Simple pneumothorax.
- Haemothorax.
- Pulmonary contusion.
- Blunt myocardial injury.
- Aortic disruption.
- Diaphragmatic injury.
- Oesophageal injury.

Tracheobronchial injury

Although uncommon, injuries to the trachea and main bronchi, caused by either blunt or penetrating trauma, may be fatal if not recognised and extensive free air in the neck, chest wall or mediastinum should always raise suspicion of damage to major airways.

Laryngeal fractures are rare and are indicated by hoarseness, subcutaneous emphysema and palpable fracture crepitus. If the airway is threatened or completely obstructed or if there is severe respiratory distress, intubation is warranted. This may be extremely difficult to achieve due to distortion of anatomy from the injury itself, subcutaneous emphysema, local haematoma or associated oropharyngeal injuries. Fibre-optic laryngoscopes or even immediate tracheotomy may be required to secure the airway, followed by surgical repair.

Penetrating injuries to trachea or bronchi are usually apparent and all require surgical repair. They may be associated with injury of adjacent structures, most commonly the oesophagus, carotid artery or jugular vein. With missile injuries, there can be extensive tissue damage to the surrounding area because of the cavitation caused by the velocity of the projectile. Transections of the trachea or bronchi proximal to the pleural reflection cause extensive deep cervical or mediastinal emphysema, which rapidly spreads to the subcutaneous tissues. Injuries distal to the pleural sheath result in pneumothoraces.

Blunt tracheal injuries may not be obvious, particularly if the patient has a depressed level of consciousness. Laboured breathing may be the only initial sign of airway obstruction. The diagnosis can be confirmed with bronchoscopy, preferably rigid, and this may be used to improve airway clearance of blood and debris. Early surgical repair is required.

The majority of blunt bronchial injuries occur within 2.5 cm of the carina. There are often severe associated injuries and most victims die at the site of the accident. For those who reach hospital, mortality is at least 30%. Signs of bronchial injury may include haemoptysis, subcutaneous emphysema, tension pneumothorax and pneumothorax with a large, persisting air leak. The diagnosis is confirmed by bronchoscopy although mucosal oedema and debris can obscure the extent of a bronchial injury, so the site should be carefully inspected. Distortion of airway anatomy by adjacent haematoma makes management more difficult, and surgery is occasionally indicated. Bronchial tears must be repaired urgently in the operating theatre via a thoracotomy.

Simple pneumothorax

A simple pneumothorax is a non-expanding collection of air in the pleural space. Classic signs of resonance to percussion and reduced breath sounds may be difficult to detect and diagnosis may only be made on chest X-ray evidence or even CT scan. Chest X-ray signs may be subtle, with increased radiolucency on one side the only evidence. In blunt trauma, the presence of rib fractures or haemothorax should raise a strong suspicion of associated pneumothorax. The diagnosis is especially important if the patient requires positive pressure ventilation or needs transfer to another hospital, as simple pneumothorax may rapidly tension.

In the trauma setting, all but trivial pneumothoraces detected on CT scan generally require intercostal drain insertion and even in the latter situation, the decision is usually influenced by the need for transfer, ventilation or general anaesthesia.

Haemothorax

Most small or moderate haemothoraces are not detectable by physical examination and will be identified on chest C-ray, CT scan or FAST. Small haemothoraces may be difficult to appreciate on chest X-ray in the supine patient and any increase in overall radio-opacity on one side of the chest, especially if associated with rib fractures or penetrating trauma, should raise the suspicion of a haemothorax. Treatment is intercostal drain insertion on the affected side.

Failure to drain haemothoraces is usually the result of failure to diagnose them. If missed, haemothoraces may become infected, leading to empyema, or may organise and fibrose, leading to permanent loss of lung volume which may impair pulmonary function.

Pulmonary contusion

Pulmonary contusion is an injury to lung parenchyma associated with blunt trauma which leads to blood and oedema accumulating in the alveoli. The resulting loss of normal architecture causes impairment of gas exchange, increased pulmonary vascular resistance and decreased lung compliance. There is associated atelectasis with shunting of blood and increased airway resistance

all contributing to hypoxia. It develops insidiously over 24 h and is usually seen in the presence of signs of blunt chest wall trauma with bruising or underlying rib fractures, complicating the clinical picture of the associated injuries. In children, severe pulmonary contusion frequently occurs without rib fractures. Around 50% of patients with significant pulmonary contusions will go on to develop acute respiratory distress syndrome (ARDS).

Pulmonary contusion is seldom diagnosed on clinical examination, but the mechanism of injury and identification of injuries associated with contusion should raise the index of suspicion. Occasionally crackles may be heard on auscultation, but initial diagnosis is frequently on chest X-ray with the presence of nodular exudates in the lung fields. X-ray appearance typically lags behind the clinical picture which is of increasing respiratory distress and hypoxia. CT scan is a sensitive investigation which helps to distinguish contusion from atelectasis or other pathology.

Treatment is supportive while the contusion resolves and many patients can be managed without the need for intubation and ventilation. However, as the condition is progressive, at-risk patients should be closely monitored over the first 24–48 h. Fluid balance must be carefully monitored as both over- and underhydration contribute to secondary lung injury. Certain patients will, however, benefit from early intubation and ventilation (Box 4.13). The majority of patients, in the absence of complications, will resolve within 3–5 days. Complications include ARDS and pneumonia.

> Box 4.13 **Relative indications for early endotracheal intubation in pulmonary contusion**
>
> - Hypoxia or worsening respiratory status.
> - Decreased level of consciousness.
> - Pre-existing chronic pulmonary disease.
> - General anaesthetic required for other injuries.
> - Extremes of age.
> - Organ failure in another organ system.
> - Necessity for transfer.

Blunt myocardial injury

Blunt myocardial injury or myocardial contusion is the most commonly undiagnosed fatal thoracic injury. It occurs when there is direct compression of the heart due to blunt trauma or rapid deceleration. Blunt cardiac injury may also lead to chamber or valvular rupture. Blunt myocardial injury is often associated with sternal fractures and in this setting, the right ventricle is most frequently damaged. Patients with blunt myocardial injury are prone to all the complications associated with myocardial infarction and may complain of chest pain which is either overlooked or attributed to the overlying chest wall injuries. Around 20% of patients experience arrhythmias, which include sinus tachycardia, supraventricular tachycardia, atrial fibrillation, ventricular ectopics, ventricular tachycardia and ventricular fibrillation. Conduction defects, ranging from bundle branch block to complete heart block, may also develop.

The diagnosis is established from the mechanism of injury, serial cardiac enzyme measurements, ECG changes such as ST elevation, two-dimensional echocardiographic evidence of ventricular wall dysfunction and pericardial effusion. A significant rise in cardiac troponin following blunt chest trauma is highly suggestive of blunt myocardial injury, but does not predict the risk of complications. Elevation of jugular venous pressure following blunt trauma may indicate right ventricular dysfunction. The presence of a completely normal ECG makes the diagnosis of significant blunt myocardial injury unlikely.

Areas of contused myocardium behave in the same way as areas of infarction, and the patient should be treated accordingly. Conduction defects may rarely require pacemaker insertion. Cardiogenic shock is rare but some patients may need temporary intra-aortic counterpulsation balloon pumping to improve the perfusion of viable myocardium. Urgent surgical repair is sometimes necessary for cardiac rupture (particularly posterior), ventricular septal rupture or valve damage.

Aortic disruption

Tears of the aorta or pulmonary arteries are associated with blunt or deceleration injuries such as road traffic accidents and falls from a height. The aorta may be completely or partially transected or may have a spiral tear. Anatomically, the aorta is firmly fixed at three points: the aortic valve, the ligamentum arteriosum and the hiatus of the diaphragm. Sudden deceleration will allow the mobile parts of the aorta to move relative to the fixed parts, creating substantial shear forces. The most common site of rupture is at the attachment of the ligamentum arteriosum, where the aorta remains tethered to the main pulmonary artery.

Aortic rupture is immediately fatal in about 90% of cases and accounts for around 15% of immediate trauma deaths due to road traffic collisions. The immediate survival of the patient depends on the development of a contained haematoma, maintained by the intact adventitia. The survival of patients after reaching hospital depends on early diagnosis followed by urgent surgical repair.

Specific signs and symptoms of aortic injury are usually absent and an index of suspicion based on mechanism of injury should be maintained. Any suspicion of aortic injury raised by the plain chest radiograph (Box 4.14) must prompt further investigation. No single radiographic sign absolutely predicts aortic rupture, but a widened mediastinum >8 cm at the level of the aortic arch is the most consistent finding. In 1–2% of cases with aortic injury, the chest X-ray may be completely normal. Contrast-enhanced spiral CT scan is becoming an investigation of choice for suspected aortic injuries, with sensitivity and specificity approaching 100%, similar to aortography. The difficulty for the clinician is that in order to obtain such investigations, patients require transfer away from the emergency department to the less safe environment of a radiology department. Instability of the patient due to other injuries or to the aortic injury itself may make this extremely difficult. Even if identified, aortic injuries that are not the cause of haemodynamic instability may be low on the list of management priorities in the multiply injured patient.

The treatment of traumatic aortic rupture is surgical repair, directly or by resection of the damaged segment and interposition of a vascular graft. All clinical situations are different, and priorities and management need to be tailored to the individual. Prior to surgery, a cautious approach to fluid resuscitation must be maintained and overvigorous volume replacement avoided at all costs (permissive hypotension). Elevations of systemic blood pressure may rupture the flimsy adventitial layer containing the rupture, causing fatal haemorrhage. Each individual situation needs to be considered on its merits and in the light of other injuries that require treatment.

> **Box 4.14 Radiographic features suggestive of aortic disruption**
>
> - Widened mediastinum >8 cm.
> - Loss of the aortic 'knuckle'.
> - Tracheal deviation to the right.
> - Oesophageal deviation to the right (NGT).
> - Filling of the aortopulmonary window.
> - Widened paratracheal stripe.
> - Pleural cap.
> - Elevation of right main bronchus.
> - Depression of left main bronchus.

Diaphragmatic injury

Penetrating injuries can cause small diaphragmatic perforations that are rarely of immediate significance, but may present months or years later. By contrast, blunt trauma produces large radial tears of the diaphragm and herniation of abdominal viscera into the chest. The right hemidiaphragm is relatively protected by the liver and left-sided ruptures are therefore more common and are more easily diagnosed because of the appearance of bowel or stomach in the chest. Bilateral rupture is rare.

The chest radiograph can be misinterpreted as showing a raised hemidiaphragm, acute gastric dilation or a loculated pneumothorax. Contrast radiography or locating an abnormal position of the stomach with plain radiography by passing and identifying the tip of a nasogastric tube confirms the diagnosis. Unless other injuries require immediate surgery, repair of the diaphragm should not be delayed. This is often performed through a laparotomy for associated abdominal injuries.

One of the main risks of diaphragmatic rupture in the acute trauma setting is the insertion of an intercostal drain into stomach or bowel. Clinical examination and correct technique should prevent this.

Oesophageal injury

Damage to the oesophagus is usually caused by penetrating trauma. The proximity of the oesophagus to major vessels and other mediastinal structures frequently means that the consequences of damage to these are a more immediate focus for the emergency physician than the oesophageal injury which may be overlooked. Blunt oesophageal injury is rare and typically associated with blunt trauma to the upper abdomen which forces gastric contents rapidly into the oesophagus, causing a linear tear with leakage of contents into the mediastinum or pleural space leading to mediastinitis or empyema. The resultant clinical picture is identical to postemetic oesophageal rupture (Boerhaave syndrome) and may have fatal consequences if not recognised (Box 4.15).

The diagnosis should be considered in any patient with severe blunt trauma to the abdomen who has a left pneumothorax or haemothorax in the absence of rib fractures. The presence of stomach contents in material draining from a correctly inserted intercostal tube is virtually diagnostic. The diagnosis is confirmed by cautious contrast study of the oesophagus or by endoscopy. Treatment is by formal surgical repair in the operating theatre, with drainage of the pleural space or mediastinum or both.

Box 4.15 **Features suggestive of oesophageal rupture**

- Blunt trauma to upper abdomen.
- Sharp, severe epigastric pain.
- Shock disproportionate to the apparent injury.
- Pneumomediastinum on chest X-ray.
- Left pneumothorax or haemothorax without rib fractures.
- Gastric contents in chest drain.

Diagnostic adjuncts to the secondary survey

Chest X-ray

Chest X-ray is typically performed as an adjunct to the primary survey, but is repeated after the insertion of endotracheal tubes, central lines and intercostal drains. It remains the default initial investigation in all forms of chest trauma.

Computed tomography scan

In the setting of thoracic trauma and indeed trauma in general, the multidetector spiral CT scan is being increasingly used as a screening adjunct to the secondary survey, providing vital information on injuries that might otherwise be overlooked and guiding management decisions and prioritisation. It has the advantage of being fast, relatively non-invasive (apart from the addition of contrast in certain settings) and yet having very high sensitivity and specificity for the majority of important intrathoracic injuries. It is increasingly replacing investigations such as aortography and may identify subtle injuries that would be overlooked on other imaging modalities. However, it must be stressed that CT scan is not a substitute for clinical assessment during the primary survey and key life-threatening injuries must be identified and treated in the emergency department. CT scanning requires the patient to be moved from the well-equipped environment of the emergency department and the potential benefits and timing of scanning must be weighed against the potential risks of transfer. It is telling that the phrase 'ring of death' has been used to describe the CT scanner. Patient safety is paramount.

Analgesia

Analgesia is an important part of the management of patients with thoracic trauma and is the mainstay of therapy for injuries such as rib fractures. Lack of adequate analgesia may even produce acid–base disturbances through rapid shallow breathing due to pain. In the acute setting of trauma, the analgesic of choice is usually administration of opiates via the intravenous route, maintaining caution regarding the potential for respiratory depression. Administration of small doses repeated as necessary is safer than large boluses. Oral and intramuscular analgesia are generally inappropriate in the acute setting of major trauma, particularly if surgery is anticipated.

Specific analgesic plans can be tailored to the individual situation. Patient-controlled opioid analgesia (PCA) may be very effective in the awake, co-operative patient recovering from trauma. For multiple rib fractures or flail chest not requiring ventilation, continuous epidural anaesthesia is extremely effective, providing complete pain relief and allowing normal inspiration, without the risks of respiratory depression associated with opiates. Intercostal nerve blocks with a long-acting local anaesthetic such as bipuvacaine are not as effective as epidural anaesthesia, but may provide relief in isolated rib fractures. Local anaesthetic injected into intercostal drains in sufficient quantities to provide pain relief may lead to toxicity.

Each case should be considered on its individual merits, but the requirement for adequate analgesia in trauma management should not be overlooked.

Summary

Thoracic trauma is common in the patient with multiple injuries and continues to be associated with a high mortality. The application of evidence-based management principles with a structured approach to assessment and management has resulted in improved outcome for a large group of patients who reach the hospital with intact vital signs.

CHAPTER 5

Hypovolaemic Shock

Jerry P. Nolan[1] and Rick Pullinger[2]

[1]Royal United Hospital, Bath, UK
[2]John Radcliffe Hospital, Oxford, UK

OVERVIEW

- After haemorrhage, the systolic blood pressure of healthy adults may not decrease until 30–40% of their blood volume has been lost.
- Stop the bleeding as rapidly as possible.
- Blood will be required rapidly if the patient is exsanguinating.
- In the severely injured patient, maintain a haemoglobin concentration in the range 8–10 g/dL depending on the specific circumstances and the patient's known co-morbidity.
- Warm all fluids: hypothermia increases mortality.
- In massive haemorrhage, give fresh frozen plasma and platelets early.

Hypovolaemic shock is a clinical state in which loss of blood or plasma causes inadequate tissue perfusion. Compensatory responses to haemorrhage are categorised into immediate, early and late. The loss of blood volume is detected by low-pressure stretch receptors in the atria and arterial baroreceptors in the aorta and carotid artery. Efferent output from the vasomotor centre triggers an increase in catecholamines, which causes arteriolar constriction, venoconstriction and tachycardia. Early compensatory mechanisms (5–60 min) include movement of fluid from the interstitium to the intravascular space and mobilisation of intracellular fluid. Long-term compensation for haemorrhage occurs by several mechanisms: reduced glomerular filtration rate; salt and water reabsorption (aldosterone and vasopressin); thirst; increased erythropoiesis.

Haemorrhagic shock causes a significant lactic acidosis; once the mitochondrial PO_2 is less than 2 mmHg, oxidative phosphorylation is inhibited and pyruvate is unable to enter the Krebs cycle. Instead, pyruvate undergoes anaerobic metabolism in the cytoplasm, a process that is relatively inefficient for adenosine triphosphate (ATP) generation. ATP depletion causes cell membrane pump failure and cell death. The aim of resuscitation, including infusion of fluid, is to restore oxygen delivery rapidly, thus preventing the onset of irreversible haemorrhagic shock and death.

Early symptoms and signs

The following are early symptoms and signs of hypovolaemic shock. They reflect the underlying pathophysiology.

- Tachycardia (caused by catecholamine release).
- Skin pallor (vasoconstriction caused by catecholamine release).
- Hypotension (caused by hypovolaemia, perhaps followed by myocardial insufficiency).
- Confusion, aggression, drowsiness and coma (caused by cerebral hypoxia and acidosis).
- Tachypnoea (caused by hypoxia and acidosis).
- General weakness (caused by hypoxia and acidosis).
- Thirst (caused by hypovolaemia).
- Oliguria (caused by reduced perfusion).

In most cases the signs and symptoms can be related to the amount of blood loss, which is classed in four groups (classes I–IV) (Table 5.1). Generally, losses up to 750 mL (class I) (15% of the circulating blood volume) do not cause pronounced signs or symptoms (Table 5.2). Further haemorrhage, amounting to 1.5 L (class II), produces cardiovascular signs of catecholamine release, thirst, weakness and tachypnoea. Systolic pressure begins to decrease as blood loss mounts to 2 L (class III) and often becomes unrecordable after 2.5–3.0 L (class IV) has been lost.

Previously healthy, young adults have remarkable compensatory capabilities and systolic pressure is often preserved despite quite appreciable blood loss (1.5–2.0 L). A narrowed pulse pressure is often the earliest sign. Eventually, however, there is a precipitous fall as the myocardium suddenly fails because of hypoxia and acidosis. In some cases, when severe haemorrhage is not accompanied by significant tissue injury, blood loss of more than 30–40% can cause a dramatic, sudden increase in cardiac vagal drive, leading to bradycardia and hypotension.

Factors affecting response to blood loss

Patients with coronary arterial disease may become hypotensive because of myocardial insufficiency after blood losses of less than 1500 mL. Patients receiving certain drugs (for example, β-blockers) may not be able to produce an appropriate sympathetic response and may also become hypotensive after modest blood loss. Other factors that may modify the response to blood loss include the

---

ABC of Major Trauma, Fourth Edition. Edited by David V. Skinner and Peter A. Driscoll.
© 2013 Blackwell Publishing Ltd. Published 2013 by Blackwell Publishing Ltd.

Table 5.1 Classification of hypovolaemic shock according to blood loss (adult).

	Class I	Class II	Class III	Class IV
Blood loss:				
Percentage	<15	15–30	30–40	>40
Volume (mL)	750	800–1500	1500–2000	>2000
Blood pressure:				
Systolic	Unchanged	Normal	Reduced	Very low
Diastolic	Unchanged	Raised	Reduced	Very low or unrecordable
Pulse (beats/min)	Slight tachycardia	100–120	120 (thready)	>120 (very thready)
Capillary refill	Normal	Slow (>2 sec)	Slow (>2 sec)	Undetectable
Respiratory rate	Normal	Tachypnoea	Tachypnoea (>20/min)	Tachypnoea (>20/min)
Urinary flow rate (mL/h)	>30	20–30	10–20	0–10
Extremities	Normal	Pale	Pale	Pale, clammy and cold
Complexion	Normal	Pale	Pale	Ashen
Mental state	Alert	Anxious or aggressive	Anxious, aggressive or drowsy	Drowsy, confused or unconscious

Table 5.2 Symptoms of hypovolaemia according to blood loss*

Blood loss (mL)	Class	Symptoms
<750	I	None
–1500	II	Cardiovascular signs due to catecholamine release: thirst, weakness, tachypnoea
–2000	III	Systolic pressure falls
>2000	IV	Systolic pressure becomes unreadable

*Assuming a 70 kg patient.

patient's age, the extent of tissue damage, and the period of time between injury and examination.

In children, normal haemodynamic values are maintained until the blood loss is relatively great. Tachycardia and skin pallor are the earliest signs, and hypotension indicates uncompensated shock with severe blood loss and inadequate resuscitation. As a rule, a child's systolic blood pressure is 80 mmHg plus twice the age in years. The diastolic pressure is about two-thirds of the systolic pressure. A systolic pressure of 70 mmHg or less in a child therefore indicates serious cardiovascular decompensation.

In elderly patients hypotension may be an early sign of blood loss. Their physiological reserves are reduced and they are less able to respond to release of catecholamines with a tachycardia. The ensuing hypotension may cause early organ failure because of hypoperfusion, and this is exaggerated in normally hypertensive patients.

Extensive tissue damage from major limb injuries is associated with early cardiovascular decompensation, not only because of blood loss and haematoma formation but also because of extravasation of fluid while oedema is developing. About a quarter of the volume of oedema fluid is contributed by lost plasma volume, and this may amount to 20–30% of the overt blood loss. Oedema formation increases as the systemic inflammatory response to trauma ensues.

Pulmonary oxygenation

To ensure optimal pulmonary oxygenation, patients with hypovolaemic shock should have a clear airway and adequate ventilation with oxygen at a high inspired concentration. Unconscious patients with severe shock will require tracheal intubation and positive pressure ventilation.

Control of haemorrhage and replacement of blood loss

Stop the bleeding as rapidly as possible; this may mean getting the patient to an operating room as soon as the airway is secured and breathing is adequate. Control peripheral haemorrhage with firm pressure. If brisk scalp bleeding persists despite adequate direct pressure, control it by closing the wound (tying off bleeding vessels with absorbable suture material if required) and applying a pressure dressing. Continuing volume loss associated with pelvic fractures may be controlled effectively with a pelvic compression device (Figure 5.1) followed by application of an external fixator (Figure 5.2). Extremity splinting using a Thomas splint, plaster of Paris and other techniques may also help limit further volume loss. Severe haemorrhage from open limb injuries may be controlled with a properly applied tourniquet. In the past, use of tourniquets in this way was discouraged, but recent military experience with blast injuries, in particular, has shown them to be a very effective. In patients at high risk of exsanguination in whom other attempts to achieve haemostasis are unlikely to be successful, early consultation with the interventional radiologist (embolisation) or thoracic surgeon (aortic cross-clamping) may save life.

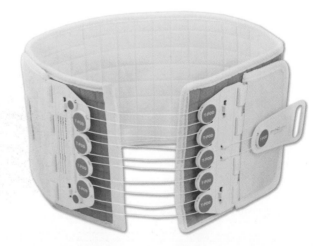

Figure 5.1 T-POD Pelvic compression device to enable immediate control of bleeding from pelvic fractures. (Pyng Medical Corp.)

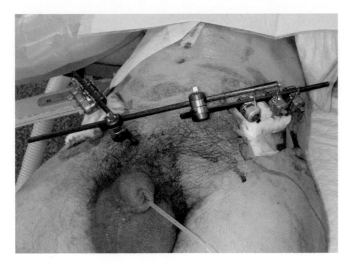

Figure 5.2 Pelvic fixator to control bleeding from complex pelvic injuries.

Attempts to gain intravenous access and infuse fluid must not delay transfer of the patient from the scene to hospital. In the presence of uncontrolled bleeding, fluid resuscitation and the accompanying increase in blood pressure may dislodge existing blood clots and increase haemorrhage. Guidance from the National Institute for Health and Clinical Excellence (NICE) indicates that in the prehospital management of trauma, intravenous fluid should not be given if a radial pulse can be felt. In the absence of a radial pulse (or a central pulse for penetrating torso injuries), NICE recommends that intravenous fluid is given in boluses of no more than 250 mL until a radial pulse is palpable. In reality, the balance between the risk of inducing organ ischaemia and the risk of accelerating haemorrhage is difficult to achieve. The head-injured patient is an exception to this principle: in this case the priority is to maintain cerebral perfusion with well-oxygenated blood (see Chapter 6).

Intravenous cannulation

In hospital, insert two short, large-bore intravenous cannulae (14 G). Take blood samples for full blood count, urea and electrolytes, and cross-match from the first cannula. The easiest site is usually the antecubital fossa, but anywhere on the upper limb is acceptable. The long saphenous vein at the ankle or the femoral vein in the groin can be used but these are not ideal if the patient has pelvic or intra-abdominal injuries. If peripheral access is impossible percutaneously, other options include central venous cannulation, cut-down on a peripheral vein or the intraosseous route. If the central route is used for rapid fluid resuscitation, insert a relatively short large-bore catheter (e.g. 8.5 F pulmonary artery introducer sheath). In the hypovolaemic patient, central venous pressure monitoring is frequently required but should not delay endeavours to limit further depletion of circulating volume. The intraosseous route (usually the proximal tibia) is particularly useful in children; the flow rates achieved via the intraosseous route have traditionally been considered inadequate for effective fluid resuscitation in adults. However, newer intraosseous infusions devices, such as the EZ-IO power driver system (www.vidacare.com), enable fluids to be infused under pressure at up to 200 mL/min, which is sufficient

for fluid resuscitation in adults. Obtain a sample for arterial blood gas analysis at an early stage.

Severely injured patients will have a marked lactic acidosis which will be reflected by a significant base deficit and high plasma lactate concentration (>2 mmol/L). Reversal of the base deficit is an indicator of adequate resuscitation. Insertion of an arterial cannula (radial, brachial or femoral) will enable continuous direct blood pressure monitoring and is convenient for repeated blood gas sampling. Patients with major injuries are critically ill and warrant invasive monitoring at the earliest opportunity.

Choice of intravenous fluid

In the exsanguinating patient, blood and blood products will be required rapidly. Crystalloids (e.g. sodium chloride or Hartmann's solution) (Figure 5.3) are typically used for initial fluid resuscitation of the trauma patient but the 2-L crystalloid fluid challenge previously recommended is no longer standard practice. Excessive quantities of normal saline will cause hyperchloraemic acidosis; this may mislead clinicians into thinking that a persisting base deficit is caused by inadequate resuscitation and may also be associated with renal impairment. Colloids (e.g. gelatin, starch; Figure 5.4) are more expensive than crystalloids, are associated with a small but well-defined risk of anaphylaxis and have no significant advantages over crystalloids in the early stages of resuscitation. Later on, when there is often considerable capillary leak caused by the systemic inflammatory response syndrome (SIRS), colloids have some theoretical advantages over crystalloid: they may reduce capillary leak and may be associated with less peripheral and pulmonary oedema. However, these theoretical advantages have never been proven in high-quality outcome studies and there is now clear evidence that starch solutions increase mortality in septic patients. In a large, randomised controlled trial of albumin versus saline in critically

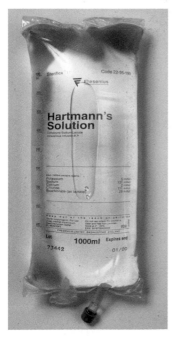

Figure 5.3 Hartmann's solution.

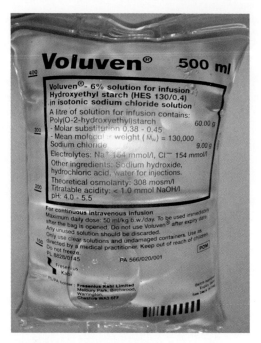

Figure 5.4 Hydroxyethyl starch.

ill patients, albumin was associated with increased mortality in a subgroup of severely head-injured patients.

Hypertonic saline solutions

Hypertonic crystalloid solutions are attractive because they provide small volume resuscitation and rapid restoration of haemodynamics with laboratory evidence of improved microcirculatory haemodynamics. They exert their effect by recruitment of interstitial volume, thus increasing circulating volume and blood pressure. However, raising the blood pressure may not always be an ideal goal, and their role in trauma resuscitation has yet to be defined. Solutions of hypertonic saline dextran and hypertonic saline with starch are now available; the addition of colloid prolongs their intravascular effect. Hypertonic saline reduces intracranial pressure and is used instead of mannitol for this purpose in some neurosurgical units. As yet, there is no evidence that use of hypertonic solutions improves survival rates for head-injured patients.

Blood and haemoglobin solutions

Once a patient has lost more than 30–40% of their blood volume, a resuscitation fluid with good oxygen-carrying capability is essential. Currently, this implies the need for a blood transfusion, which unfortunately has several disadvantages (Box 5.1).

> Box 5.1 **Disadvantages of blood transfusion**
>
> - Requires at least 45 min for full cross-match.
> - Expensive and in relatively short supply.
> - Limited shelf-life and requires a storage facility.
> - Small but definite risk of disease transmission .
> - Immunosuppressive effect, although reduced by leucodepletion.

Having overcome several problems related to toxic stroma, short intravascular half-life and high colloid osmotic pressure, several haemoglobin-based oxygen carriers (HBOCs) are at advanced stages of development. One HBOC (HBOC-201) is licensed for clinical use in South Africa. Unfortunately, these solutions are still associated with significant adverse effects: a trial of a diaspirin cross-linked haemoglobin solution (DCLHb) in trauma patients was stopped prematurely because of increased mortality in those receiving DCLHb. One of the reasons for the increased mortality may have been vasoconstriction caused by the DCLHb binding nitric oxide, a property shared by some of the other HBOCs.

What is the optimal haemoglobin concentration in the acute trauma patient?

Normovolaemic patients with good cardiopulmonary function will tolerate a haemoglobin concentration down to at least 7 g/dL. As long as normovolaemia is restored, the reduction in viscosity induces a significant increase in cardiac output and tends to improve tissue oxygenation. The problem is that during the resuscitation of the acute trauma patient, a history of ischaemic heart disease or significant respiratory disease may not be available. Furthermore, the haemoglobin concentration of a haemorrhaging patient undergoing resuscitation will be changing rapidly. Under these conditions the margin of safety is very small if the haemoglobin concentration is reduced as low as 7 g/dL. Thus, the haemoglobin concentration of the severely injured patient should be targeted in the range 8–10 g/dL depending on the specific circumstances and the patient's known co-morbidity.

Fluid warming

All intravenous fluids should be warmed adequately. A high-capacity fluid warmer, such as the Level 1 H1000 (www.smiths-medical.com), will be required to cope with the rapid infusion rates used during trauma patient resuscitation (Figure 5.5). Hypothermia (core temperature less than 35°C) is a serious complication of severe trauma and haemorrhage; it is caused by exposure, tissue hypoperfusion and infusion of inadequately warmed fluids. In trauma patients hypothermia is an independent predictor of survival. Hypothermia has several adverse effects (Box 5.2).

> Box 5.2 **Adverse effects of hypothermia**
>
> - Hypothermia contributes to the coagulopathy accompanying massive transfusion.
> - The oxyhaemoglobin dissociation curve is shifted to the left by a decrease in temperature, thus impairing peripheral oxygen delivery.
> - Shivering may compound the lactic acidosis which typically accompanies hypovolaemia.
> - Increased incidence of infection.
> - Causes a gradual decline in heart rate and cardiac output while increasing the propensity for myocardial dysrhythmias and other morbid cardiac events.
> - Hyperglycaemia.

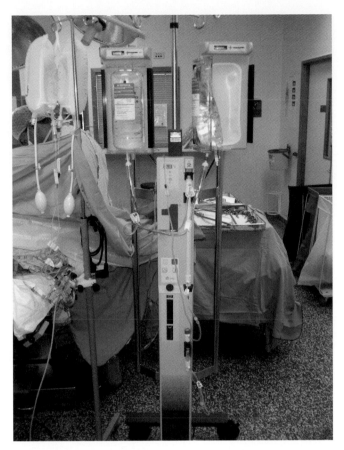

Figure 5.5 High-capacity fluid warmer.

Coagulation

The combination of hypothermia and massive transfusion will cause a profound coagulopathy. Until recently, fresh frozen plasma (FFP), platelets and cryoprecipitate have been given on the basis of abnormal clotting tests as well as clinical evidence of coagulopathy. But in the presence of massive haemorrhage, the results of clotting studies will lag far behind the clinical condition of the patient.

Observational data from both military and civilian settings have documented increased survival rates associated with earlier use of platelets and FFP, particularly when given with blood in ratios approximating 1:1:1. Despite significant methodological weaknesses associated with these non-randomised studies, many clinicians have adopted this transfusion strategy in the presence of massive haemorrhage. There is good evidence that tranexamic acid (1 g over 10 min given within 3 h of injury and then an infusion of 1 g over 8 h) reduces mortality from bleeding in trauma patients. A multicentre, randomised, placebo-controlled phase III trial failed to show benefit for activated recombinant factor VII in severely injured trauma patients with bleeding refractory to standard treatment. The use of recombinant factor VII may still be considered if coagulopathy persists despite adequate treatment with other blood products, but the initial enthusiasm for this expensive product is waning.

Monitoring progress and treatment

The status of the patient's intravascular volume is best determined by observing the change in vital signs and other monitored variables (see factors in Box 5.3) after a fluid challenge. Failure to improve the patient's vital signs suggests exsanguinating haemorrhage (associated with major thoracic, abdominal or pelvic injuries) and the need for immediate surgery and transfusion of blood. Group O blood can be obtained immediately, group-confirmed blood can be issued in 10 min, and a full cross-match will take 45 min. A transient response to the initial fluid challenge suggests that the patient may have lost 20–40% of their intravascular volume and has ongoing bleeding; they will require immediate surgical assessment and are likely to need blood. A sustained reduction in heart rate and increase in blood pressure suggest only moderate blood loss (<20% blood volume); in the absence of ongoing bleeding, these patients may be effectively resuscitated with clear fluids only. Once haemorrhage has been controlled, continue fluid resuscitation to produce an adequate arterial pressure and a urine output of 1 mL/kg/min. A normal serum lactate and reducing base deficit indicate adequate oxygen delivery.

Box 5.3 **Variables to monitor**

- Oxygen saturation by pulse oximetry (SpO_2).
- Respiratory rate.
- Pulse rate.
- Arterial blood pressure.
- Pulse pressure.
- Central venous pressure.
- Urine output.
- Base deficit and/or lactate.
- Temperature.
- Mental state.
- Changes in the electrocardiogram.

A rising central venous pressure associated with a low blood pressure, tachycardia and a reduced urine output indicates tension pneumothorax, cardiac tamponade or cardiac failure (secondary to cardiac contusion or ischaemic heart disease). Cardiac failure may be confirmed by echocardiography, which will demonstrate a poorly contracting myocardium; treatment with an inotropic drug such as dobutamine may be appropriate.

Analgesia

Analgesia is given not only for its compassionate value but also because it reduces the catecholamine secretion associated with hypovolaemic shock. Give an opioid (e.g. morphine or fentanyl) intravenously in increments.

Summary

The priority in treating haemorrhagic shock is to stop the bleeding. Before haemorrhage is controlled, fluid resuscitation should be individualised: the decision to give fluid is determined by the risk of organ ischaemia versus the risk of increasing the bleeding. Fluid resuscitation may be initiated with crystalloid and blood is given to achieve a haemoglobin concentration of 8–10 g/dL. Adequate warming of all fluid is essential and coagulopathy is common. In the presence of massive haemorrhage, early infusion of FFP and platelets, as well as blood, may increase survival.

Further reading

American College of Surgeons Committee on Trauma. (2008) *Advanced Trauma Life Support Program For Doctors: Student Course Manual*, 8th edn. Chicago: American College of Surgeons.

CRASH-2 trial collaborators. (2010) Effects of tranexamic acid on death, vascular occlusive events, and blood transfusion in trauma patients with significant haemorrhage (CRASH-2): a randomised placebo-controlled trial. Lancet 376:23–32.

Finfer S, Bellomo R, Boyce N, *et al.* (2004) A comparison of albumin and saline for fluid resuscitation in the intensive care unit. N Engl J Med 350: 2247–56.

National Institute for Health and Clinical Excellence. (2004) *Pre-Hospital Initiation of Fluid Replacement Therapy for Trauma*. London: National Institute for Health and Clinical Excellence.

CHAPTER 6

Head Injuries

Lisa E. Munro-Davies

University Hospitals Bristol NHS Foundation Trust, Bristol, UK

OVERVIEW

At the end of this chapter the reader should be able to:

- appreciate the range of incidence, causes and severity of head injuries
- understand the pathophysiology of head injury
- assess the severity of a head injury
- appreciate the role of radiological investigations in the head-injured patient
- understand the appropriate initial management in head injuries of all severities
- assess which patients require discussion with and possible transfer to a neurosurgical unit.

In 400 BC Hippocrates said that 'No head injury is too severe to despair of or too trivial to ignore'. This aphorism remains true today and reflects the difficulty facing clinicians who treat head-injured patients; how do you identify those with a head injury who may go on to develop life-threatening complications?

The search for an assured answer to this question has over recent years lead to the development of several sets of evidence-based guidelines aimed at helping the assessing clinician to identify such patients and also outline advice on appropriate initial management and disposal of head-injured patients. All these guidelines share similar principles and their implementation is often determined by local factors such as the availability of specialist resources.

The majority of head injuries within the UK are managed within general hospitals, with the emergency department being the first and often only point of contact. Less than 1% of all head-injured patients presenting to hospitals in the UK are admitted to a neurosurgical unit. Therefore the majority of head injury care in the UK is performed by doctors working within non-neuroscience areas (emergency physicians, general practitioners (GPs), orthopaedic/general surgeons) and it is these practitioners that such guidelines are intended to assist.

ABC of Major Trauma, Fourth Edition. Edited by David V. Skinner and Peter A. Driscoll.
© 2013 Blackwell Publishing Ltd. Published 2013 by Blackwell Publishing Ltd.

Advice given in this chapter accords with guidelines recommended by the National Institute for Health and Clinical Excellence (NICE) and the Scottish Intercollegiate Guidelines Network (SIGN) on the management of patients with head injuries.

Epidemiology and causes of head injury

Blunt head injury is a leading cause of death and disability both in the UK and worldwide, the socioeconomic cost of which is estimated to be in the order of hundreds of millions of pounds per annum in the UK alone.

The published incidence rates of emergency department attendances with a presenting complaint of head injury vary widely, depending on a number of geographical and social factors, but in the UK can be approximated to 500 per 100,000 of the population (although published figures have varied between 300 to nearly 2000 per 100,000). This represents approximately 4% of all emergency department attendances and has a preponderance of young males where there has been alcohol involved and the mechanism of injury is a road traffic accident (RTA). There are multiple associated factors in head injury, summarised in Table 6.1, of which alcohol is the most common. There are also multiple mechanisms of injury (Table 6.2) and there have been shown to be reliable correlations between these two (e.g. young/male/alcohol/RTA or child/fall/lower socioeconomic class).

In terms of acute prognosis, head-injured patients are typically classified as minimal, minor, moderate or severe according to features in the history and their Glasgow Coma Score on initial presentation (Table 6.3). The vast majority of presentations are within the minimal to minor groups with only around 10% being in the moderate to severe head injury group (MSHI).

Table 6.1 Factors associated with attendance at emergency departments with a presenting complaint of head injury.

Factor	Association
Alcohol	Increased risk
Age	Peak incidence 15–24 years
Gender	Male ×2 rate of female
Geography	USA ×2 rate UK
Environment	Higher rate in urban versus rural areas
Affluence	Increased rate with decreased affluence

Table 6.2 Most common mechanisms of injury in head injury presentations to emergency departments in UK (listed in decreasing order of incidence).

Mechanism of injury	Notes
Road traffic accidents (most common mechanism)	Account for only 25% of all head injuries but 60% of all deaths from head injury
Domestic accidents	
Assaults	
Falls	May be from trips, syncope, seizures, suicide or other causes. More common in children
Sports	Horse riding most frequent cause in adults, golf most frequent cause in children
Industrial accidents(least common mechanism)	

Table 6.3 Classification of head injury by presentation and Glasgow Coma Score.

Head injury group	Features of presentation	Glasgow Coma Score on presentation (3–15)
Minimal	No loss of consciousness, amnesia, disorientation	15
Minor	Loss of consciousness or amnesia or disorientation (need only be 1 of above)	13–15
Moderate		8–12
Severe		<8

Pathophysiology of head injury

Damage to the brain from a head injury can occur either at the time of impact, *primary brain injury*, or as a result of events that may occur subsequent to the impact, *secondary brain injury*. There is nothing that can be done to limit primary brain injury other than pre-emptive accident prevention measures. However, secondary brain injury can be prevented and this is where the focus of head injury management lies.

The clinical manifestation of primary brain injury can range from a minor concussional injury with brief loss of consciousness to severe brain injury with focal neurological deficits or prolonged coma. Primary brain injury may be closed or penetrating. In the United Kingdom the majority of head injuries result from blunt force trauma and penetrating head injuries are relatively rare.

Primary brain injury

The impact damage of primary brain injury may result in two types of brain damage which may co-exist.

- *Contusions and/or lacerations to the cortical tissue*: these may be single or multiple and may be at the point of impact or opposite (contre-coup). The presence of a contusion may not in itself depress the level of consciousness, but this may develop if bleeding into the area creates a haematoma or if significant oedema develops, having a mass effect (Figure 6.1).

- *Diffuse axonal injury*: this is a deceleration injury which causes shearing of the neuronal axons. Macroscopically the brain may appear 'normal' but microscopic areas of haemorrhage will be present in areas such as the corpus callosum and the superior cerebellar peduncle. The clinical effects range from mild confusion to coma and even death. As neuronal regeneration is limited the effects of repeated minor injury are cumulative.

A further type of primary impact injury of consequence is a fracture of the skull. If this is a closed linear fracture then its importance is in the increased risk of intracerebral injury that is associated with the presence of a fracture. If the injury is compound and depressed then it requires prompt surgical treatment for debridement and elevation. Such injuries carry a high risk of causing epilepsy particularly if the dura mater has been breached when intracerebral infection is also a significant possible complication.

Secondary brain injury

Secondary brain injury may occur at any time following the impact episode and may be the result of several mechanisms in isolation or conjunction.

Intracerebral haematoma (Table 6.4)

Bleeding may occur outwith (extradural; Figure 6.2) or within the dura (subdural; Figure 6.3).

Subdural bleeding occurs from rupture of the bridging veins running from the cortical surface to the venous sinuses. This

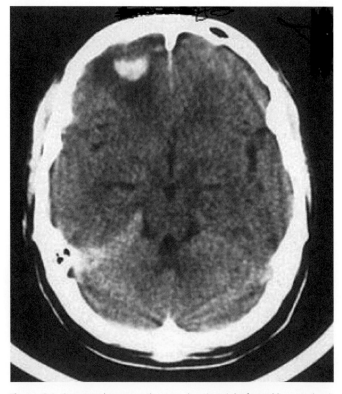

Figure 6.1 Computed tomography scan showing right frontal haemorrhagic contusion.

Table 6.4 Incidence of intracerebral haematomas by location.

Type of haematoma	Incidence
Pure extradural	27%
Pure subdural	26%
Subdural + intracerebral	38%
Extradural + subdural	9%

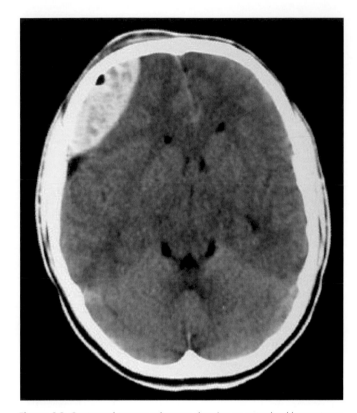

Figure 6.2 Computed tomography scan showing an extradural haematoma.

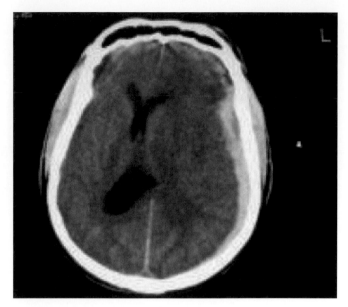

Figure 6.3 Computed tomography scan showing a subdural haematoma.

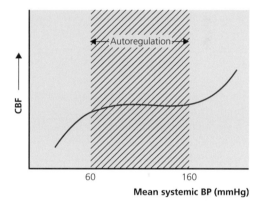

Figure 6.4 Autoregulation of cerebral blood flow. BP, blood pressure; CBF, cerebral blood flow.

can occur in isolation but more frequently it will co-exist with intracerebral haemorrhage from underlying damaged cortex. In the frontal and temporal areas this may result in necrotic brain tissue mixed with subdural haemorrhage, which may be referred to as a 'burst lobe'. The high incidence of underlying cortical damage gives a poor prognosis for traumatic subdural haemorrhage.

Bleeding may also occur from vessels outside the dura, which may be in the presence or absence of a skull fracture. Most common would be from the middle meningeal vessels although occasionally extradural haematomas are caused by damage to the transverse or sagittal sinuses. The bleeding from these vessels may occur slowly and give the 'lucid period' post injury associated with such injuries. If evacuated promptly, extradural haematomas can have a good outcome as the underlying cortical tissue is intact.

Intracerebral haematomas cause brain damage directly or indirectly as a result of tonsillar or tentorial herniation.

Cerebral swelling

This occurs with or without haematomas and results from vasodilation and oedema through poorly understood mechanisms.

Cerebral ischaemia

Cerebral ischaemia can be caused either by hypoxia or by impaired cerebral perfusion. Cerebral perfusion pressure (CPP) is related to mean arterial pressure (MAP) and intracranial pressure (ICP):

$$CPP = MAP - ICP$$

Normally a compensatory mechanism known as 'autoregulation' ensures that fluctuations in MAP and therefore CPP do not significantly alter cerebral blood flow (CBF). This mechanism works between pressures of 60 and 160 mmHg. In damaged brain autoregulation is impaired and the relationship between CPP and CBF becomes linear, i.e. if CPP/MAP drops, CBF drops; if CPP/MAP rises, CBF rises (Figure 6.4). So, an increase in ICP following head injury (from swelling, haematoma) will result in decreased CBF with the situation being further worsened by any decrease in MAP secondary to systemic hypotension. Glutamate excess and free radical accumulation may cause further neuronal damage.

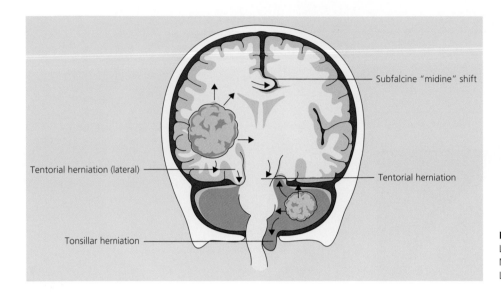

Subfalcine "midine" shift

Tentorial herniation (lateral)

Tentorial herniation

Tonsillar herniation

Figure 6.5 Types of brain shift. (Adapted from Lindsay & Bone (1997) Neurology and Neurosurgery Illustrated, 3rd Edition, Churchill Livingstone.)

Brain shift

The brain is contained in an inelastic box and any increase in the pressure in that box (haematoma formation, swelling) will result in the contents being forced into other parts of the box through openings: 'brain shift'. Four types of brain shift can occur and if pressure rises are unchecked they can occur sequentially (Figure 6.5).

- **Subfalcine shift**: occurs early with unilateral pressure increase. Seldom produces any clinical effect.
- **Lateral tentorial/uncal herniation**: further unilateral pressure increase herniates the medial edge of the temporal lobe (uncus) through the tentorial hiatus. The oculomotor nerve runs beneath and is stretched, leading to dilation of the ipsilateral pupil.
- **Central tentorial herniation**: follows if pressure increases further. The midbrain and diencephalon are vertically displaced through the tentorial hiatus. Both pupils may dilate and ischaemia of the brainstem with progressive dysfunction occurs from mechanical distortion and stretching of the perforating vessels.
- **Tonsillar herniation**: may follow central tentorial herniation or occur in isolation as the result of an expanding subtentorial mass. The cerebellar tonsils herniate through the foramen magnum. A degree of upward herniation may also occur. Clinically the effects are of midbrain/brainstem dysfunction.

Infection

Both compound depressed or basal skull fractures may be associated with a dural tear. In such instances there is a potential route for intracranial infection (meningitis/abscess). This seldom occurs within 48 h of injury but may develop after several months or even years.

Assessment and treatment of head injuries are aimed at the prevention of secondary brain injury with early recognition of the signs of rising ICP and appropriate interventions to reverse/minimize these effects and to maintain adequate CBF.

Initial assessment of head injuries

In severely injured patients with multiple injuries, the 'ABCDE' principles of trauma assessment and resuscitation as outlined in the American College of Surgeons Advanced Trauma Life Support (ATLS) courses remain unchanged in the presence of a depressed level of consciousness or significant head injury. Standard assessment and resuscitation with interventions to support airway, breathing and circulation will in such patients identify any significant primary brain injury and also include the appropriate initial steps in limiting secondary brain injury by preventing hypoxia and supporting MAP and therefore CBF.

However, the majority of head-injured patients reviewed in primary care and emergency departments do not have such severe injury patterns and their assessment should focus on features in the history and examination which allow risk stratification and facilitate decision making regarding the need for further investigation and/or observation.

Table 6.5 lists features in the history which must be sought when assessing a head-injured patient and, for those in the prehospital setting, the presence of any of these features necessitates referral to hospital for further assessment. Where no history is available from the patient, every effort should be made to interview any observers for a record of events surrounding the injury.

As well as eliciting key features in the history, the assessing clinician must also perform specific examinations on patients following head injury, summarised in Table 6.6. As with features in the history, the presence of these signs necessitates referral for further assessment.

Conscious level must be recorded using the Glasgow Coma Scale (GCS), a scoring system combining eye opening with verbal and motor responses initially developed as a research tool for assessing efficacy of head injury management in neurosurgical centres (Table 6.7). It assigns a score of 3–15 according to graded responses to voice and pain. Serially performed, it is a reliable predictor of worsening intracranial injury and any deterioration in GCS in the head-injured patient under observation

Table 6.5 Features in the history that must be recorded and if present necessitate referral to hospital for further assessment.

Feature	Additional information
Significant mechanism of injury	High energy (RTA, fall from a height) Possible penetrating head injury Possible non-accidental injury in a child
Loss of consciousness	GCS <15 at any time
Post-traumatic amnesia (PTA, i.e. amnesia for the incident or subsequent events)	The period of PTA relates to the severity of the injury. However, retrograde amnesia (i.e. amnesia for events before the injury) bears no relation to the severity of the injury and may improve with time
Neurological symptoms	Severe and persistent headache Persistent nausea and vomiting Altered behaviour/irritability Seizure Alterations in vision Weaknesses or altered sensations
Medical co-morbidity	Anticoagulant therapy Bleeding tendency Previous neurosurgery Alcoholism
Adverse social factors	Acute intoxication with alcohol Concurrent use of social drugs No-one to supervise patient at home

GCS, Glasgow Coma Score; PTA, post-traumatic amnesia; RTA, road traffic accident.

indicates the need for immediate investigation and action where necessary.

All head-injured patients should also be assessed for possible injury to the cervical spine. If the mechanism of injury makes this likely (hyperextension, axial loading) or if there is any clinical suspicion of this (C-spine pain/tenderness, neurological signs) then the patient must be immobilised appropriately and referred for further assessment.

Radiological assessment in head injuries

Most head-injured patients require minimal or no investigation. The main consideration is whether a computed tomography (CT) scan, which is now the primary investigation for the diagnosis or exclusion of significant intracerebral injury in head-injured patients, is required. This should only be performed following appropriate assessment and if certain criteria which have been shown to be indicative of an increased risk of intracerebral injury are met. This may involve imaging of the head only but may also include the cervical spine. Where required, the cervical spine may often be adequately imaged using plain radiographs (lateral, anteroposterior [AP] and peg views). Where the whole C-spine is not visualised on plain films or where injury is suspected on these, further assessment by CT scanning is required. Criteria for who should be scanned are outlined in Boxes 6.1 and 6.2.

The role of plain radiographs of the skull (SXR) in head injury management is much reduced in modern practice and some would

Table 6.6 Physical signs to be sought in head injury.

Examination features	Additional information
Scalp injury	Lacerations: should be explored for evidence of fracture or foreign body Haematomas: may overlie a fracture/depressed injury **NB**: Intracranial haematomas can occur in the absence of any external evidence of injury
Basal skull fracture	Anterior fossa: CSF rhinorrhoea/bilateral periorbital haematoma/subconjunctival haemorrhage without posterior limit Petrous fracture: CSF otorrhoea/haemotympanum/bruising over mastoid (Battle's sign: may take 48 h to develop)
Conscious level	GCS must be recorded in its component parts rather than as a single score (e.g. E4 V5 M6 = 15)
Pupil response	Light reflex tests optic (II) and oculomotor (III) cranial nerve function. Tentorial herniation due to raised pressure dilates the ipsilateral pupil due to pressure on cranial nerve III
Limb weakness	Pronator drift is the most sensitive test for a mild hemiparesis. Hemiparesis usually occurs contralateral to the side of an expanding lesion. It may also occur on the ipsilateral side due to indentation of the contralatral cerebral peduncle by the edge of the tentorium cerebelli (Kernohan's notch)
Cranial nerves	Basal skull fracture can result in damage to cranial nerves and a full examination should be recorded where possible
Vital signs	Cushing's reflex (hypertension with bradycardia) is a late sign of raised ICP

CSF, cerebrospinal fluid; GCS, Glasgow Coma Score; ICP, intracranial pressure.

Table 6.7 Components of the Glasgow Coma Score (3–15).

Component	Response	Score
Eye opening	Spontaneous	4
	To speech	3
	To pain	2
	None	1
Best verbal response	Orientated	5
	Confused	4
	Inappropriate words	3
	Incomprehensible sounds	2
	None	1
Best motor response	Obeys commands	6
	Localises to pain	5
	Withdraws from pain	4
	Flexion to pain	3
	Extension to pain	2
	None	1

suggest that it is obsolete. However, if the patient is GCS 15 and a CT is not being performed then SXR should be considered particularly if a depressed skull fracture cannot be excluded. The diagnosis of a fracture on SXR indicates the need for CT to further evaluate injury.

Box 6.1 **CT head should be performed in a head-injured patient who has any of the following**

- Glasgow Coma Score (GCS) less than 13 at any point since injury.
- GCS 13 or 14 at 2 h post injury.
- Suspected compound or depressed skull fracture.
- Any sign of base of skull fracture.
- Post-traumatic seizure.
- Focal neurological deficit.
- Persistent severe headache or vomiting.
- Irritability or altered behavior.
- Post-traumatic amnesia >30 min.
- Impaired clotting (warfarin therapy or bleeding disorder).
- Dangerous mechanism of injury (ejected from vehicle, pedestrian struck by vehicle, fall >1 metre or 5 stairs).

Box 6.2 **Cervical spine imaging (CT or X-ray) should be performed in a head-injured patient who has any of the following**

- Glasgow Coma Score <15 at the time of assessment.
- Paraesthesia in the extremities.
- Focal neurological deficit.
- Not possible to test range of movement in the neck.
- Not possible to actively rotate neck to 45° left and right (if assessment possible).

Admission or discharge?

Only a small minority of head-injured patients require admission to hospital, usually for one of the following reasons.

- The severity of their primary brain injury.
- Risk stratification identifies them as being at high risk of developing a worsening secondary brain injury.
- Social reasons.

The majority of patients admitted undergo a brief (24 h) period of observation which may or may not involve further investigation prior to their discharge.

Indications for admission to hospital following head injury are listed in Box 6.3.

A patient may be safely discharged for observation at home if GCS 15 and if none of the features noted in Box 6.3 are present. If discharged, then certain social criteria must be met prior to discharge (Box 6.4). One of these criteria is that verbal and written advice must be given to patients and carers about observations and actions in the event of any concerns. The suggested wording for such advice is outlined in national guidelines and summarised in Box 6.5. The patient should also be advised that they may experience some symptoms lasting up to 2 weeks such as mild headache and nausea, dizziness, irritability, poor concentration and memory,

Box 6.3 **Indications for admission to hospital following head injury**

- Impaired level of consciousness (Glasgow Coma Score [GCS] <15).
- GCS 15 but any of the following risk factors:
  - Post-traumatic amnesia
  - Persistent nausea/vomiting
  - Seizure
  - Focal neurological sign
  - Irritability/altered behaviour
  - Clinical or radiological evidence of skull fracture
  - Suspected penetrating injury
  - Abnormal computed tomography scan
  - Severe headache or other neurological symptom
  - Significant medical problems.
- Bleeding tendency (warfarin therapy or clotting disorder).
- Cannot be supervised by a responsible adult for 24 h following discharge.
- Under the influence of social drugs or alcohol.

Box 6.4 **Social criteria that must be met prior to discharge from hospital following a head injury**

- A responsible adult is available and willing to supervise the patient for 24 h.
- Verbal and written instructions about observations to be made and action to be taken are given to and discussed with the responsible adult.
- There is easy access to a telephone.
- The home is within a reasonable distance of medical advice.
- Transport home is available.

tiredness, lack of appetite and sleeping problems. These are all features of a concussional injury.

Inpatient management

The mainstay of management in the small proportion of patients admitted to hospital following head injury is careful repeated observations aimed at prompt detection of any neurological deterioration which may necessitate further action. Observations should be performed by suitably trained staff to ensure consistency and reliability and must include recording of GCS, pupil responses, limb power, respiratory rate, pulse and blood pressure. These are all features included on a standard neurological observation chart. How frequently such observations should be made has not been rigorously studied but should relate to the estimated risk of clinically influential findings. The risk of significant deterioration is greatest in the first 6 h and reduces thereafter. A suggested frequency of observations is outlined in Box 6.6. Certain patterns of deterioration in observations should prompt immediate reappraisal by a doctor (Box 6.7).

Box 6.5 **Information to be contained in discharge advice following a head injury**

Indications for returning to hospital following a head injury.

- Any decrease in level of consciousness.
- Any confusion.
- Any drowsiness when you would normally be awake.
- Any problems understanding or speaking.
- Any loss of balance or problems walking.
- Any weakness in limbs.
- Any altered vision.
- Very painful, persistent headaches.
- Any vomiting.
- Any fits.
- Clear fluid from nose or ears.
- Bleeding from one/both ears.

Advice following a head injury

- **DO** stay within easy reach of a telephone and medical help.
- **DO** have plenty of rest and avoid stressful situations.
- **DO NOT** stay at home alone for the first 48 h.
- **DO NOT** take alcohol or other social drugs.
- **DO NOT** take sedatives, sleeping tablets or tranquillisers unless on a doctor's instructions.
- **DO NOT** play contact sports for at least 3 weeks.
- **DO NOT** return to school, college, work until you feel you have completely recovered.
- **DO NOT** drive a car, motorbike or bicycle or operate machinery unless you feel you have completely recovered.

Box 6.6 **Frequency of observations in head-injured patients requiring hospital admission**

- $1/2$ hourly for 2 h then
- 1 hourly for 4 h then
- 2 hourly for 6 h then
- 4 hourly thereafter until fit for discharge.

Box 6.7 **Examples of neurological deterioration prompting immediate review by a doctor**

- The development of agitation or altered behavior.
- A sustained decrease in conscious level of at least one point in the motor or verbal response or two points on the eye opening responses of the Glasgow Coma Score.
- The development of severe or increasing headache or persistent vomiting.
- New or evolving neurological symptoms or signs, such as pupil inequality or asymmetry of limb or facial movements.

The second aim of admission is to provide optimal conditions for recovery from primary brain injury and to prevent worsening of any secondary brain injury. Paramount in this is the prevention of hypoxia, maintenance of adequate CBF and control of ICP.

Hypoxia

Ensure that the airway is patent and administer supplemental oxygen. This may involve use of facemask oxygen only or may require airway adjuncts in the obtunded patient or even endotracheal intubation (Box 6.8). Intubation should be by rapid-sequence induction (RSI) and with inline C-spine immobilisation unless injury can be definitely excluded. Ventilation should aim at maintaining normocarbia and good oxygenation.

Box 6.8 **Indications for endotracheal intubation in head-injured patients**

- Glasgow Coma Score <9.
- Absent gag reflex on suctioning in unconscious patient.
- Threatened airway compromise: facial fracture, oropharyngeal bleeding.
- Inadequate ventilation or oxygenation: low PO_2/high PCO_2 with supplemental oxygen. (**NB**: Look for and treat any underlying chest injury, e.g. pneumothorax).

Maintainence of cerebral blood flow

Intravenous (IV) fluids should be administered as required to resuscitate the patient and to maintain normovolaemia or slight hypervolaemia whilst being careful not to overload the patient. Hypotonic or glucose-containing fluids should be avoided as they may worsen cerebral oedema and result in harmful hyperglycaemia. Normal saline or Ringer's lactate should be used.

Intracranial pressure control

Diuretics (mannitol and furosemide) can be used for the management of elevated ICP. They should only be used in response to a clear neurological deterioration (e.g. unilateral dilating pupil) and ideally in discussion with a neurosurgical centre as such patients are likely to require transfer for further management of their raised ICP. In such instances, a bolus dose of 1 mg/kg of mannitol should be given over 5 min. If CT scanning has not been performed, it should be done immediately if the patient's condition allows safe transfer to the scanner. Furosemide may be used in conjunction with mannitol at a dose of 0.3–0.5 mg/kg IV. Both drugs should be avoided in the hypovolaemic patient and repeated doses are not recommended in the acute setting. Titrated aliquots of hypertonic saline may be administered intravenously as an alternative to these diuretics for the same indications and with the same caveats to it's use. Barbiturates are also effective in reducing ICP but they are not indicated in the acute management of raised ICP and their use is retained for further management in the intensive care setting. Steroids have been shown to have no beneficial effect in controlling raised ICP and should not be used in head injury management.

Further management of patients with persistently elevated ICP should be undertaken in an intensive care setting and those with an expanding intracranial mass will require transfer to a neurosurgical centre for a definitive surgical procedure to assist in the treatment of their ICP problems. This may involve any or all of: insertion of an ICP monitoring device, external ventricular drainage and craniotomy.

Management of seizures

Seizures occur in about 5% of closed head injuries requiring admission to hospital and in 15% of those with severe head injury. If they occur within the first week, they carry a low risk of future epilepsy but in the acute setting they require prompt treatment as they may worsen hypoxia and elevate ICP further. Phenytoin should be used to prevent and treat seizures (18 mg/kg IV over 20 min with ECG monitoring) as a loading dose and maintenance therapy thereafter. If seizures persist following phenytoin loading, titrated doses of suitable IV benzodiazepines (clonazepam, lorazepam) may be used but respiratory depression should be avoided. Persistent seizures may need a general anaesthetic to resolve.

Antibiotics

Empirical antibiotics should be given according to local protocols in compound skull injuries. In the case of basal skull fractures, there is no conclusive evidence that their use reduces the incidence of meningitis and there is a concern that their use may promote the growth of resistant organisms. In such instances advice should be taken from the regional neurosurgical unit.

Transfer to a neurosurgical unit

As already stated, less than 1% of head-injured patients require admission to a neurosurgical unit in the UK. Those who do are the most severely injured with the highest risk of complications and death. Their admission may be to undergo a surgical procedure or for specialist monitoring and treatment of persistently raised ICP or other complications of head injury.

Many more head-injured patients than will require admission to a neurosurgical unit will have their care discussed with surgeons at such a unit. Patients who should be discussed with a neurosurgeon include those:

- in whom CT shows a recent intracranial lesion
- fulfilling the criteria for CT scanning but this cannot be done within an appropriate period
- in whom the clinical features suggest that neurosurgical assessment, monitoring or management are appropriate irrespective of CT findings (Box 6.9).

For patients requiring transfer, this should follow the guidelines set out by the Neuroanaesthesia Society of Great Britain and Ireland and the Association of Anaesthetists of Great Britain and Ireland. Good communication and documentation are essential to ensure patient safety in such transfers.

Box 6.9 **Features suggesting that neurosurgical assessment, monitoring or management is appropriate**

- Persisting coma (Glasgow Coma Score [GCS] <9) after initial resuscitation.
- Confusion persisting more than 4 h.
- Deterioration in level of consciousness following admission (a sustained drop of 1 point on the motor or verbal scores or 2 points on the eye opening score of the GCS).
- Progressive focal neurological signs.
- Seizure without full recovery.
- Compound depressed skull fracture.
- Definite or suspected penetrating injury.
- Cerebrospinal fluid leak or other sign of basal skull fracture.

Paediatric head injuries

All the principles of head injury assessment and management outlined already apply to injuries in the paediatric population. Table 6.8 outlines additional specific practice points to be considered when dealing with a paediatric head injury.

Delayed effects of head injury

The majority of people sustaining a head injury will make an uncomplicated recovery. There are, however, a number of sequelae of varying significance which may follow a head injury (Table 6.9).

All patients discharged from hospital following a head injury should have a letter sent to their GP and should be advised to seek review with the GP for any continuing concerns or symptoms.

Table 6.8 Additional points to remember when managing paediatric head injuries.

Stage of management	Paediatric point
Assessment	Paediatric version of GCS should be used Assess the fontanelle in infants (? tense) Non-accidental injury (NAI) must be considered and local protocols followed Assessment should be performed by staff experienced in assessing children Resuscitation should follow standard APLS protocols
Imaging	Skull fractures are less of a discriminator of severity of injury than in adults SXR may be required if NAI suspected
Admission versus discharge	Admit for observation if assessment difficult to complete in full (e.g. <3 years old) Admit if suspicion of NAI
Observation	Observation should be undertaken by staff experienced in paediatric care
Transfer	Should be performed by staff experienced in the transfer of the critically ill child

APLS, Advanced Paediatric Life Support; GCS, Glasgow Coma Score; SXR, plain radiograph of the skull.

Table 6.9 Delayed effects of head injury.

Effect	Significance
Post-traumatic epilepsy	
Early epilepsy (occurs <1 week post HI)	Occurs in 5% HI admitted to hospital Generalised or focal seizures Risk factors: age less than 5 years, prolonged PTA, intracranial haematoma, compound depressed fracture
Late epilepsy (occurs >1 week post HI)	Occurs in 5% HI admitted to hospital Generalised or complex partial seizures Usually presents within 1 year post HI Risk factors: early epilepsy (25%), intracranial haematoma (35%), compound depressed fracture (17%)
CSF leak	Persistent otorrhoea, rhinorrhoea, headache or 'salty taste' Surgical repair to decrease risk of meningitis
Postconcussional symptoms	Headache, dizziness, irritability, poor concentration and memory, fatigue lasting >2 weeks post HI. No specific treatment, symptom control and HI support services follow-up
Cumulative brain damage	Repeat 'minor' trauma has a cumulative effect from non-recoverable primary injuries. Eventually fixed deficits develop, e.g. boxer's dementia/parkinsonism
Chronic subdural haematoma	May present with non-specific features: dementia, headache, vomiting, occasionally focal weakness. Predisposing factors: cerebral atrophy, alcoholism, coagulation disorder, low CSF pressure (e.g. shunted) Can be evacuated through burr holes

CSF, cerebrospinal fluid; HI, head injury; PTA, post-traumatic amnesia.

Further reading

Advanced Life Support Group. (2005) *Advanced Paediatric Life Support Student Course Manual*, 4thedn. London: BMJ Publishing.

American College of Surgeons. (2004) *Advanced Trauma Life Support for Doctors. Student Course Manual*, 7th edn. Chicago: American College of Surgeons.

National Institute for Health and Clinical Excellence. (2003) *Head Injury. Triage, Assessment and Early Management of Head Injury in Infants, Children and Adults. Clinical Guideline 4*. London: National Institute for Health and Clinical Excellence. Partial Update CG56 September 2007.

Scottish Intercollegiate Guidelines Network. (2000) *Early Management of Patients with a Head Injury. A National Clinical Guideline. SIGN Publication 46*. Edinburgh: Scottish Intercollegiate Guidelines Network.

Working Party of the Neuroanaesthesia Society and Association of Anaesthetists. (1996) *Recommendations for the Transfer of Patients with Acute Head Injuries to Neurosurgical Units*. London: Neuroanaesthesia Society of Great Britain and Ireland and the Association of Anaesthetists of Great Britain and Ireland.

CHAPTER 7

Maxillofacial Trauma

Steve R. Watt-Smith,[1,2] Sarah J. Wilson[3] and Karen A. Eley[2]

[1]Oxford University Hospitals NHS Trust, Oxford, UK
[2]University of Oxford, Oxford, UK
[3]Wexham Park Hospital, Slough, UK

OVERVIEW

Priorities when managing maxillofacial trauma

- Airway control with cervical spine immobilisation: consider sitting the patient more upright if there is significant facial trauma.
- Adequate ventilation.
- Haemorrhage control (see Box 7.1).

Other considerations

- Assess visual function and globe position.
- Check facial sensation.
- Look for cerebrospinal fluid leaks.
- Check dentition.
- Accurate documentation is essential.

Severe injuries to the head and neck region may deter the unwary from the absolute goals of securing the airway and correcting life-threatening haemorrhage. On initial presentation, injuries may seem trivial, but may be life or sight threatening, requiring a high index of suspicion to make the correct diagnosis. Knowledge of the mechanism of injury and the anatomy involved enables the maxillofacial team to correctly identify injuries and be alert for potential complications.

Primary survey

Airway problems

All severely injured patients with maxillofacial damage will experience degrees of hypoxia. It is the first priority to clear the airway of debris. Removal of foreign bodies should be performed under direct vision. Adequate lighting and suction are essential, and if vomiting is continuing then the trolley needs to be tilted head down. One of the difficulties experienced is that patients who are laid flat for the Advanced Trauma Life Support (ATLS) optimum position may compromise their airway. To avoid potential vomiting, a Guedel airway should be restricted to those with an absent gag reflex. This is a temporary method of bringing the tongue forward to create a patent oropharynx in the unconscious patient, prior to definitive airway protection with an endotracheal tube. A laryngeal mask is unlikely to seat correctly in a damaged and traumatised upper airway.

It must be assumed that the cervical spine is fractured in any patient with head trauma, and the neck must be fully immobilised throughout. Life-saving oxygenation by needle or surgical cricothyroidotomy, which can be followed by surgical tracheostomy in the more controlled environment of an operating theatre, is an option where the cervical spine is at significant risk. For less severely damaged and conscious patients without spinal injury, it may be much easier to protect the airway in an upright position.

Severe haemorrhage from the facial skeleton and neck can be potentially fatal. Severe comminuted fractures of the maxilla result in displacement of the middle third of the facial skeleton posteroinferiorly which may impact on the posterior pharyngeal wall. Apart from the airway being compromised, this can be associated with torrential haemorrhage, and a simple manoeuvre is to manipulate the maxilla and fragments anterosuperiorly (Figure 7.1) and to use ribbon gauze packs, posterior nasal packs or Epistat balloons to tamponade the bleeding. By reducing the bony fractures, the rate of blood loss is significantly quelled. For open facial and neck wounds, direct digital pressure will usually stem the flow of blood and sutures and vascular clips may be useful adjuncts to stemming blood flow from identifiable vessels (Box 7.1).

Box 7.1 **Haemorrhage control options**

- Seek expert help.
- Manipulate maxilla forwards (see text and Figure 7.1).
- Pack with gauze or balloons.
- Direct pressure if possible.
- Vascular clips or sutures.
- Fluid resuscitation as appropriate.

Fractures

Fractures of the maxillofacial skeleton can be associated with profuse bleeding. Repositioning the maxilla anterosuperiorly as described above may require the placement of postnasal packs to maintain

ABC of Major Trauma, Fourth Edition. Edited by David V. Skinner and Peter A. Driscoll.
© 2013 Blackwell Publishing Ltd. Published 2013 by Blackwell Publishing Ltd.

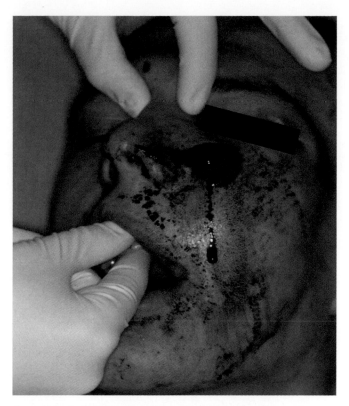

Figure 7.1 Manipulation of maxilla. Used to either reduce fracture for haemorrhage control or to assess stability. (Courtesy of S.R. Watt-Smith.)

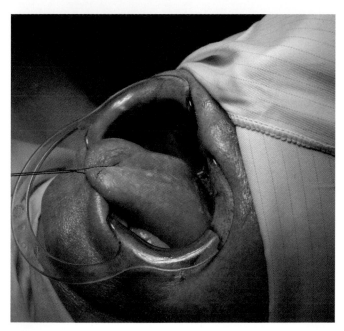

Figure 7.2 Tongue stitch. (Courtesy of S.R. Watt-Smith.)

the new position. Nasal fractures may also require posterior and anterior nasal packing or the use of Epistat balloons.

Mandibular fractures must always be assumed to be open fractures. Bilateral fractures can be associated with an unstable tongue, resulting in severe and rapid airway obstruction. A tongue stitch (Figure 7.2) secured through the body of the tongue with

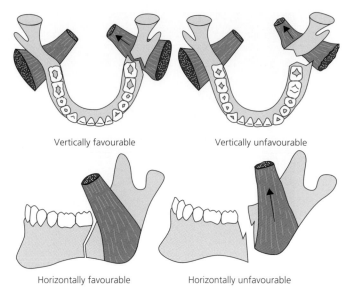

Vertically favourable   Vertically unfavourable

Horizontally favourable   Horizontally unfavourable

Figure 7.3 Diagrammatic representation of mandibular fracture favourability related to the pull of local musculature. (Courtesy of S.R. Watt-Smith.)

anterosuperior traction will improve airway patency. Mandibular fracture stability is related to the pull of the local musculature on the bony fragments (Figure 7.3). The majority of mandibular fractures will require maxillofacial assessment for consideration of fixation.

Tracheal/laryngeal trauma

Oedema and bruising of the neck, a history of blunt trauma plus surgical emphysema and a hoarse voice would all suggest possible direct tracheal and laryngeal trauma. There is usually significant swelling and oedema of the associated soft tissues. Fractures of the hyoid bone (Figure 7.4), thyroid cartilages and trachea are all possible.

Secondary survey

The securing of an adequate airway with the control of problematical haemorrhage permits treatment for life-threatening injuries to occur. In some instances it is appropriate to combine treatments such as cranial or neurosurgical procedures with maxillofacial surgery.

Specific craniomaxillofacial injuries

It is essential to conduct a thorough examination of the cranium, face and neck. It is easy to miss scalp (Figure 7.5) and posterior neck lacerations and shaving of hair-bearing skin may be necessary for the margins to be adequately delineated. Palpation for fractures and foreign bodies is essential. The cranium must be diligently palpated, mentally comparing left with right. Obvious deformities, fractures and brain herniation need to be noted and recorded on accurate diagrams.

The frontal sinus is frequently breached with craniomaxillary trauma. Fine cut computed tomography (CT) images are required to assess the integrity of the inner and outer sinus walls. Where the

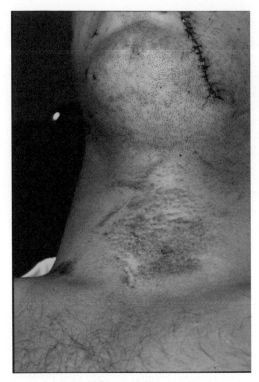

Figure 7.4 Hyoid fracture from a seatbelt injury. (Courtesy of S.R. Watt-Smith.)

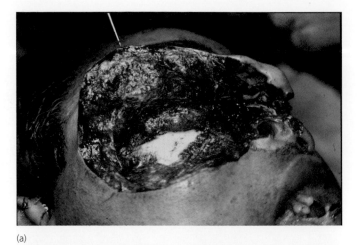

(a)

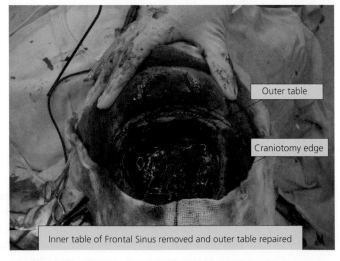

(b)

Figure 7.5 Obvious facial laceration (a), but the scalp wound (b) was missed initially. (Courtesy of S.R. Watt-Smith.)

overlying skin is breached and bony sinus walls are comminuted, it is important to consider antibiotics in conjunction with a neurosurgical opinion. Cranialisation of the frontal sinus (Figure 7.6) removes the inner table of bone, allowing the damaged frontal lobes to expand. A pericranial vascularised flap is used to line the inner surface of the frontal bone to aid healing.

The craniotomy will be held in correct position using bone plates, and the facial skeleton is repaired systematically, again using bone plates and screws, from the skull downwards to the mandible.

Children

Children suffer craniomaxillary trauma, but the incidence of facial damage is less than that to the cranium due to the relative smaller size of the face.

The dental bearing areas are complicated by the numerous teeth and tooth buds, which prevent the use of bone screws for fixation. Fortunately, many such fractures are 'greenstick' and heal with minimal intervention. However, the mandibular condyles and nasoethmoid regions are looked upon as growth centres, and fractures in these areas can result in reduced growth potential.

Nose

Examination of the nose includes palpation and assessment of the air passages. Deformity and pain are frequently evident. Significant bleeding may require anterior and posterior packing of the nasal cavities, and bending forward may provoke seepage of cerebrospinal

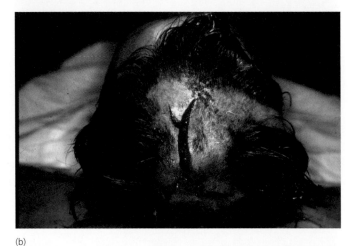

Outer table

Craniotomy edge

Inner table of Frontal Sinus removed and outer table repaired

Figure 7.6 Cranialisation of the frontal sinus, viewed from above. (Courtesy of D. Dhariwal.)

fluid (CSF) (Figure 7.7). This would suggest an anterior cranial fossa fracture at the level of the cribiform plate.

Direct blunt trauma to the nasoethmoid complex can result in traumatic telecanthus (with an increased intercanthal distance

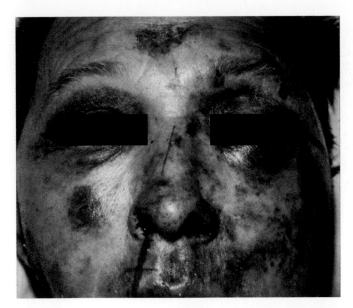

Figure 7.7 Facial injuries with cerebrospinal fluid rhinorrhoea. (Courtesy of S.R. Watt-Smith.)

>35 mm). Such injuries are frequently associated with fractures of the outer table of the frontal sinus from which air can escape into the periorbital tissues.

Retrobulbar haemorrhage

Haemorrhage within the bony orbital cavity or within the cone causes significant pain, ever-decreasing visual acuity, reduced colour vision, proptosis and oculoplegia. Medical management requires administration of mannitol 10%, acetazolamide and dexamethasone followed by urgent surgical decompression.

Ruptured globe

Loss of turgor of the globe is frequently associated with rupture and any mechanism that raises intraocular pressure should be avoided in such circumstances including intubation and systemic administration of anticholinergic drugs.

Ears

The pinnas need to be examined diligently to exclude foreign bodies, subdermal haematomas and lacerations involving cartilage.

Bleeding and leakage of CSF from the auditory canal may be due to posterior wall and middle ear damage indicating middle cranial fossa skull base fractures. Tears of the anterior external auditory meatus are frequently associated with fractures of the mandibular condyle and neck. Late presentation of mastoid bruising is associated with skull base fractures (Battle's sign).

Soft tissues

The principle of managing damaged soft tissues of the face and neck is to be as conservative as possible (Figure 7.8; Box 7.2). Delicate treatment of damaged tissues is important, especially on the face, to preserve as much facial nerve function as possible. Gaping wounds should be temporarily sutured, blood vessels tied or clipped, and special tissues such as parotid ducts should be left alone in the first instance, so that definitive repair is unimpeded.

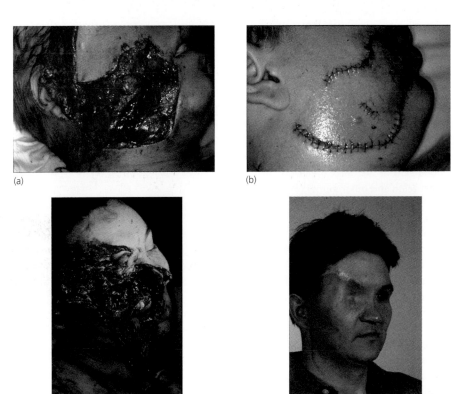

(a)

(b)

(c)

(d)

Figure 7.8 Preserve as much soft tissue as possible to optimise cosmetic outcome. Patient 1, (a) and (b). Patient 2, (c) and (d). (Courtesy of S.R. Watt-Smith.)

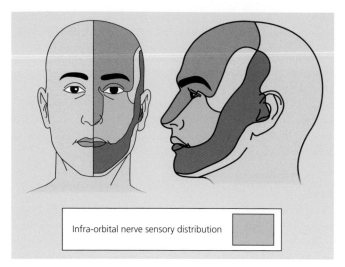

Infra-orbital nerve sensory distribution

Figure 7.9 Sensory supply of face by Trigeminal nerve (V). The green colour depicts the area of sensory loss following a malar fracture affecting the infra-orbital nerve (part of V(ii)). (Courtesy of S.R. Watt-Smith.)

Foreign bodies including glass and grit will need to be removed to prevent long-term tattooing of the soft tissues. Gunshot wounds can create significant tissue damage and specialist assessment is essential.

Box 7.2 **Soft tissue management: key points**

- Preserve as much tissue as possible.
- Superficial foreign bodies require removal (e.g. glass or grit).
- Use a temporary suture if the wound is gaping.
- Check and document skin sensation .
- Beware of special structures, e.g. parotid duct, facial nerve.
- Ask about tetanus status.
- Consider need for antibiotics.

The trigeminal nerve innervates the soft tissue of the face and direct trauma to these tissues will result in areas of paraesthesia or anaesthesia. Frequently zygomatic complex fractures are associated with altered sensation in the infraorbital nerve distribution (ipsi-lateral skin of the nose, upper lip, lower eyelid, cheek tissues and upper teeth and outer gums) (Figure 7.9).

Facial bones

Examination of the facial skeleton is mandatory, feeling for asymmetry, crepitation, loss of bony continuity and step deformities. A systematic examination should include the apex of the cranium, skull, forehead, supraorbital and infraorbital rims, zygoma and middle face, dentition, mandible and spine. Intraoral examination must include running of fingers around the dentition and associated alveolar bones, and palpation and visualisation of the palate.

Examination of the maxilla requires gentle pulling on the anterior maxilla downwards and forwards whilst restricting head movement with the contralateral hand (see Figure 7.1). Fractures of the maxilla

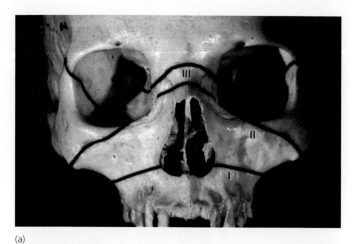

(a)

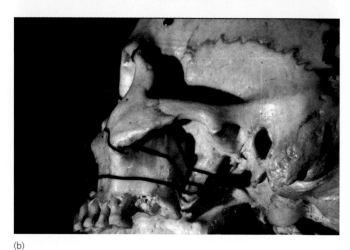

(b)

Figure 7.10 (a,b) Le Fort fracture lines viewed on anteroposterior and lateral skull. Le Fort I, most inferior line; Le Fort III, most superior line. (Courtesy of S.R. Watt-Smith.)

may be at the Le Fort I, II or III level (Figure 7.10) and can be present either bilaterally or unilaterally and be perceived as movement with crepitation.

Midfacial fractures

The occipitomental (OM) radiographs (10° and 30°) are used to evaluate damage to the zygomatic and maxillary complexes. These images can only be taken after the cervical spine has been cleared. Occipitomental views should be systematically examined looking for breaches in bony continuity at the supraorbital level, infraorbital level, Le Fort I level, interdental level and fractures of the inferior mandible and odontoid peg (Figures 7.11 and 7.12). Opacity in the maxillary sinus is usually blood and frequently associated with fractures of the zygomatic complex, maxilla or nose.

Eyes

The eye examination should include assessment of visual acuity, utilising a pinhole if a patient has lost their spectacles. Limitation of eye movements resulting in diplopia (Figure 7.13) or hypoglobus

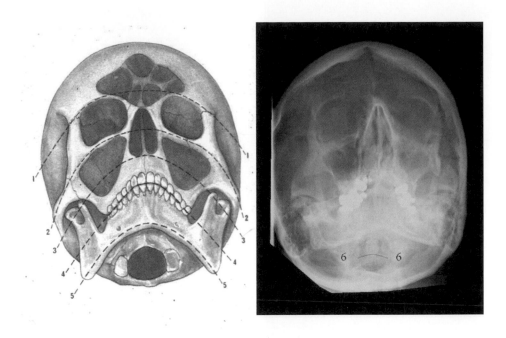

Figure 7.11 Schematic diagram and X-ray showing the six lines to look at on a facial view. (Courtesy of S.R. Watt-Smith.)

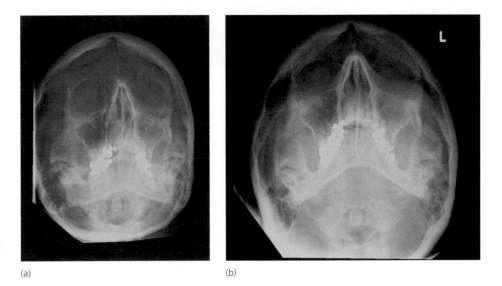

Figure 7.12 Occipitomental (a) 10° and (b) 30° X-rays showing fractured left zygoma and fluid level in right maxillary antrum. (Courtesy of S.R. Watt-Smith.)

(a)   (b)

may be associated with orbital floor or medial orbital wall fractures. The initial deformity needs to be documented in the contemporaneous notes and will require fine cut CT or MRI images with sagittal and coronal reformats for diagnosis. Direct consensual and accommodation reflexes of the pupils should be assessed and documented. Loss of such reflexes can be associated with direct traumatic mydriasis or raised intracranial pressure.

Dentition

Teeth are frequently missing or displaced following maxillofacial trauma (Box 7.3). All dental fractures should be treated as open

fractures (Figure 7.14). If subluxed, they may be pushed gently back into the socket using local anaesthesia prior to splintage. If appropriate, teeth may be stored in milk prior to reinsertion. Expert help is advisable to ensure the teeth are reinserted in the correct orientation. Missing teeth and fragments need to be excluded from the air passages and a chest X-ray is essential to exclude aspiration. Malocclusion of the teeth is assessed by asking a patient to clench their teeth together. If the patient states that this feels abnormal or the teeth are clearly malaligned, then this is strongly suggestive of an alveolar or jaw fracture until proven otherwise.

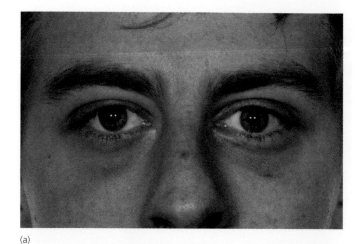

(a)

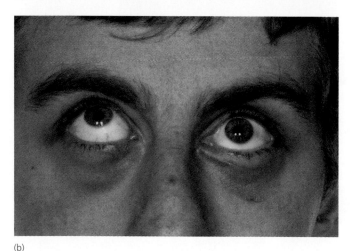

(b)

Figure 7.13 (a) Neutral gaze and (b) upgaze restriction causing diplopia. (Courtesy of S.R. Watt-Smith.)

Box 7.3 **Teeth**

- Reinsert as soon as possible in correct orientation: seek expert help if any doubt. **NB**: Don't reinsert deciduous teeth.
- Store in milk or normal saline until reinsertion is possible. If prehospital, consider storage in the patient's own mouth adjacent to the buccal mucosa.
- Replace gently in socket with local anaesthesia. Avoid touching the root of the tooth at all times.
- Missing teeth require a chest X-ray.

Penetrating injuries

Knife wounds are frequently seen in assaults and can be involved in craniomaxillofacial trauma (Figure 7.15). Removal of deeply imbedded objects must be completed in theatre, having fully evaluated the likely risk of haemorrhage and damage to other vital structures. Appropriate imaging including angiography is mandatory to assess the damage. Typically, the removal may require a multidisciplinary surgical team.

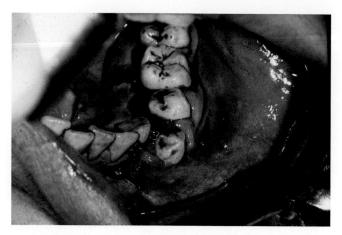

Figure 7.14 All mandibular and dental fractures are compound. (Courtesy of S.R. Watt-Smith.)

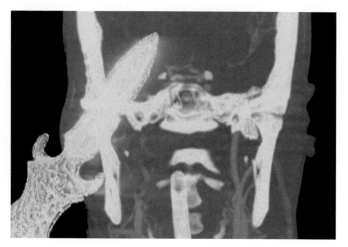

Figure 7.15 Scan showing deeply imbedded knife requiring careful multidisciplinary assessment and surgical management. (Courtesy of D. Dhariwal.)

Imaging: brain and facial trauma

Computed tomography for head injuries requires image acquisition angled parallel to the skull base to restrict unnecessary radiation to the eyes. CT scans for facial damage require contiguous fine cut images from above the damaged area to below damaged tissues. This can mean two separate scans if the face and brain are involved. Orthogonal and three-dimensional rendering techniques have made interpretation of difficult anatomy easier and more intuitive (Figure 7.16).

Medication

For the conscious and alert patient in pain, it is appropriate to administer analgesia. Grating bony fractures will be painful and, in the mandible particularly, can be managed in the first instance by injection of local anaesthetic and stabilising of segments using wire loops around teeth.

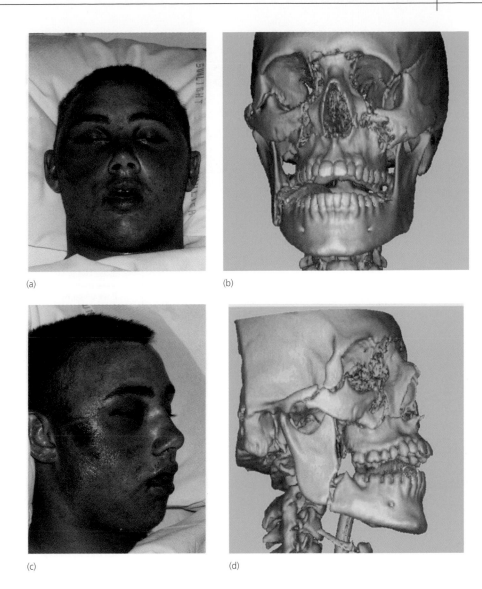

(a)

(b)

(c)

(d)

Figure 7.16 (a–d) Three-dimensional computed tomography reconstruction demonstrating significant underlying injuries in this patient. (Courtesy of S.R. Watt-Smith.)

Tetanus status must be assessed and contaminated wounds may require a booster of tetanus toxoid or immunoglobulin.

All fractures involving the dental bearing areas of the mouth should be considered open, requiring prophylactic antibiotics. For the majority of patients, intravenous co-amoxiclav and metronidazole would be appropriate. For those who are allergic to penicillin, an intravenous cephalosporin or clindamycin may be used.

The use of steroids in maxillofacial trauma is commonplace with the aim of reducing soft tissue swelling, particularly around the eyes and pharynx. A dose of 8 mg dexamethasone 8 hourly (for three doses) would be appropriate.

Potential or actual CSF leaks may be isolated or associated with facial fractures. Discussion with the neurosurgical team is important, especially if maxillary fractures are to be treated surgically.

Further reading

Ceallaigh PO, Ekanaykaee K, Beirne CJ, Patton DW. Diagnosis and management of common maxillofacial injuries in the emergency department.

Advanced trauma life support. *Emerg Med J* 2006; 23: 796–7.

Dentoalveolar injuries. *Emerg Med J* 2007; 24: 429–30.

Mandibular fractures. *Emerg Med J* 2006; 23: 927–8.

Orbital floor and midface fractures. *Emerg Med J* 2007; 24: 292–3.

Orbitozygomatic complex and zygomatic arch fractures. *Emerg Med J* 2007; 24: 120–2.

Ward Booth P, Eppley B, Schmelzeisen R. (2003) *Maxillofacial Trauma and Esthetic Reconstruction*. Edinburgh: Churchill Livingstone.

CHAPTER 8

Spine and Spinal Cord Injury

Andrew Swain[1] and Andre Cromhout[2]

[1]University of Otago, Wellington, New Zealand
[2]Wellington Hospital, Wellington, New Zealand

OVERVIEW

- In patients suffering major trauma, significant spinal injury cannot be excluded without appropriate imaging of the whole spine and completion of a normal neurological examination.
- Until spinal injury is excluded, the spine needs to be maintained in the anatomical position using whatever splintage is appropriate and available.
- The need for airway maintenance always over-rides that of optimal positioning of the spine.
- The priorities of airway, breathing and circulation are as important for spinal cord nutrition and perfusion as they are for other vital organs.
- Spinal cord injury can occur in the absence of any significant radiological abnormality. Rectal and peripheral neurological examinations must therefore be undertaken and repeated as necessary until partial or complete spinal cord injury can be confirmed or excluded.
- Experimental work on spinal cord regeneration and remyelination is a developing field and functional electrical stimulation of paralysed muscles continues to advance.

A patient with serious multiple injuries is rarely able to provide a coherent history. Potential injuries that carry the risk of death or severe disability must therefore be suspected from the outset so that correct early management can be instituted. Any force that results in impaired consciousness should be assumed to have injured the cervical spine until proven otherwise, as half of all spinal injuries involve the neck. The thoracolumbar spine must also be managed carefully. Approximately 10% of patients with one spinal injury have a co-existing injury at a different level. The most common reason for failing to detect an important spinal injury is failure to suspect one, particularly in patients with multiple trauma.

In patients who sustain spinal injury, the cord is most often damaged in the cervical region but it is also particularly at risk near the thoracolumbar junction (Table 8.1). The thoracic spine is splinted by ribs and sternum but the spinal canal is narrower

ABC of Major Trauma, Fourth Edition. Edited by David V. Skinner and Peter A. Driscoll.
© 2013 Blackwell Publishing Ltd. Published 2013 by Blackwell Publishing Ltd.

Table 8.1 Incidence of neurological injury in patients with fractures or dislocations of various parts of the spine

Part of spine	Incidence (%)
Any	14
Cervical spine	40
Thoracic spine	10
Thoracolumbar junction	35
Lumbar spine	3

in this region and the blood supply to the cord is relatively poor. For these reasons, the thoracic cord is more susceptible to trauma. Partial cord injuries are now more common and the potential for neurological improvement or deterioration is correspondingly greater. Although the primary injury to the spine is irreversible, the spinal cord is susceptible to secondary mechanical, hypoxic and hypotensive damage and these risks have a major influence over early management of the trauma patient.

Management at the scene of the accident

Spinal trauma may be suspected from a witness's description of an accident (e.g. rollover or ejection from a vehicle, diving into shallow water). It cannot, however, be excluded without a definitive examination, even in the fully conscious casualty who may be intoxicated or distracted by other injuries.

Particular care must be taken moving unconscious casualties, those who complain of pain in the back or neck, and those who describe altered sensation or loss of power in the limbs. Provided that the neck is not locked and that it can be moved without precipitating neurological symptoms, the head must be aligned in the neutral position, avoiding longitudinal compression or distraction. Correctly aligning the neck will improve the airway and reduce spinal deformity, helping to relieve pressure on the spinal cord or arteries. If the patient is a motorcyclist wearing a full-face helmet, access to the airway is achieved with one rescuer immobilising the neck from below while another carefully pulls the sides of the helmet outwards and eases it off the head from above (Figure 8.1). The neck is now splinted with a rigid collar of appropriate size to grip the chin (Figure 8.2). Collars alone are inadequate and they should be supplemented by manual stabilisation of the head or lateral support using sandbags or bolsters held in position by tape applied across the forehead and collar. Be wary of swelling

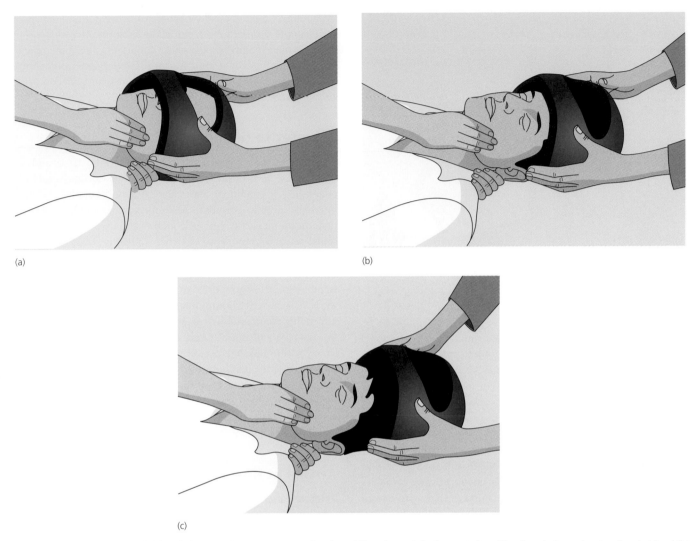

(a)

(b)

(c)

Figure 8.1 Safe removal of a full-face helmet requires two rescuers. One immobilises the neck in the neutral position from below using two hands (a), whilst the other removes the jaw strap, spreads the lateral margins of the helmet apart and gently eases the helmet upwards (b,c). Tilting the helmet forwards helps to avoid flexion of the neck as the occiput rides over the posterior lip of the helmet but care must be taken not to trap the nose.

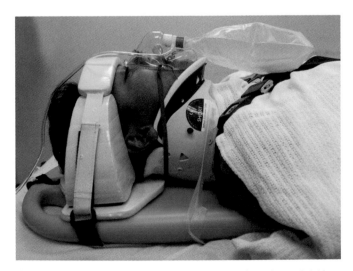

Figure 8.2 Patient on spinal board: close-up view to show the semi-rigid collar, bolsters and positioning of straps.

under the collar which may develop from a haematoma or surgical emphysema. Small children who cannot accommodate a collar may be padded and taped to a removable car seat or immobilised within an adult lower-limb vacuum splint.

In the unconscious patient, the airway should be opened by chin lift or jaw thrust without extending the neck and airway adjuncts can then be used in the normal way. The supine position facilitates examination of the patient, resuscitation, respiratory movements and control of the neck but tracheal intubation is required to prevent aspiration. Alternatively, the unconscious patient can be rolled into the lateral position with the trunk aligned but tilted forwards approximately 20°, allowing secretions to discharge freely from the mouth. The three-quarter prone or coma position cannot be recommended as it rotates the cervical spine and splints the diaphragm, causing hypoventilation. However, modifications of the latter position are taught on first aid courses where the importance of airway maintenance and ease of positioning over-rides that of cervical alignment.

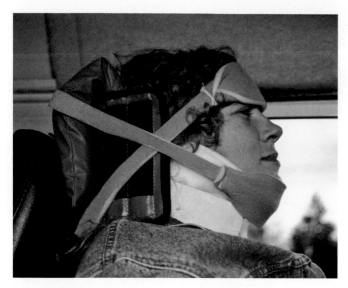

Figure 8.3 Patient with semi-rigid collar and spinal immobiliser (Kendrick extrication device) in position.

The presence of thoracolumbar injury must also be assumed and treated by carefully straightening the trunk and correcting rotation. During turning or lifting, it is vital that the whole spine is maintained in the neutral position. This process of 'log rolling' should ideally be undertaken by four assistants. The neck and back can be protected simultaneously by placing supine casualties on a spinal board incorporating a head immobiliser. For sitting casualties (e.g. car occupants), the same goal can be achieved by using a spinal immobiliser such as a Kendrick or Russell extrication device (Figure 8.3). However, physically unco-operative casualties are exempt from full splintage of the spine as they may sustain more harm struggling against the restraints used. Verbal restraint, use of a rigid collar and treatment of hypoxia and shock should be attempted initially in such cases. Doctors should familiarise themselves with the splints available in their locality.

It is important to note that in the flexion-extension axis, the neutral position of the cervical spine varies with the age of the casualty. The relatively large head and prominent occiput of small children push their neck into flexion when they lie on a flat surface such as a spinal board. On paediatric spinal boards, this is corrected by the insertion of padding under the thoracic spine (Figure 8.4). Conversely, elderly patients may have a thoracic

kyphosis and require a pillow between the occiput and the spinal board to prevent the head from falling back into hyperextension. In ankylosing spondylitis and other conditions, the spine may be deformed and its curvature abnormal. Cervical extension should not be enforced on such patients. The aim is to achieve normal cervical curvature for the individual.

Transfer to hospital

Once the airway is protected, oxygen is administered and the casualty has been positioned, an intravenous infusion should be established. If conditions allow, the casualty should be examined briefly before transportation. A scoop stretcher can be assembled underneath a casualty who is lying free and used for transfer to a spinal board or ambulance stretcher. Casualties fitted with spinal immobilisers must be supported in and not lifted by the splint. In the absence of life-threatening injury, casualties at risk of spinal trauma should be transported carefully to hospital and hard objects should be removed from any anaesthetic parts of the body. If there is impending regurgitation or vomiting, the casualty who is strapped to a spinal board can be safely tilted head down or turned into a lateral position by one person using the board. This is safer than a hurriedly attempted and unco-ordinated turn of an unsplinted casualty into the lateral position.

If spinal cord injury is present, peripheral vasodilation exposes the casualty to greater heat loss. It is important that body temperature is maintained as close to normal as possible during transit.

Arrival at hospital

Primary survey

Safe transfer of the patient from the ambulance stretcher to a trauma trolley can be achieved with the patient strapped to a spinal board. This should be removed within 30 min of arrival to avoid unnecessary pain or pressure sores. Alternatively, a scoop stretcher may be used (Figure 8.5). If a patient slider is employed, transfer from the ambulance stretcher in the trauma room can be safely accomplished by four people, the person in charge grasping the head and neck whilst assistants keep the chest, pelvis and legs in line. The primary survey is then commenced in the standard manner. The sections that follow focus on aspects of care that are of specific relevance to patients with spinal injury.

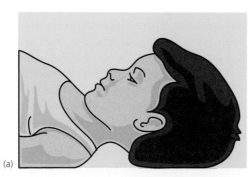
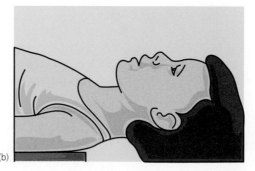

(a)   (b)

Figure 8.4 (a) Cervical flexion on a spinal board attributable to the relatively prominent occiput that is characteristic of smaller children. (b) The flexion can be relieved by inserting padding under the thoracic spine.

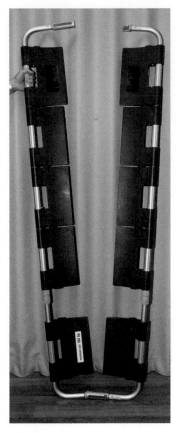

Figure 8.5 A scoop stretcher.

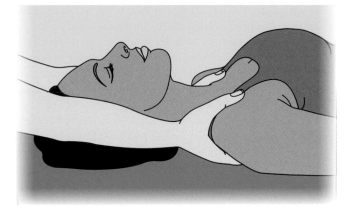

Figure 8.6 Manual immobilisation of the neck.

Airway with protection of the cervical spine

Trauma patients are invariably kept supine during resuscitation unless regurgitation occurs and the airway is unprotected. In such an emergency, the patient may be tipped head down and oropharyngeal suction applied. In patients with cervical cord injury, laryngeal stimulation by vigorous suction, manipulation of an oropharyngeal airway or intubation may result in unopposed vagal discharge and cardiac arrest. This can be prevented by administration of atropine.

Many seriously injured patients require intubation which is not contraindicated in patients with an unstable cervical injury. However, the procedure should be performed whenever possible by an experienced intubator and an assistant who holds and stabilises the head to minimise neck movement (Figure 8.6). Alternative intubation techniques exist that do not require the neck to be moved (e.g. fibre-optic intubation, blind tracheal intubation) but should be employed only by those experienced in their use. A naso- or orogastric tube is required in these patients as ileus develops after spinal cord injury. Occasionally, suspicion of an injury to the upper cervical spine may be aroused by the presence of a retropharyngeal haematoma seen through the mouth; the trachea may then be deviated.

Breathing

This is assessed and managed in accordance with standard ATLS principles. However, it is important to note that chest injuries are common in patients sustaining spinal trauma. Serious respiratory complications resulting from spinal injury tend to be either immediately fatal or of relatively slow onset. They are therefore included in the secondary survey. See Box 8.1.

Box 8.1 Causes of respiratory insufficiency

In tetraplegic patients

- Intercostal paralysis
- Partial phrenic nerve palsy:
  - Immediate
  - Delayed

In paraplegic patients

- Variable intercostal paralysis according to level of injury
- Associated chest injuries:
  - Rib fractures
  - Pulmonary contusion
  - Haemopneumothorax

Circulation

Haemorrhage is the most common cause of post-traumatic shock. However, patients with injury to the cervical or high thoracic cord may have reduced sympathetic outflow between T1 and L2 segments causing bradycardia, hypotension and peripheral vasodilation. This condition is referred to as neurogenic shock. Bradycardia with hypotension is not a classic feature of hypovolaemic shock and in a traumatised patient, it should increase suspicion of spinal cord injury, especially if the peripheries are well perfused. The degree of bradycardia and hypotension in neurogenic shock depends on the level and extent of neurological injury. All trauma patients must be connected to a cardiac monitor on admission. Tetraplegic patients with bradycardia should be given atropine if their pulse rate drops below 50 beats per minute. If the systolic blood pressure falls below 80 mmHg, inotropic support is necessary. Bradycardic shock is also seen in elderly patients and those taking β-blockers.

In recent years, the importance of maintaining adequate tissue perfusion and oxygenation in patients with spinal cord trauma has been emphasised. Episodes of hypotension or hypoxaemia often lead to irreversible neurological deterioration. Patients with spinal trauma are likely to have hypovolaemia from other injuries. Circulatory volume must be restored but aggressive fluid replacement is detrimental in patients with purely neurogenic hypotension as it can precipitate pulmonary oedema. Therefore, traumatised patients with bradycardia and hypotension should be subjected to a fluid challenge and the response observed and monitored by measuring central venous pressure. For this, cannulation of the subclavian vein is preferred as access to the internal jugular vein is difficult to obtain without rotating the neck.

Secondary survey

Any injury to the spinal cord carries a high risk of early and late medical complications. Important early complications include respiratory failure resulting from intercostal paralysis or partial phrenic nerve palsy, impaired ability to expectorate and ventilation-perfusion mismatch. The patient's respiratory state may also deteriorate shortly after admission as a result of ascending oedema in the traumatised cervical cord. Care must be taken administering narcotic analgesics as these will further impair ventilation and reversal may be necessary. Cardiac arrest usually results from respiratory failure. The level of consciousness, rate and depth of respiration, and oxygen saturation must be monitored and blood gas tensions checked. End-tidal carbon dioxide monitoring is helpful if available.

Abdominal trauma is not easily assessed in tetraplegic patients as the abdominal wall is anaesthetic, flaccid and areflexic, and ileus results from the neurological injury (Box 8.2). A useful positive sign is pain at the tip of the shoulder aggravated by abdominal palpation. Abdominal ultrasound or computed tomography (CT) are useful diagnostic aids in patients with cervical or thoracic cord injury.

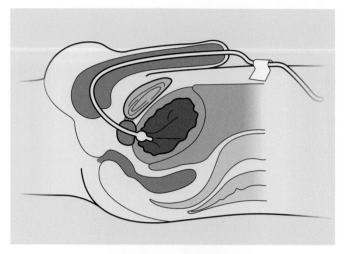

Figure 8.7 Method of catheterisation in patients with spinal cord injury.

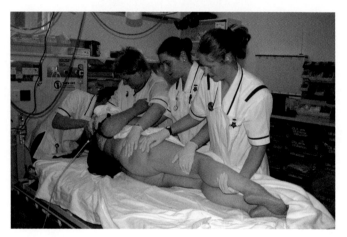

Figure 8.8 Log roll.

sepsis (Figure 8.7). Alternatively, a suprapubic catheter can be inserted.

Spinal examination

Examination of the whole length of the spine must be performed in all unconscious patients with multiple trauma. In the supine position, the cervical and lumbar lordoses may be palpated by sliding a hand under the patient. Unless there is an urgent need to inspect the back, it is usually examined near the end of the secondary survey. A co-ordinated log roll, maintaining spinal alignment, is performed by a team of four led by the person who is holding the patient's head (Figure 8.8). Another doctor then examines the back for specific signs of injury, including bruising or deformity of the spine, vertebral tenderness, malalignment of spinous processes or an increased interspinous gap. The whole length of the spine must be palpated and a rectal examination is usually undertaken at this time to assess anal tone and sensation.

Neurological examination

This normally follows the log roll but it is materially influenced by the patient's state of consciousness.

> Box 8.2 **Influence of cervical or high thoracic spinal cord injury on abdominal examination**
>
> - Loss of internal and external sensation.
> - Loss of power and tone in abdominal wall.
> - Loss of abdominal reflexes.
> - Ileus.
> - Referred pain to shoulder.

Acute urinary retention will develop in paraplegic and tetraplegic patients unless the sacral segments are spared. Measurement of urine output is important in trauma patients and the bladder will usually require drainage, particularly if the patient has been drinking. In the absence of urethral trauma, a narrow-gauge catheter with a small (5 mL) balloon is passed under strictly aseptic conditions and taped to the anterior abdominal wall to prevent unnecessary movement of and injury to the urethra which can lead to

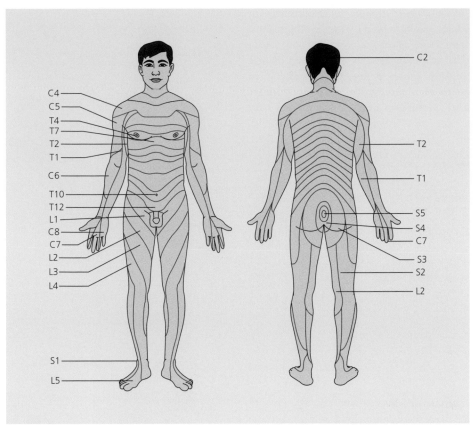

Figure 8.9 The sensory dermatomes.

The conscious patient

Sensory loss or motor symptoms should never be disregarded, no matter how unimportant they seem. Diagnosis of spinal cord injury relies on symptoms and signs of pain in the spine with sensory loss and disturbances in motor function distal to a neurological level (Box 8.3). The pain may radiate owing to nerve root irritation. A full neurological examination must be performed, including testing of cranial nerves, sensation to fine touch and pinprick in each dermatome (Figure 8.9), proprioception, power in each myotome, tone, co-ordination and reflexes. Anal sensation, tone and voluntary contraction must be checked. By examining the dermatomes and myotomes, the level and completeness of the spinal cord injury can be assessed.

The highest segment of normal spinal cord function is referred to as the neurological level of the lesion. This does not necessarily correspond with the level of bony injury so the neurological and skeletal diagnoses should both be recorded.

Box 8.3 **Clinical features of spinal cord injury**

- Pain in the neck or back, often radiating because of nerve root irritation.
- Sensory disturbance distal to neurological level.
- Weakness or flaccid paralysis below this level.

Incomplete spinal cord lesions have traditionally been defined as those in which some sensory or motor function is preserved below the level of neurological injury. The definition now requires there to be some demonstrable sensory or motor function within the anal canal (Box 8.4). If there is no such function, any dermatomes or myotomes that exhibit function below the main neurological level are referred to as zones of partial preservation (ZPP).

Box 8.4 **Reflexes and their nerve supply**

Biceps jerk	C5, 6
Supinator jerk	C6
Triceps jerk	C7
Abdominal reflex	T8–12
Knee jerk	L3, 4
Ankle jerk	L5, S1
Bulbocavernosus reflex	S3, 4
Anal reflex	S5
Plantar reflex	

'Spinal shock' is a state of shutdown following spinal cord injury which manifests as generalised muscle flaccidity and loss of reflexes below the neurological level. This must not be confused with neurogenic shock. However, it is rare for all reflexes to be absent (except in lower motor neurone lesions) and the description of spinal shock as a state of areflexia is erroneous. Almost a third of patients with spinal cord injury have intact reflexes below the neurological level during the first 3 h after injury (Box 8.5). This has caused the diagnosis of spinal cord trauma to be dismissed in some cases. Clinicians may also be misled by the delayed plantar response which resembles a normal plantar response and is seen in patients with complete cord injuries. In the delayed plantar response, the normal stimulus causes the toes to flex and relax in delayed sequence. This has been misinterpreted as a reassuringly normal plantar response, resulting in delayed diagnosis of cord injury (Box 8.6).

Box 8.5 Spinal reflexes after cord injury

Note: almost one-third of patients with spinal cord injury examined within 1–3 h of injury have reflexes.

Box 8.6 Plantar reflex after cord injury

Distinguish between:

- Delayed plantar response – present in all complete injuries.
- Normal plantar response.

Great care must be taken in conscious patients as symptoms and signs may be dismissed if they do not demonstrate a clear neurological level. In partial cord lesions, preserved function may follow a different pattern. If the zone of injury lies centrally within the cord, the cervical tracts supplying the arms are most affected so there is a flaccid (lower motor neurone) weakness of the arms but spastic (upper motor neurone) function in the legs (Figure 8.10). This central cord syndrome is usually seen in older patients whose spinal canal is narrowed by degenerative changes. It frequently occurs in the absence of any detectable bony injury. Trauma to the anterior part of the spinal cord can damage the anterior spinal artery, causing ischaemia in the corticospinal and spinothalamic tracts leading to weakness and impaired pain and temperature sensation below the lesion (Figure 8.11). If the posterior columns are contused, ataxia results from loss of proprioception. In the Brown–Sequard syndrome, one side of the cord is damaged, resulting in reduced ipsilateral power but reduced contralateral loss of pain and temperature sensation because the spinothalamic tract crosses to the opposite side of the cord.

The unconscious patient

There are no truly pathognomonic features of spinal cord injury but important signs in the unconscious patient are flaccid paralysis, diaphragmatic breathing, priapism, neurogenic shock and upward movement of the umbilicus on tensing the abdomen (Beevor's sign, indicating a neurological level of T10). The neurological examination in unconscious patients is usually limited to completing the Glasgow Coma Chart, fundoscopy and the assessment of tone and reflexes, including those of the abdomen and anal canal (Figure 8.12). Baseline sacral reflexes (bulbocavernosus and anal) should be checked if spinal cord injury is suspected. The sensory

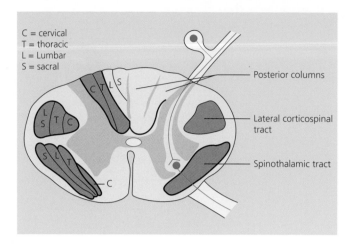

Figure 8.10 Cross-section of spinal cord, with main tracts.

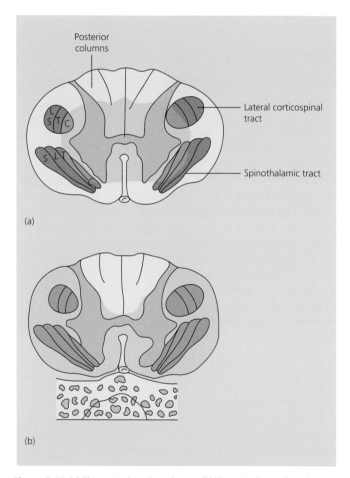

Figure 8.11 (a) The central cord syndrome. (b) The anterior cord syndrome.

response to pain is routinely assessed in patients with depressed consciousness and the presence of spinal cord injury may be suggested by different responses above and below a neurological level. Beware of flaccidity and areflexia in an arm as this may result from brachial plexus injury or spinal cord trauma (or both), particularly in motorcyclists.

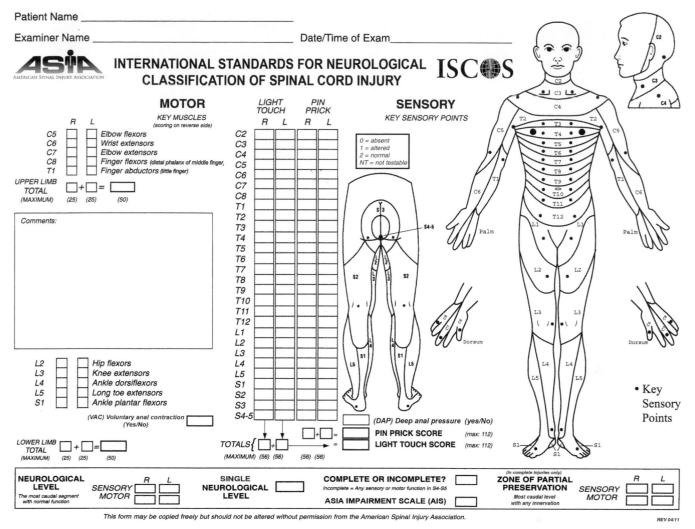

Figure 8.12 Standard neurological classification of spinal cord injury. (Reproduced from American Spinal Injury Association: International Standards for Neurological Classification of Spinal Cord Injury, revised 2011; Atlanta, GA. Reprinted 2011.)

Although the initial injury to the spinal cord is mechanical, there is usually an associated ischaemic lesion that may progress rapidly, producing cord necrosis. Superior extension of this ischaemic zone in the cervical region may result in increasing respiratory impairment whereas inferior spread produces signs of a lower motor neurone lesion below the level of injury.

Radiology

Good-quality radiographs are essential for accurate diagnosis of spinal injury. However, radiology sometimes has to be deferred until emergency surgery for life-threatening injuries has been completed. This is not a problem as long as the spine is maintained in neutral alignment during the operative phrase. In physiologically stable patients, films are best obtained in the radiology department and if spinal injuries are suspected or neurological symptoms are present, the examination should be supervised by a doctor to ensure that there is no unnecessary movement of the patient. Collars, sandbags and splints are not always radiolucent and they may need to be removed once preliminary films have been obtained.

The radiographic appearances of the spine after injury represent the recoil position of the vertebrae and are not necessarily a reliable guide to the severity of underlying neurological damage.

Riggins found that there was no radiological evidence of trauma in 17% of adult patients with spinal cord injury. Spinal cord injury without radiological abnormality (SCIWORA) may result from central disc prolapse, pure ligamentous instability or narrowing of the spinal canal from cervical spondylosis. SCIWORA is also relatively more common in children because greater mobility of the developing spine affords less protection to the spinal cord. So when in doubt, a radiological opinion should always be sought.

Plain lateral and anteroposterior films are fundamental to the diagnosis of spinal injuries. Special views, CT and magnetic resonance imaging (MRI) permit further evaluation.

Cervical spine

In patients sustaining major trauma, radiographs of the cervical spine, chest and pelvis are mandatory (Figure 8.13). Most radiologically detectable abnormalities of the neck are shown in a standard

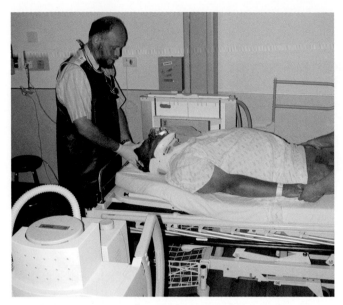

Figure 8.13 Lateral cervical spine radiograph being taken. Note traction on the arms.

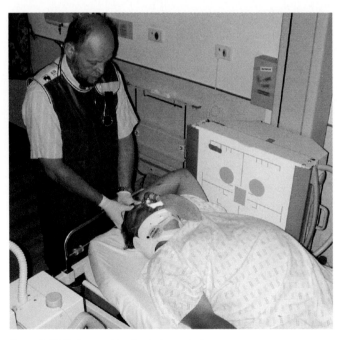

Figure 8.14 Patient position for Swimmer's view.

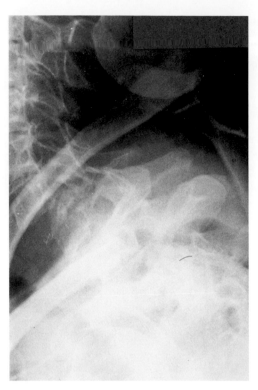

Figure 8.15 Swimmer's view radiograph.

this region. Computed tomograms of the cervical spine are often obtained as part of a more extensive CT examination of the head and trunk.

The interpretation of cervical spine radiographs may pose problems for the inexperienced. A recommended approach is the acronym 'ABCS'.

- A for alignment
- B for bones
- C for cartilages
- S for soft tissues

A for alignment

Follow the four lines on the lateral radiograph (Figure 8.16). From anterior to posterior, the lines represent the anterior longitudinal ligament, the posterior longitudinal ligament, the ligamentum flavum and the tips of the spinous processes. The anterior arch of C1 lies in front of the anterior line of alignment, unless the odontoid process is fractured and displaced posteriorly.

B for bones

The outline of each individual vertebra should be checked for any steps or breaks.

C for cartilages

The intervertebral discs and facet joints should be checked for displacement. The disc space may be widened if the annulus fibrosis is ruptured or it may be narrowed in degenerative disc disease.

supine lateral radiograph which must display all seven cervical vertebrae and the C7T1 junction if injuries are not to be missed. This can usually be achieved by applying traction to both arms whilst the radiograph is obtained; traction must be released if it precipitates any pain in the neck or exacerbation of neurological symptoms. If the lower cervical vertebrae are still not adequately demonstrated, a swimmer's view (Figure 8.14) or CT scan can be requested. The swimmer's view is not always easy to interpret and it does not produce clear bony detail but usually allows assessment of spinal alignment at the cervicothoracic junction (Figure 8.15). Oblique supine radiographs can also provide helpful views of

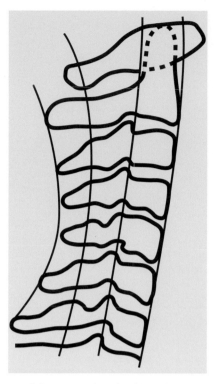

Figure 8.16 Lines of alignment on lateral radiograph.

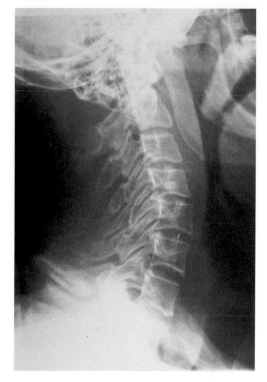

Figure 8.17 Prevertebral swelling.

S for soft tissues

The soft tissue shadow anterior to the spine may be widened, denoting the presence of a prevertebral haematoma (Figure 8.17). Similarly, widening of bony interspaces (e.g. those between spinous processes) results from ligamentous injury.

If anterior or posterior displacement of one cervical vertebra on another exceeds 3.5 mm, this must be considered abnormal. Anterior displacement of less than half the diameter of the vertebral body suggests unilateral facet dislocation which is associated with a rotational deformity at the level of injury (Figure 8.18). Forward displacement greater than this is consistent with bilateral facet dislocation. Rupture of the transverse ligament of the atlas (causing atlantoaxial subluxation) may be identified by an increased gap between the odontoid process and the anterior arch of the atlas (more than 3 mm in adults or 5 mm in children).

Many patients present with more subtle signs of an unstable injury. A chip fracture of the lower anterior margin of the vertebral body ('teardrop' fracture) is associated with unstable flexion injuries and retropulsion of disc material into the spinal canal (Figure 8.19). There may be widening of the interspinous gap, loss of normal lordosis and minor subluxation.

Always look for a prevertebral haematoma which is indicated by an increased gap between the nasopharynx or trachea and the cervical spine. The width of the retropharyngeal soft tissue space (at C2) should not exceed 7 mm in adults or children whereas the retrotracheal space (C6) should not be wider than 22 mm in adults or 14 mm in children (the retropharyngeal space widens in a crying child).

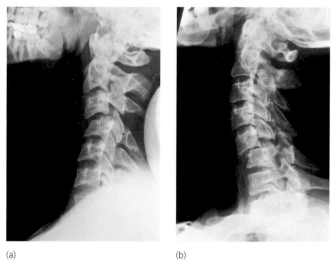

(a)   (b)

Figure 8.18 (a) Unilateral and (b) bilateral facet dislocations, the former with rotation on AP view.

Beware of inadequate lateral C spine views (you must see the first to the seventh cervical vertebra and the cervico-thoracic junction) (Figure 8.20).

After the lateral radiograph has been scrutinised, an open-mouth view of the odontoid process and an anteroposterior radiograph must be obtained to complete the basic series of cervical films. The former assists with the diagnosis of fractures of the odontoid and atlas (e.g. Jefferson fracture) but the odontoid and atlantoaxial

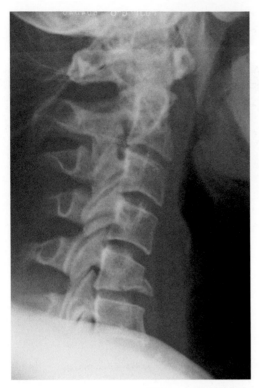

Figure 8.19 Tear drop fracture.

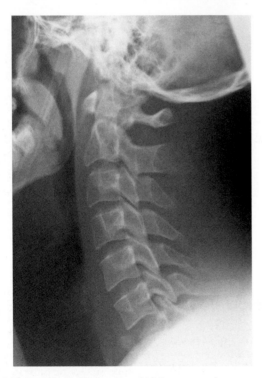

Figure 8.20 Inadequate C spine view which happens to show a compression fracture C7.

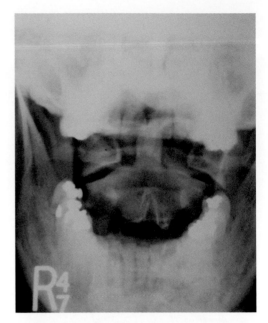

Figure 8.21 Jefferson fracture.

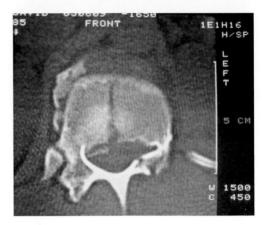

Figure 8.22 Computed tomography.

joints must not be obscured by overlying teeth or skull shadows (Figure 8.21). In the anteroposterior radiograph, the upper thoracic vertebrae and ribs should be examined as severe trauma is required to injure these structures. Lateral displacement of spinous processes on the anteroposterior view may result from a unilateral facet dislocation or fracture.

When standard radiographs of the cervical spine appear normal but cervical injury is still suspected because of severe pain, radiological signs of ligamentous injury or the mechanism of trauma, flexion and extension views can be obtained if the patient has no neurological symptoms or signs. To obtain these views, flexion and extension of the whole neck must be performed as far as the patient can tolerate under the supervision of a doctor. Movement must cease if it precipitates neurological symptoms. However, flexion and extension views are rarely appropriate in the acute situation or in the context of major trauma so if there is any doubt about the integrity of the cervical spine on plain radiographs, CT should be performed (Figure 8.22). CT provides much greater bony detail and is particularly useful in assessing the cervicothoracic junction, the upper cervical spine and any suspected fracture or malalignment. Many trauma patients already require CT of the head, chest or abdomen.

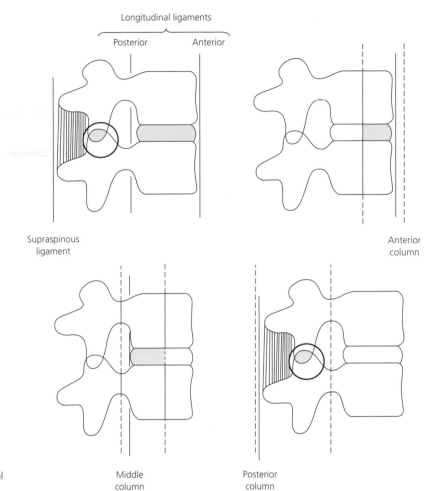

Figure 8.23 The three (anterior, middle and posterior) spinal columns.

Thoracolumbar spine

Anteroposterior and lateral radiographs represent the standard views of the thoracolumbar spine but the first indication of a

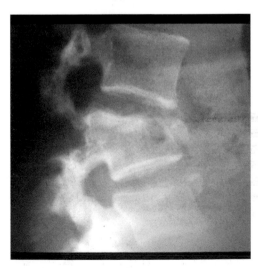

Figure 8.24 A Chance fracture of L4 in a 17-year-old backseat passenger wearing a lap belt. There is a horizontal fracture of the upper part of the vertebral body extending into the posterior elements. There is also wedging of the body of L4 and more minor wedging of L5.

thoracolumbar injury may be an abnormality seen on the patient's chest X-ray. Views of this part of the spine should be requested for all victims of major trauma as studies have shown that injuries are common but not all patients exhibit symptoms or signs of spinal injury. Radiography of the thoracolumbar spine is also indicated in the presence of cervical spine trauma because of the frequency with which injuries at more than one level co-exist. However, if CT of the chest and abdomen is to be undertaken for other reasons, radiography of the thoracolumbar spine can be deferred.

A significant force is normally required to damage the thoracic, lumbar and sacral segments of the spinal cord and the skeletal injury is usually evident on the standard anteroposterior and lateral radiographs. Burst fractures that encroach on the spinal canal and those that involve the facet joints or pedicles are unstable and more easily seen on the lateral radiograph. Instability requires at least two of the three columns of the spine (Figure 8.23) to be disrupted. In simple wedge fractures, only the anterior column is disrupted and the injury remains stable. However, all spinal fractures should be considered unstable if there is any uncertainty. The lateral view of the thoracic spine often fails to demonstrate detail, particularly of the upper four vertebrae, and CT is often required.

In the thoracolumbar region, any paravertebral haematoma is more readily seen on the anteroposterior radiograph. A similar

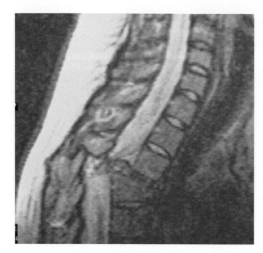

Figure 8.25 Magnetic resonance imaging.

through the vertebral body and usually results from forced flexion across a lap seatbelt during severe deceleration. The fracture is frequently associated with retroperitoneal and intra-abdominal injuries.

Magnetic resonance imaging

Magnetic resonance imaging is the investigation of choice for visualising the spinal cord and surrounding soft tissues (Figure 8.25). It normally reveals the cause of cord compression, whether from bone, prolapsed disc, ligament damage or intraspinal haematomas. This is an asset when other investigations demonstrate no bony injury. The nature and extent of cord injury and oedema can also be evaluated with MRI and this has prognostic value. Pathological changes in the spine, such as ankylosing spondylitis or rheumatoid arthritis, increase susceptibility to injury after relatively minor trauma and MRI may be helpful in such patients.

appearance can result from traumatic aortic dissection and if there is any uncertainty, further imaging is indicated.

A particular type of fracture, the Chance fracture (Figure 8.24), may involve one of the upper lumbar vertebrae. It runs transversely

Treatment

Cervical injuries

Orthopaedic surgeons should participate in the patient's management at an early stage. Unstable cervical injuries may be immobilised

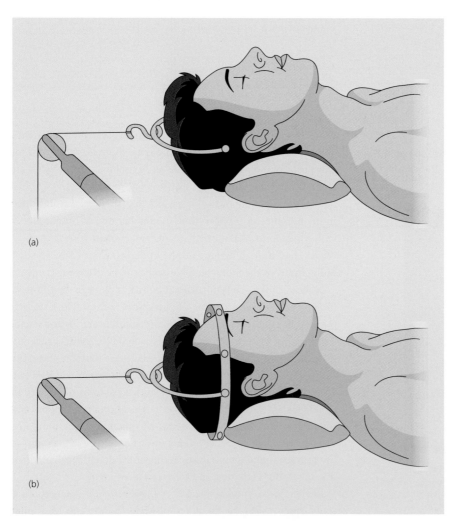

(a)

(b)

Figure 8.26 (a) Skull traction using Gardner–Wells calliper with neck roll in position to maintain postural reduction. (b) Halo applied with bale arm – an alternative approach to skull traction if early mobilisation into a halo brace is being considered.

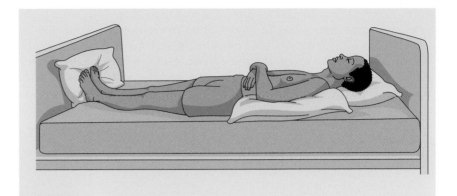

Figure 8.27 Conservative treatment for thoracolumbar injuries (postural reduction).

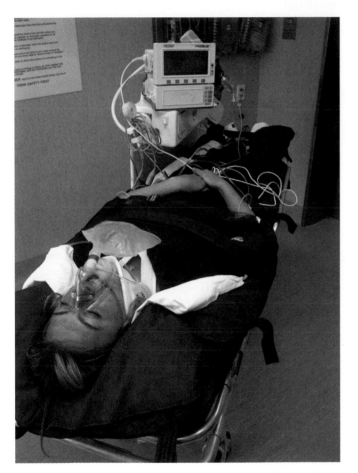

Figure 8.28 Patient on a vacuum mattress. For secure immobilisation during transportation, forehead and collar tapes should be applied.

using a firm collar (supplemented by sandbags and tape) or skeletal traction, depending on the nature of the injury. All treatment should be supervised by a specialist. Skull traction helps to correct the alignment of the injured spine, reduce fractures and dislocations, decompress the cord and nerve roots, and stabilise the injury.

Various skull callipers are available but spring-loaded types such as the Gardner–Wells or University of Virginia models are easily applied and carry a low risk of complications. Padding should be placed behind the cervical spine to maintain the normal lordosis. Halo traction has become more popular as the halo may be incorporated into a brace to allow the patient to mobilise (Figure 8.26).

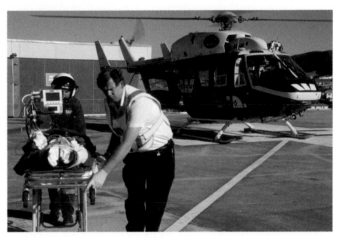

Figure 8.29 Helicopter transfer of a spinally injured patient.

Care must be taken not to overdistract injuries of the upper cervical spine and for some of these, traction is contraindicated. For interhospital transfer, immobilisation of the head with a semi-rigid collar, sandbags and tape provides effective spinal protection.

Thoracolumbar injuries

These may be treated by 'postural reduction' which consists of bedrest on a lumbar support to maintain the normal lordosis and help reduce the fracture or dislocation (Figure 8.27). However, surgery is often performed on unstable injuries to facilitate nursing care and enable mobilisation of the patient without significant delay.

Spinal injury associated with paraplegia or tetraplegia

Early referral and transfer to a spinal centre allow the medical complications associated with paraplegia or tetraplegia to be managed promptly by appropriate experts and the patient will receive better overall care. Staff are experienced in dealing with complicated cases and if the patient is not fit to travel, the specialist in spinal injury will be able to advise on management. Referral is normally the responsibility of the orthopaedic or neurosurgical team. The administration of mannitol in these patients is of no proven benefit whilst treatment with methylprednisolone remains controversial and is not without complications (e.g. pneumonia). A policy regarding pharmacological therapy should be agreed with the local spinal injury centre. Transfer of a patient with a cervical or high thoracic cord injury to a spinal centre must be supervised by an experienced doctor with anaesthetic skills in case respiratory problems develop *en route*. The use of a vacuum mattress provides good splintage and low interface pressures during transfer, minimising the risk of pressure sore development (Figure 8.28).

There is no conclusive evidence that urgent surgery improves neurological outcome but it is undertaken when there are signs of deteriorating neurological function and it can also prevent deformity. The neurological prognosis is always uncertain and patients should therefore be treated actively (Figure 8.29).

The future

In the past decade, there have been many scientific breakthroughs in the field of spinal cord regeneration and remyelination. Work is still in the experimental stage but the results are encouraging and they have greatly expanded the therapeutic possibilities for spinal cord injury. Some examples of therapies that may stimulate regeneration are axonal growth inhibitor blockade, cell adhesion molecules, cell transplants and electrical currents, while Schwann cell and stem cell transplants may stimulate remyelination.

Further reading

Bracken MB, Shepard MJ, Collins WF, *et al.* (1990) A randomized, controlled trial of methylprednisolone or naloxone in the treatment of acute spinal cord injury: results of the second national acute spinal cord injury study. N Engl J Med 322: 140–51.

Denis F. (1988) Thoracolumbar spinal injuries: classification. Curr Orthopaed 2: 214–17.

Riggins R. (1977) The risk of neurologic damage with fractures of the vertebrae. J Trauma 17: 126–33.

CHAPTER 9

Abdominal Trauma

Munawar Al-Mudhaffar and Philip Hormbrey

John Radcliffe Hospital, Oxford, UK

OVERVIEW

- The resuscitation of abdominal trauma patients should follow the ABCDE pathway to identify and treat life-threatening injuries.
- The shocked multiple trauma patient who fails to respond to fluid therapy and in whom there is no obvious bleeding source in the thorax, and no pelvic or long bone fracture is identified, should be presumed to have bleeding in the abdomen until proved otherwise.
- While focusing on resuscitation, the aim in abdominal trauma should be to identify patients who need immediate laparotomy.
- Establishing the mechanism of injury, meticulous physical examination and appropriate use of special investigations such as ultrasound, diagnostic peritoneal lavage and computed tomography will help to avoid missing abdominal injuries.
- A high index of suspicion should be maintained to avoid missing perineal and retroperitoneal injuries.

Evaluation of the abdomen in trauma is a challenge because of the physical extent of the abdominal cavity, the paucity of clinical signs and the difficulties associated with the main modes of investigation. Death secondary to uncontrolled and sometimes unrecognised haemorrhage is common. To avoid missing significant injuries, one must assume that every major trauma patient has suffered an abdominal injury unless the patient is awake, has no abdominal pain or distracting injuries and has normal vital signs. Abdominal trauma needs surgical expertise. Call for surgical aid as soon as you suspect abdominal trauma.

Anatomical considerations

The abdomen extends anteriorly from the nipple line (at the fourth intercostal space) down to the inguinal creases and posteriorly from the inferior border of the scapulae down to the gluteal creases. The flanks lie between the anterior and posterior axillary lines from the sixth intercostal space to the iliac crests. The abdominal cavity is divided into the peritoneal cavity and the retroperitoneal spaces and therefore abdominal trauma could be classified into:

- *intraperitoneal*: blood here collects in the peritoneal cavity. Structures injured could be the diaphragm, liver, spleen, gallbladder, small bowel and transverse and sigmoid colon
- *retroperitoneal*: trauma here is more difficult to recognise because it causes fewer physical signs. Structures injured could be the aorta, inferior vena cava, most of duodenum, pancreas, ascending and descending colon and upper urinary tract.

Box 9.1 summarises the anatomical considerations in abdominal trauma.

Box 9.1 **Anatomical considerations in abdominal trauma**

- Anterior extent from the fourth intercostal space to the inguinal creases.
- Posterior extent from inferior scapulae to gluteal creases.
- Remember the retroperitoneal space which is difficult to assess.
- Remember to assess the pelvis.

Mechanism of injury

Blunt

Blunt injuries are difficult to diagnose, particularly in the context of multiple trauma, and physical signs can be unreliable. Abdominal injuries should be considered in any trauma patient with unexplained shock. Common causes are road traffic accidents, falls and assaults. Direct trauma usually causes solid organ injury while deceleration forces (high-speed road traffic accidents and high falls) tear tissues and vessels. The organs most frequently injured are the spleen and liver followed by small bowel and retroperitoneal structures.

Penetrating

Penetrating wounds are caused by knives, handguns or rifle bullets and shrapnel from bombs or blasts. Visceral injury occurs in 30% of stab wounds, with the liver being the most common organ injured. Penetrating wounds are easy to identify, but

ABC of Major Trauma, Fourth Edition. Edited by David V. Skinner and Peter A. Driscoll.
© 2013 Blackwell Publishing Ltd. Published 2013 by Blackwell Publishing Ltd.

it is difficult to determine whether peritoneal penetration has occurred.

Assessment

The primary survey, associated with simultaneous resuscitation and treatment, should be followed by a comprehensive secondary survey.

Primary survey

Attend to life-threatening airway and breathing issues before moving onto circulation. Beware the patient with the dull sounding chest who has a ruptured diaphragm rather than a haemothorax. However, most findings related to abdominal trauma will be first encountered when assessing the circulation.

There are three components to the circulatory assessment. The first is the clinical assessment of the circulation, using skin colour, pulse, capillary refill and blood pressure. The second is the initial treatment of any detected shock and the third and most difficult component, is the determination of the site of blood loss including abdominal assessment. Ideally, these three tasks should be performed simultaneously with different personnel obtaining observations, resuscitating with fluid and performing the abdominal assessment.

All patients with suspected abdominal trauma should receive two large-bore intravenous cannulae. Blood should be taken for cross-matching, full blood count and coagulation screen with other tests as indicated. A fluid challenge of warmed crystalloid should be commenced. The size of the challenge will depend on the perceived extent of the shock but can range from 500 mL to 2 L. See Chapter 5 for the role of hypovolaemic shock.

Abdominal treatment

Inspect the abdomen and look for signs such as the bruising associated with seatbelt marks or entry and exit wounds associated with gunshot injuries. Palpation may reveal tenderness associated with organ injury or peritoneal irritation after visceral damage. Abdominal examination may change with time and therefore should be repeated at regular intervals.

If abnormal vital signs continue despite a normal examination of the anterior abdomen, the patient should be log rolled to assess the posterior abdomen and perineum. The opportunity should be taken to perform a rectal examination at the same time. This is to check the integrity of the rectal wall and assess for the presence of blood. A high-riding prostate indicates urethral damage. Vaginal examination may also be necessary to check the integrity of the vaginal vault.

Adjuncts to the primary survey

Consideration should be given to insertion of a urethral catheter and a nasogastric tube. The urethral meatus should be inspected for blood. If present, a urinary catheter should be deferred to avoid worsening urethral trauma. A nasogastric tube should be considered to decompress the stomach. If there are severe facial injuries or there is the suspicion of a basal skull fracture, tube insertion should be oral to avoid the risk of inadvertent cranial placement.

The initial haemoglobin may be normal and does not reflect the amount of blood lost as at least several hours are required for haemodilution to alter the result. Nevertheless, this can serve as a baseline value. If blood is needed urgently, group O negative can be requested; otherwise type specific may be available more quickly than a full cross-match. Urea and electrolytes, glucose, liver function tests, amylase, urinalysis and pregnancy test (when appropriate) are also requested. The standard trauma series of X-rays should also be done.

Specific investigations include ultrasound (US) scanning or diagnostic peritoneal lavage (DPL) in the haemodynamically unstable patient and computed tomography (CT) scanning in the stable patient. Diagnostic laparoscopy is becoming popular especially in penetrating injuries as it can avoid unnecessary laparotomy.

Ultrasound scan

The focused abdominal sonography in trauma (FAST) scan is the bedside sonographic assessment for fluid in the peritoneal cavity (Figure 9.1). A major use of this highly sensitive and rapid scan is to exclude free fluid in the abdomen. Ultrasound scans (US) can also establish pregnancy status and fetal viability. However, it does not reveal the initial injury and has the disadvantage of being operator dependent.

Computed tomography scan

The major advantage of CT scanning is the specificity of the achievable diagnosis (Figure 9.2). However, this must be weighed against the disadvantages. The move to CT necessitates a transfer with its inherent dangers. The patient may need to be anaesthetised and for accuracy of diagnosis contrast may be necessary, which can be time consuming. Furthermore, CT does not identify all potential intra-abdominal injuries, the retroperitoneal area and small bowel perforations being particularly difficult. Nevertheless, the diagnostic

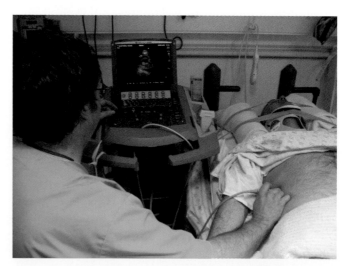

Figure 9.1 FAST scan being performed in the emergency department.

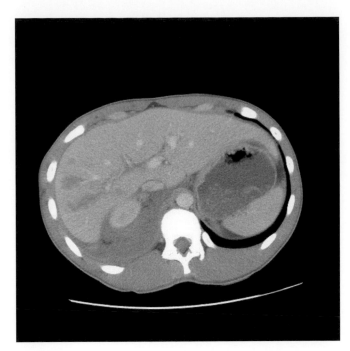

Figure 9.2 Computed tomography scan of abdomen showing liver contusion.

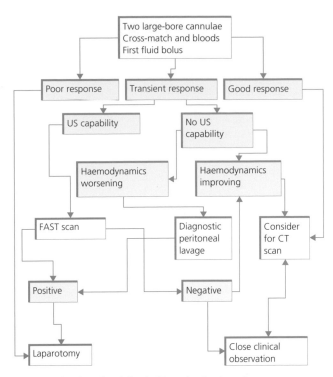

Figure 9.3 Flowchart for abdominal investigation in major trauma. CT, computed tomography; FAST, focused assessment with sonography in trauma; US, ultrasound.

accuracy of CT has prompted many centres to perform a CT from head to pelvis in all patients who are stable enough to go to the scanner. This allows effective and rapid clearing of the neck and more accurate chest and abdominal assessment.

Diagnostic peritoneal lavage

The prime use of DPL is to exclude intraperitoneal bleeding in the patient who has major trauma. As this can now be accurately performed by ultrasound, the need for DPL has receded. It is still of use in centres with no FAST scan when a decision has to be made about the need for laparotomy. It is an invasive procedure and is relatively contraindicated in pregnancy or where there have been previous laparotomies. Positive indicators for a DPL are highlighted in Box 9.2. A positive DPL should result in laparotomy.

Box 9.2 **Indicators for a positive diagnostic peritoneal lavage**

- 5 mL of fresh blood on initial aspiration.
- Presence of bile, enteric contents or bacteria.
- Red blood cells >100,000/mm³ or white blood cells >500/mm³ of aspirate.
- Exit of lavage fluid out of catheters (e.g. chest drain).

Other investigations

The choice of further investigation is often the most difficult decision that needs to be made in the early management of abdominal trauma. A decision algorithm that is suitable in all situations is demonstrated in Figure 9.3. The trauma victim's response to IV fluid resuscitation is graded as shown (good, transient, poor).

History

Using the mnemonic AMPLE from the Advanced Trauma Life Support Course, the attending doctor should inquire about Allergies, Medication, Past history, Last meal, and Events preceding the injury. The patient may have limited recall of the injury owing to loss of consciousness, alcohol or hysteria, so relatives and friends can provide valuable information. When considering road traffic accident victims, the police and ambulance crew may have extensive details and photographs of the accident. Knowledge of the speed of the vehicle, the nature of the impact, steering wheel injury, whether seatbelts were worn and the condition of other victims can help delineate the patient's pattern of likely injuries. In penetrating injuries, the position of the victim when shot or stabbed and the length of the blade or the type of gun and the range of shots fired provide similarly useful information.

Treatment

The first decision that should be made after the immediate resuscitation of the patient is the need for immediate laparotomy. These indications are summarised in Box 9.3.

Haemodynamically stable patients can be investigated further. In patients with solid organ injuries (liver and spleen) identified by CT scan, there is an increasing tendency toward conservative treatment (i.e. observation). Even if all investigations are normal, patients with suspicion of blunt abdominal injury should be admitted for observation and repeat serial examination as hollow organ injury may only become apparent with time.

Box 9.3 **Indications for immediate laparotomy**

- Poor responders.
- Clinical or radiological evidence of perforated viscus.
- Evisceration of peritoneal contents.
- Ruptured diaphragm.
- Gunshot wounds.
- Positive diagnostic peritoneal lavage.
- Transient responders with positive FAST scan.

In the case of stab wounds, if the object used is still visible it should be left in place and only removed in theatre. If the patient is haemodynamically stable, a stab wound could be explored under local anaesthesia and if it does not penetrate the peritoneum, it can be closed and the patient admitted for observation. However, if the peritoneum is breached then the patient can be assessed by any or a combination of DPL, CT, laparotomy or repeat physical examinations.

Further reading

American College of Surgeons Committee on Trauma. (2004) *Advanced Trauma Life Support Course Student Manual*, 7th edn. Chicago: American College of Surgeons.

CHAPTER 10

The Urinary Tract

Jaskarn Rai,[1] Ajith Malalasekera,[1] Timothy Terry[1] and Anthony Deane[2]

[1]Leicester General Hospital, Leicester, UK
[2]William Harvey Hospital, Ashford and Buckland Hospital, Dover, UK

OVERVIEW

- Renal trauma is commonly associated with other intra-abdominal injuries, especially in penetrating renal trauma.
- The imaging method of choice to investigate such patients is contrast-enhanced computed axial tomography (CAT) scan.
- Most renal injuries can be managed non-operatively, with specific indications for renal exploration.

Upper urinary tract

Ten percent of abdominal trauma leads to renal injury and most of these injuries are mild and can be managed non-operatively. Over the last decade, indications for surgical intervention have been clarified with early use of contrast-enhanced computed axial tomography (CAT) scan imaging. The outcome has been decreased nephrectomy rates using initial conservative management, without any increase in morbidity.

Epidemiology

Renal trauma is an affliction mainly of young men (Box 10.1), the male-to-female ratio being 3:1. Blunt trauma accounts for over 90% of renal injuries in the UK. Important associated intra-abdominal injuries occur in about 40% of patients with blunt renal trauma. Penetrating injuries cause more renal damage in comparison to blunt trauma and are also more commonly associated with multiorgan involvement (up to 80%).

Box 10.1 **Typical victims of urinary tract trauma**

- Young men while performing sporting activity (55%).
- People in road traffic accidents (25%).
- Victims of domestic or industrial accidents (15%).
- Victims of assault (5%).

Mechanism of injury

The mechanism of renal injury in blunt trauma can be due to either direct or indirect transmission of forces (Figure 10.1). In direct trauma the injury results from impact of the lower ribs and anterior abdominal wall with the kidney (e.g. run over injuries). Rapid posterior movement of the kidney can cause a second impact with the lumbar spine and paravertebral muscles.

Indirect injury occurs when a deceleration injury is applied to the renal pedicle (e.g. falling from a height) which can tear or avulse the renal vessels or the pelviureteric junction.

Penetrating injury is usually due to stab wounds or gunshot injuries. Stab wounds anterior to the anterior axillary line have more potential to cause injury to the renal pelvis, hilum and pedicle because these structures are directed towards the midline of the abdomen. Wounds posterior to this line are therefore less injurious to the kidney. Gunshot wounds of low velocity cause tissue injury by direct injury while high-velocity missiles have the potential to cause more tissue damage due to the temporary cavity formation. High-velocity missiles tend to carry in contaminated substances from the surface of the body and cause more devitalisation.

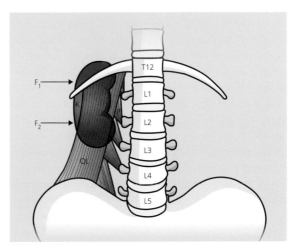

Figure 10.1 Mechanism of direct blunt renal trauma. An external force (F1) may crush the kidney (K) between the 12th rib and the vertebral column, or a force (F2) may crush the kidney against the paravertebral muscles (quadratum lumborum, QL, or psoas major in position P but deleted from diagram). (Adapted from Moore EE, Shackford SR, Pachter HL, *et al.* (1989) Organ injury scaling: spleen, liver, and kidney. J Trauma 29(12): 1664–6.)

ABC of Major Trauma, Fourth Edition. Edited by David V. Skinner and Peter A. Driscoll.
© 2013 Blackwell Publishing Ltd. Published 2013 by Blackwell Publishing Ltd.

Table 10.1 American Association for the Surgery of Trauma (AAST) organ injury severity scale

Grade	Type	Description	
I	Contusion	Microscopic or gross haematuria, urological studies normal	
	Haematoma	Subcapsular, non-expanding without parenchymal laceration	
II	Haematoma	Non-expanding perirenal haematoma confined to renal retroperitoneum	
	Laceration	<1.0 cm parenchymal depth of renal cortex without urinary extravasation	Initial conservative treatment
III	Laceration	>1.0 cm parenchymal depth of renal cortex without collecting system rupture or urinary extravasation	
IV	Laceration	Parenchymal laceration extending through renal cortex, medulla and collecting system	
	Vascular	Main renal artery or vein injury with contained haemorrhage	
V	Laceration	Completely shattered kidney	Early surgical intervention
	Vascular	Avulsion of renal hilum which devascularises kidney	

Adapted from Moore EE, Shackford SR, Pachter HL, *et al.* (1989) Organ injury scaling: spleen, liver, and kidney. J Trauma 29(12): 1664–6.
Advance one grade for bilateral injuries up to grade III.

Classification of renal trauma

Renal injury classification is beneficial in selecting appropriate therapy, predicting outcomes and conducting trauma research. The American Association for the Surgery of Trauma (AAST) severity scaling system for renal trauma has been validated and usefully predicts the need for renal repair or nephrectomy (Table 10.1).

Clinical evaluation

Clinical evaluation is summarised in Box 10.2. Initial assessment of trauma patients should be a primary survey according to ATLS protocols. Patients who are haemodynamically unstable due to major renal injury will require resuscitation with or without early surgical intervention. Stable patients with trauma need to be further evaluated regarding the possibility of renal injury. Conscious patients can be directly interviewed while accompanying persons can provide valuable information in unconscious patients. The mechanism of the injury and forces involved should be ascertained. Those who have sustained a direct blow will complain of flank pain and have gross haematuria in up to 90% of cases. The haematuria may be subsequently accompanied by ureteric colic caused by the passage of blood clots. Rapid deceleration injuries to the renal pedicle may be caused by falls from a height or motor vehicle accidents. Caution must be exercised as renal pedicle injuries and pelviureteric junction disruptions may not be associated with gross haematuria.

Clinical examination may show skin abrasions or bruises overlying the upper abdomen, loin or lower thoracic area (Figure 10.2). Rigidity of the anterior abdominal wall and local loin tenderness over the affected kidney are invariably elicited. A flattening of loin contour together with a palpable mass indicate the presence of a perinephric haematoma with or without urinary extravasation. In such cases paralytic ileus may be present.

In penetrating trauma, details of the weapon used are relevant in gauging the potential of the injury. Entry and exit wounds as well as any missile trajectory should be identified.

Patients with pre-existing renal abnormalities and solitary kidneys should be identified.

Box 10.2 **Clinical evaluation**

- Primary survey (ATLS).
- Haemodynamic stability.
- Mechanism of the injury obtained from concious patients, witness and rescue team including times and settings of incident.
- Symptoms and signs:
  - Flank pain
  - Gross haematuria ± clot colic
  - Skin abrasions or bruises
  - Rigidity of the anterior abdominal wall and local loin tenderness
  - Flattening of loin contour and/or palpable mass
  - Entry and exit wounds
  - Missile trajectory.
- Pre-existing renal abnormalities (pelvi-ureteric junction obstruction, large cysts, lithiasis, past renal surgery) and solitary kidneys should be recorded.

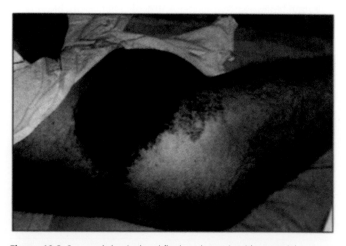

Figure 10.2 Severe abdominal and flank ecchymosis with potential urological injury (caused by seatbelt).

Investigations

Box 10.3 summarises the investigations that may be carried out. Urinalysis will identify microscopic haematuria. As the haematuria may be transient, it is important to evaluate the first obtained sample. Creatinine levels measured especially within the first hour can be useful to identify any pre-existing renal dysfunction.

Box 10.3 Investigations

- Urinalysis and gross inspection for visible haematuria.
- Serum creatinine within first hour often indicates pre-existing renal injury.
- Serial haematocrit can indicate blood loss (not necessarily renal).
- Imaging:
  - Spiral contrast CT scan
  - Intravenous urography
  - Ultrasound scanning
  - Magnetic resonance imaging
  - Renal arteriography.

Imaging is carried out in selected individuals to assist in the decision of conservative versus operative management (Box 10.4). It is useful to stage an injury, record the presence and function of the opposite kidney, identify pre-existing renal pathology and any associated injury/injuries. As most renal injuries are minor and can be managed conservatively, there are clear guidelines on when imaging is required.

Box 10.4 Indications for imaging in renal trauma

- Gross haematuria.
- Microscopic haematuria and shock (systemic blood pressure <90 mmHg).
- Presence of major associated injuries.
- History of rapid deceleration injury with clinical indicators of renal trauma or associated injuries.
- Renal injury is clinically suspected on the basis of an entry or exit wound.

In haemodynamically stable patients helical CT with intravenous contrast has become the imaging method of choice in the primary imaging of patients with probable major renal injuries (Figure 10.3). It has proven to be more sensitive and specific than intravenous urography, ultrasound scanning and angiography.

Special protocols with scanning from the diaphragm to the ischial tuberosities and to include delayed films which better identify collecting system injuries have been defined. On-table one-shot intravenous urography is indicated in haemodynamically unstable patients requiring early surgical intervention. A rapid bolus of contrast (2 mL/kg) is given and a single plain abdominal film taken 10 min afterwards. This can help to identify a functioning contralateral kidney and any injuries of the traumatised kidney. Ultrasonography has advantages in the follow-up of renal injury, e.g. assessing urinomas. Magnetic resonance imaging may be used instead of contrast-enhanced CAT when there is a history of contrast allergy. Renal arteriography is now only indicated after the identification of a vascular injury with CAT scanning and as a preliminary to embolisation of a well-defined bleeding renal vessel.

Management

The principle underlying the management of patients with renal trauma is conservation of the maximum number of functioning nephrons with minimal morbidity and mortality. The immediate management of any individual patient is invariably determined more by the patient's general clinical state and the presence of important associated injuries than by the mode and type of renal injury. Less than 5% of all renal injuries are by themselves life threatening, and hypovolaemic shock in a patient with renal trauma is nearly always secondary to the presence of concomitant injuries. The initial general assessment of the patient is thus all-important in deciding a plan of supportive and definitive treatment (Box 10.5).

The majority of renal injuries are minor and may safely be managed non-operatively (Box 10.6). This involves strict bedrest, appropriate fluid input, analgesia, prophylactic antibiotics and frequent serial clinical observations of vital signs. Monitoring should be continued until haematuria resolves. A clear understanding that conservative management leads to more renal preservation has led to surgical intervention being reserved for a minority of patients. Indications for renal exploration are given in Box 10.7.

Box 10.5 Management of renal trauma

- Treat hypovolaemic shock.
- Stage renal injury radiologically.
- Treat patients with stable minor and major renal injuries (up to 95%) expectantly.
- Operate on patients with critical and unstable major renal injuries.

Box 10.6 Non-operative management of renal injuries

- Institute strict bedrest.
- Appropriate fluid input.
- Give analgesia.
- Give appropriate prophylactic antibiotics.
- Make frequent serial clinical observations of vital signs.

Box 10.7 Indications for surgery/renal exploration

- Persistent, life-threatening haemorrhage believed to stem from renal injury.
- Renal pedicle avulsion (grade V injury).
- Some grade IV and rarely grade III injuries which fail initial conservative treatment.
- Expanding, pulsatile or uncontained retroperitoneal haematoma (thought to indicate renal pedicle avulsion).
- Pelviureteric junction avulsion.
- Failed interventional radiological management of renovascular injuries.

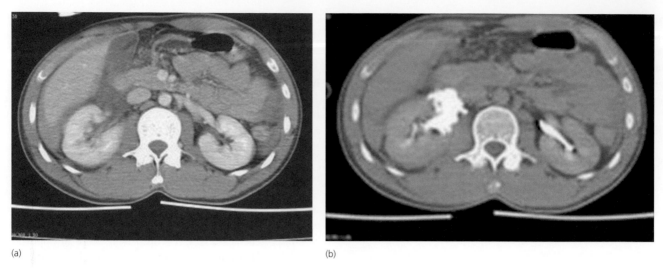

(a)   (b)

Figure 10.3 (a) Spiral CAT scan of abdomen showing a right-sided perirenal fluid collection following blunt trauma. (b) Delayed images showing the fluid collection to be due to urinary extravasation. (Reproduced with kind permission from Dr Raman Tyagi and Dr Arumugam Rajesh, Consultant Radiologists, University Hospitals of Leicester.)

When surgical intervention is required a generous midline abdominal incision is advocated. This provides good access to the kidneys, the entire length of the ureters and the vascular pedicles. It also allows a full laparotomy for associated injuries. Controlling the renal artery and vein prior to opening Gerota's fascia is recommended when conservative renal surgery is contemplated (Figure 10.4). Renorrhaphy or partial nephrectomy is attempted whenever possible. Higher rates of nephrectomy are associated with penetrating injuries, especially those arising from high-velocity missiles. Grade V injuries are invariably treated by simple nephrectomy. Disruption of the pelviureteric junction is treated by spatulation and reanastomosis over a ureteric stent. Conservative renal arterial surgery is not indicated in those with a normal contralateral kidney due to poor nephron survival with this procedure. Incomplete arterial lacerations may be suitable for repair. Renal vein injuries, especially on the right side, can be debrided and sutured. Those on the left, if close to the inferior vena cava, can be safely ligated as collateral venous drainage is via the proximal adrenal and gonadal veins.

Selective angioembolisation may occasionally be successful in managing renovascular injuries in haemodynamically stable patients.

Complications of renal injury

The complications of renal injury are shown in Box 10.8.

> **Box 10.8 Complications of renal injury**
>
> - *Early*: bleeding, infection, urinoma formation, perinephric abscess, urinary fistula, hypertension and sepsis.
> - *Delayed*: bleeding, hydronephrosis, calculus formation, chronic pyelonephritis, hypertension, arteriovenous fistula, hydronephrosis and pseudoaneurysm.
>
> Adapted from Guidelines on Urological Trauma, European Association of Urology, 2012.

Follow-up management

Patients who have sustained a significant renal injury should be followed up with further imaging within 36–72 h, to identify complications. A repeat spiral CT scan or ultrasound is indicated especially in grade III–V injuries.

After discharge, regular follow-up is necessary in the first year for all major renal trauma patients. This should include clinical examination, blood pressure assessment, urinalysis, imaging of the urinary tract (principally ultrasound) and quantification of renal recovery by nuclear isotope studies.

Ureteral injuries

The ureters are small mobile conduits draining each ipsilateral kidney. They are rarely involved in urological trauma (1%) and

Figure 10.4 (*Left*) Retroperitoneal incision sited over the aorta medial to the inferior mesenteric vein to isolate the renal vessels before opening Gerota's fascia. (*Right*) The left renal vein crosses anterior to the aorta. With this vein retracted superiorly, the left and right renal arteries may be located arising from the aorta.

most ureteral injuries are Iatrogenic (75%) with most of these occurring in gynaecological surgery followed by general surgery. The lower third of the ureter is the most common area to be injured. Traditionally, intravenous urethrograms have been used to diagnose a ureteral injury but, if the injury occurs in the context of a major trauma, a CT will most likely be performed. Delayed imaged with contrast entering the ureter (30 min post injection) gives excellent images of any ureteric injury.

The American Association of Surgery of Trauma (AAST) have classified ureteral injuries as Grade I–V with I haematoma, II lacerations <50% circumference, II laceration >50% circumference, IV Complete tear <2 cm of devascularisation and Grade V >2 cm of devascularisation.

Management

Partial injuries can be managed by endoscopic placement of a ureteric stent across the injured ureter to allow drainage of urine and the injury to heal. A nephrostomy can be placed percutaneously to divert urine but a stent is superior as it allows canalisation of the ureter whether placed antegrade or retrograde using fluoroscopy. An initial urinary catheter for 2 days to prevent stent reflux allows the mucosa to heal and the stent can be removed at 6 weeks with a follow up intravenous urogram at 3–6 months with a renogram to check kidney function and that a stricture has not formed. If a grade II or III injury is noticed intra-operatively then the primary repair of the ureter over stent is the preferred option with a non-suction drain placed adjacent the the injury site.

For complete injuries there are different approaches for those in the upper, middle and lower third of the ureters and these depend on surgeons choice and the nature of injuries. Recommendations for upper third: uretero-ureterostomy, transuretero-ureterostomy or ureterocalycostomy. For middle third: uretero-ureterostomy, transuretero-ureterostomy and Boari flap and reimplantation. For lower third: direct reimplantation, Psoas hitch and Blandy cystoplasty are the choices. In a complete ureteral injury where there is not enough length to do any of the above then ileal interposition or transplant of the affected kidney to the pelvis and a neoureterocystotomy can be fashioned.

Lower urinary tract

Injuries of the lower urinary tract cause more confusion than those of the upper urinary tract as their management is controversial. The rule in patients with suspected urethral injuries, especially with urethral haemorrhage, and major pelvic fractures is not to pass a urethral catheter without first seeking advice from a urologist. Even though monitoring urinary output is very important in patients with major injuries, a catheter should not be passed without careful thought. Urinary extravasation is not dangerous in the short term. CT scanning is replacing IVP as the investigation of choice. The investigations in patients with lower urinary tract injuries are shown in Box 10.9.

Bladder injuries

Bladder injuries may be associated with a pelvic fracture – that is, they may be caused by penetration by a bony fragment or a direct blow to the lower abdomen, especially when the bladder is full.

> **Box 10.9 Investigations in patients with lower urinary tract injuries**
>
> - Inspect the urinary meatus for blood.
> - Examine the abdomen for peritonism, perineal bruising, and a high-riding prostate.
> - Perform intravenous urography to detect bladder perforation, displaced bladder, upper urinary tract injuries.
> - Perform cystography to exclude bladder perforation if patient has a catheter in place.
> - Perform ascending urethrography (aqueous contrast) to exclude urethral injury (controversial).

The condition may be missed in patients intoxicated with alcohol or those with a head injury. Patients with a bladder injury may have lower abdominal peritonism and not be able to pass urine. A catheter may have been passed by the receiving clinicians and the urine may contain blood.

Investigation begins by obtaining a plain radiograph to exclude pelvic fractures. Disruption of the pelvic symphysis alerts the clinician to the possibility of urethral injury and delayed rupture of the bladder due to stretching of the anterior bladder wall. An intravenous urogram or CT scan may show an extravasation from a bladder injury. If there is no pelvic fracture and no urethral haemorrhage, a urethral catheter may be passed, and cystography with 10% dilute contrast agent will show any important bladder injury. If an intraperitoneal bladder rupture is suspected, then cystography (Figure 10.5) should be done before diagnostic peritoneal lavage because a laparotomy will be required to repair such a lesion, if present, making lavage unnecessary. In patients with serious pelvic fracture, especially if it affects the pubic symphysis, upward dislocation of the bladder on CT urography should be excluded first, although this would usually be accompanied by urethral haemorrhage.

Treatment

Patients with significant intraperitoneal rupture and peritonism are best treated by laparatomy and drainage by suprapubic catheter as well as by urethral catheter for about seven days. Broad spectrum antibiotics should be given. Extraperitoneal injuries are managed

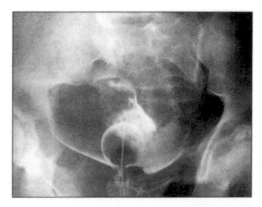

Figure 10.5 Cystogram of a bladder full of haematoma with extravasation of contrast due to a torn anterior bladder wall. The patient required 30 units of blood before bleeding was controlled by selective internal iliac embolisation.

by drainage by catheter without irrigation for about 10 days. A catheter of at least 20F is necessary and cystography to confirm healing is advisable before withdrawal of the catheter.

Bulbar injuries

Bulbar injuries occur by direct trauma – for example by falling into onto a bicycle crossbar. Occasionally they can be caused by penetrating trauma. Patients with bulbar injuries have perineal bruising and blood at the urinary meatus. A urethral catheter must not be passed as it may aggravate the injury and introduce infection. The patient should be treated expectantly and, if he or she passes urine, should be given antibiotics and followed up. Patients with urinary retention should be treated by inserting a suprapubic catheter of small calibre percutaneously, as heavy haematuria is not usually a problem. Antibiotics are given and urethrography can be performed after about five days. The patient will need urological follow-up to exclude stricture formation. See Box 10.10 for the management of patients with bulbar injuries.

> Box 10.10 **Management of patients with bulbar injuries**
>
> - Do not pass a urethral catheter.
> - If the patient passes urine give antibiotics and follow up.
> - If the patient has urinary retention insert a suprapubic catheter with a small calibre and give antibiotics. Perform urethrography after about 5 days and follow up.

Urethral injuries caused by pelvic fractures

The membranous urethra below the prostrate is damaged in about 10% of men with pelvic fractures. Serious injuries, though rare, are devastating, as impotence and stricture are common sequelae. Damage usually comprises a partial tear but, occasionally, complete disruption and upward dislocation of the bladder and prostate occurs. The prostate is fixed to the pubic symphysis by the puboprostatic ligaments and any severe disruption of the pubic symphysis is liable to tear the prostate off the membrane urethra, which is attached to the pelvic floor (Figure 10.6).

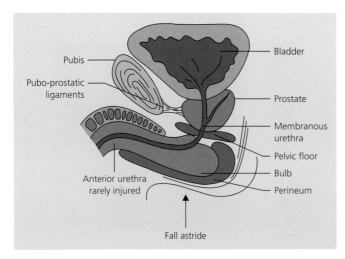

Figure 10.6 The puboprostatic ligaments carry the prostate with them in patients with pelvic fracture, tearing the urethra off the pelvic floor.

The signs of urethral injury caused by pelvic fracture are blood at the meatus, perineal bruising and inability to pass urine (Box 10.11). A urethral catheter must not be passed as it may aggravate the injury, even if it passes the tear: the urethra is often traumatised and devascularised and may be eroded by the catheter or disintegrate around it; the catheter will prevent the haematoma from draining and introduce infection with possible fistulation on its withdrawal and, worst of all, the catheter may pass out of the tear and drain blood and urine below the prostate. Balloon inflation may convert a partial disruption into a complete one.

> Box 10.11 **Signs of membranous urethral injury**
>
> - Pelvic fracture.
> - Perineal bruising.
> - Blood at the meatus.
> - Inability to pass urine.
> - High-riding prostate.

The safest way to treat urethral injuries caused by pelvic fractures is to pass a suprapubic catheter of adequate calibre either percutaneously, or by cystotomy if the patient requires a laparatomy for other reasons, if the bladder is impalpable. CT scan or intravenous urography should be performed to exclude total disruption with a high-riding bladder above the pubic symphysis – an indication for exploration and repositioning. Some authorities advise performing ascending urethrography to delineate the extent of the injury and plan its management but this can be difficult in the emergency room. In general, a urethral catheter can be passed in a patient with a pelvic fracture if there is no blood at the meatus or if the pubic symphysis is not severely disrupted on radiography. If any difficulties are encountered, urological help should be summoned and an ascending urethrogram considered or suprapubic catheterisation performed. If there is a severe disruption of the pubic symphysis, orthopaedic help should be requested as early fixation may assist in management and reduce morbidity.

Later treatment of these injuries entails urethroscopy but late strictures are very common.

In women, the urethra is injured only rarely, and usually a catheter can easily be passed in those with pelvic fractures and, if necessary, cystography performed to exclude the possibility of bladder injuries.

The urological management of men with serious pelvic fractures is summarised in Figure 10.7.

Practical points

Attempts may already have been made to pass a catheter and failed. These patients should go straight on to CT or IVP and a suprapubic catheter placed, plus realignment if the bladder is high-riding.

Ascending urography: contrast (water soluble) should be flushed up the urethra via syringe and catheter. This investigation is useful in difficult cases with a minor amount of urethral haemorrhage and an impalpable bladder.

Suprapubic catheterisation: this is a potentially hazardous procedure. Percutaneous sets, such as Lawrence Add-A-Cath system, are only suitable if urine can be easily aspirated by suprapubic needle puncture. Bladder volume should be at least 350 ml. A *small*

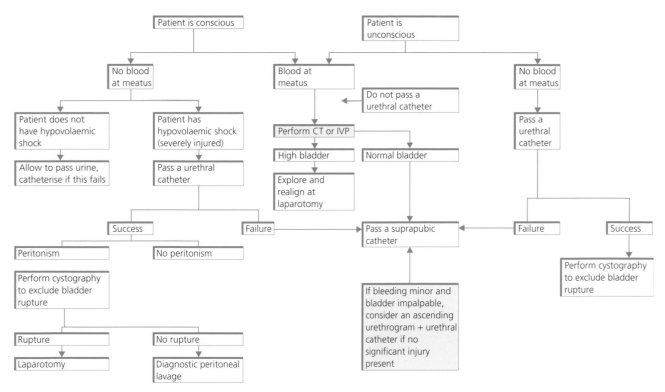

Urological management of men with serious pelvic fractures.

Figure 10.7 Algorithm for urological management of men with serious pelvic fractures.

calibre catheter is suitable for bulbar injuries whereas a *large calibre* (at least 16F) is required for pelvic fracture injuries as bleeding will block a small one.

Open suprapubic catheterisation with a 20F – 22F catheter may be needed via a suprapubic incision if percutaneous methods are impossible. This is the method of choice if the patient requires a laparatomy anyway.

External genitalia

Serious injuries to the penis and scrotum are unusual. The mobile scrotal skin can be used to cover penile defects and has good powers of recovery. Scrotal tears heal well without suturing. The erectile mechanism should always be repaired if torn with monofilament non-absorbable sutures or polydioxanone suture (PDS).

The testicles can be damaged by direct trauma – usually a blow or a kick. If bleeding is confined to the scrotal skin, no active treatment is required (Figure 10.8). Tense haematoceles should, however, always be explored as these usually indicate that the testis is torn and needs repair. Severe damage may require orchidectomy.

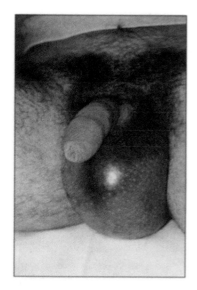

Figure 10.8 Scrotal haematoma.

Acknowledgements

Figure 10.2 is reproduced from the advanced trauma life support (ATLS) slide set by kind permission of the American College of Surgeons' committee on trauma. Figure 10.8 was provided by Mr Andrew Cope, St Bartholomew's Hospital. The line drawings were originally prepared by the Department of Education and Medical Illustration Services, St Bartholomew's Hospital.

Further reading

Dobrowolski Z, Kusionowicz J, Drewniak T, *et al.* (2002) Renal and ureteric trauma: diagnosis and management in Poland. BJU Int 89(7):748–51.

Djakovic E, Plas l, Martínez-Piñeiro TH, *et al.* (2012) Imaging of renal trauma: a comprehensive review. RadioGraphics 21:557–74.

Lynch D, Martinez-Piñeiro L, Plas E, Serafetinidis E, Turkeri L, Hohenfellner M. (2003) *Guidelines on Urological Trauma.* Arnhem, The Netherlands: European Association of Urology.

Santucci RA, Wessells H, Bartsch G, *et al.* (2004) Evaluation and management of renal injuries: consensus statement of the renal trauma subcommittee. BJU Int 93:937–54.

CHAPTER 11

Limb Injuries

Rohit Kotnis[1], Nigel Rossiter[2] and Keith Willett[1]

[1]John Radcliffe Hospital, Oxford, UK
[2]Basingstoke General Hospital and Royal Defence Medical College, Basingstoke, UK

OVERVIEW

- Limb assessment in the multiply injured patient.
- Management of wounds and open fractures.
- Early management of pelvic fractures and injuries.
- Compartment syndrome.
- Joint dislocations: immediate management.

Up to 70% of multiply injured patients have injured limbs and fractures or dislocations of the appendicular skeleton. Severe limb injuries must not distract the resuscitation team from the ABC principles of establishing an airway, optimising ventilation, and restoring circulatory volume. The exception is limb injuries that may cause exsanguination which may be immediately life threatening, in which case a 'military' tourniquet must be employed immediately. A compressive pad should control external bleeding and any wounds covered with a sterile dressing.

Careful thorough examination, after the primary survey is complete, must identify injuries, particularly those threatening the overall mortality or morbidity of the patient. Apparently minor injuries, often overlooked in the face of multiple trauma and only discovered some days later, must not be neglected; they may result in long-term disability or disfigurement.

Prehospital care

Doctors attending the scene of an accident should confine themselves initially to personal safety, assessment of the scene and management of the patient's airway with cervical spine immobilisation, breathing and circulation. Attention can then be directed towards the injured limbs. When moving a patient with a fractured limb, the pain is reduced by supporting the limb on either side of the fracture and applying gentle traction along the axis of the limb. All unnecessary handling of the injured part without splinting should be avoided as this may increase pain and bleeding from the fracture site. The exceptions to this rule are when severe deformity or ischaemia distal to the fracture threatens survival of the soft tissues;

reduction is then indicated. This is achieved by gentle traction and restoration of the normal anatomical alignment. Perfusion of the distal limb must be assessed before and after any manipulation, to ensure restoration of distal blood supply and prevent any further soft tissue injury that may have resulted from the manipulation.

Profuse haemorrhage from limb injuries, particularly complete or incomplete amputation, can result in life-threatening blood loss. In these circumstances military tourniquets are life saving and must be applied at the earliest opportunity, prior to transfer.

Splints are mandatory before the victim is evacuated. Anything rigid can be used, such as pieces of wreckage and wooden sticks. Strapping to the opposite leg is useful in solitary lower limb injuries, and 'bulk' splints can be produced by bandaging blankets or pillows around the limb. Rapid transfer to a hospital with resuscitation facilities and appropriate staff is then required.

Hospital care

Haemorrhage

Blood loss from limb wounds and occult bleeding from fractures contribute to hypovolaemic shock in patients with multiple injuries. Haemorrhage from multiple fractures may result in exsanguination, particularly when the pelvis and femora are involved. Patients with hypovolaemic shock should be resuscitated immediately along the lines described in Chapter 5

Total blood loss can be estimated (Table 11.1), and blood for transfusion should be cross-matched urgently. Blood loss from open fractures may be two or three times greater than that from closed fractures. Fractures of the long bones should not be assumed to be responsible for any hypovolaemic shock; occult bleeding into visceral cavities must be excluded first. These include the chest cavity, the abdomen and the retoperitoneal space and in association with disruption of the pelvic ring. Blood loss from wounds can be reduced by a compressive bandage or hand pressure over a sterile pad. A tourniquet is indicated only for unmanageable life-threatening haemorrhage or after traumatic amputation with exsanguinating haemorrhage (see earlier regarding the military tourniquet).

Assessment

Evaluation of limb injuries is not started until life-threatening conditions have been treated. Careful examination is complemented

ABC of Major Trauma, Fourth Edition. Edited by David V. Skinner and Peter A. Driscoll.
© 2013 Blackwell Publishing Ltd. Published 2013 by Blackwell Publishing Ltd.

Table 11.1 Estimated blood loss caused by fractures

Site of the fracture	Estimated blood loss (litres)
Humerus	0.5–1.5
Tibia	0.5–1.5
Femur	1–2.5
Pelvis	1–4

by suspicions raised by knowledge of the mechanism of injury. One of the best sources of information on this is the ambulance personnel at the scene who will give important clues even before the patient reaches the resuscitation room. Witnesses should not be discharged until at least the mechanism, environment, time and immediate care of the injury have been established. For victims of road traffic accidents, it is important to determine whether they were vehicle occupants, whether they were restrained by a seatbelt, the direction of impact and degree of damage to the vehicle. It is also important to find out whether other people were involved, their clinical injuries and whereabouts. Ejection from a vehicle, death and serious injury of others involved in the accident suggest a high-energy mechanism of injury.

Certain injury patterns are common. For instance, a direct blow to the knee in a seated occupant of a car may produce not only knee injury and femoral fracture but is commonly associated with hip dislocation or fractures of the acetabulum or both. These injuries are also seen in motorcyclists who receive axial trauma along the horizontal femur. The femoral neck is injured in 10% of incidents of this type and should be carefully studied, as the injury is often initially missed, with significant morbidity resulting. A victim falling from a height and landing on his or her feet may sustain compression fractures of the calcaneum, ankle, tibial plateau and one or more vertebrae at the thoracolumbar junction or in the lower cervical spine.

Full exposure of the patient is essential for a thorough secondary survey. Assessment should begin with a comparison of the injured limb with the uninjured limb if possible. Look at the attitude of the limb, any shortening or rotational abnormalities, which may indicate proximal fractures or dislocations.

A clear appreciation of the mechanism of injury is vital in understanding the potential for injury. In addition, a wound seen close to a joint may well have communicated with the joint at the moment of impact which then mandates joint exploration and washout.

As clinical signs are often subtle, particularly in the unconscious patient, careful inspection of the whole circumference of each limb for local swelling and bruising is necessary. Gently palpate along the axes and the bony prominences for tenderness, fracture crepitus (grating) and abnormal inter-fragmentary mobility.

Carefully examine adjacent joints so that co-existing injuries are not overlooked. Co-operative patients may indicate the active ranges of joint movement. Passive ranges of motion should be assessed cautiously in a limb that is suspected of being fractured.

Vascular state

Of prime importance to limb survival is the competence of the vasculature distal to any injury. Local contusion, penetrating injuries, fractures and particularly major joint dislocations may occlude or disrupt blood vessels.

In the haemodynamically stable patient, examination of tissue perfusion distal to the injury is essential. Markers of this include the skin colour and temperature, distal pulses, capillary return and pulse oximetry. Skin pallor or a blue-grey colour should arouse suspicion. Similarly, a low skin temperature indicates inadequate perfusion. It may be useful to compare pulse oximetry on the digits of the affected limb and a normal limb in the same patient. A sensitive indicator is capillary return: the normal prompt pink flush of the nail bed seen after transient compression which should return in less than 2 sec. This response will be slowed if the circulation is inadequate. Diminished or absent pulses strongly suggest vascular disruption. More proximal pulses should also be checked.

Even if the above parameters suggest satisfactory tissue perfusion, a diagnosis of arterial spasm should never be made. Any suggestion of vascular compromise must be accounted for and managed promptly.

Any joint dislocation or major deformity must be reduced and splinted. This will lead to restoration of tissue perfusion in the majority of cases. It is important to make sure that the splint device is checked for local compression. If the above measures do not lead to an improvement, an urgent vascular opinion must be sought.

Doppler ultrasonography may be useful in evaluation of limb perfusion, but if a vascular injury is suspected, urgent arteriography remains the gold standard. Treatment should result in a restoration of circulation within 6 h of injury.

Neurological state

Peripheral nerves are sensitive to ischaemia and sensation is lost early. Therefore, total insensibility in a hand or foot suggests ischaemia because, with the exception of a brachial plexus or spinal cord injury, it is unlikely that all of a limb's nerve trunks would have been damaged.

Evidence of nerve injury may be difficult to obtain in the unconscious or multiply injured patient. There is a higher incidence of neurological damage with dislocations than with fractures. Simple tests to assess touch, motor function and sweating are sufficient to determine nerve integrity. When testing distal motor function, the more proximal innervation of the muscle bellies must be appreciated. Injury to a peripheral nerve must be assumed if there is altered sensation in the distribution of that nerve and a wound overlying its course. Neurological function should be documented to allow later comparison. In such cases, an early specialist referral is appropriate.

Wound management

Fifty percent of patients with open fractures will have multiple injuries. The extent of soft tissue damage, which is related to the energy of the injury, will determine the outcome. An antiseptic-soaked sterile dressing applied to an open wound at the site of an accident should not be disturbed; repeated examinations outside the operating theatre increase the risk of infection. Instant or digital photography of the wound is recommended. Splintage of the fracture is required prior to theatre. Intravenous antibiotic prophylaxis with a cephalosporin (for example, cefuroxime 1.5 g) should be commenced in the emergency department. This should be continued in intravenous form for at least 48 h with subsequent oral preparation. With heavy contamination and farmyard injuries, it is appropriate to give gentamicin and metronidazole.

Tetanus prophylaxis must not be forgotten and depends on the patient's immunisation status. An immunised patient with a contaminated wound prone to tetanus requires a booster of tetanus toxoid if more than 10 years have elapsed since his or her last dose. In addition, tetanus immunoglobulin is required if no immunity exists or the immunisation state is unknown.

An open wound should be extended and debrided in the operating theatre (surgical toilet with removal of dead tissue and foreign material) within 6 h of the injury. This timeframe is based on the multiplication of contaminating bacteria. An early consult with the plastic surgeons is important and they should be present at the time of the wound debridement if soft tissue reconstruction is anticipated. Open fractures are graded according to the Gustilo and Anderson classification after debridement (Table 11.2). Internal fixation is encouraged in stable patients with early tissue flap coverage by a plastic surgeon.

Pelvic injuries

Pelvic fractures must be sought clinically and radiologically (Figure 11.1) in all patients with multiple injuries. They are relatively common in this group and if missed can have disastrous consequences with respect to morbidity and mortality. The pelvic spring test should be performed only once to avoid clot displacement from a potential bleeding point.

Any pelvic displacement seen on a radiograph is usually considerably less than that present at the time of impact, because of the inherent elasticity of the pelvic structures (see Chapter 13). Considerable force is necessary to disrupt the pelvic ring and associated extensive soft tissue and visceral damage may result in life-threatening haemorrhage. In cases of persistent hypovolamia despite resuscitation (grade IV shock), stabilisation of the pelvis is appropriate to control further blood loss during movement of the

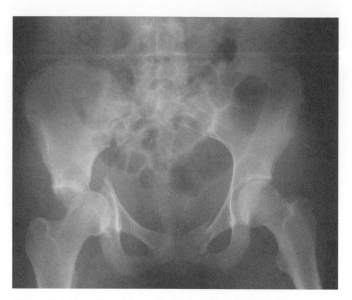

Figure 11.1 Disruption of the pelvic ring including acetabular fracture.

patient. The rationale is no different from that outlined for other fractures, but action is more urgent in the case of the pelvis.

Stabilisation of the pelvis in the emergency department is easily and rapidly achieved with the use of a folded sheet. This can be placed on a trolley before the arrival of a patient, folded to about 20 cm wide and positioned to lie under the patient's buttocks. If unstable pelvic disruption is suspected or shown radiologically, the sheet can be wrapped tightly around the front of the pelvis and secured with a sponge forceps. (Custom-made devices are available.) This will not interfere with access to the abdomen, perineum or genitalia, further radiological investigations or patient transfer. To avoid skin pressure necrosis, the sheet should be removed after 6–8 h and replaced with definitive pelvic fixation if appropriate. In the absence of hypovolaemic shock, emergency pelvic external fixation is not necessary.

The placement of an external fixator on the pelvis may be part of the initial stabilisation (Figure 11.2). This is ideally applied in the theatre environment but may be done in the emergency department. All resuscitation rooms should have access to a pelvic external fixator. A surgeon experienced in the rapid application of a frame and the correct positioning of pins should perform this. A poorly applied external fixator and pins may limit further management options.

If, despite this, bleeding is not controlled and other causes have been excluded, urgent angiography or pelvlic packing is required to arrest the bleeding points. Disruption of the pelvic ring with extensive damage to the pelvic blood vessels is an important cause of death in multiple trauma.

Open pelvic fractures are almost always fatal unless dealt with properly. This includes diverting the bowel and washing out the distal segment. The stoma should be sited in the upper quadrants, well away from any iliac crest pin sites, to reduce pin site/pelvic infection and so increase the options for definitive pelvic fixation. Close co-operation between orthopaedic and general surgeons is critical to avoid unnecessary deaths.

Table 11.2 The Gustilo and Anderson classification of open fractures

Grade	Mechanism	Description
I	Low energy	Clean wound, <1 cm, simple fracture, no skin crushing
II	Moderate energy	>1 cm laceration, no significant soft tissue injury, more complex fracture
III	High energy	Complex fracture with extensive soft tissue injury. Injuries >8 h, farmyard injuries
IIIA	High energy	Adequate soft tissue cover of the fracture after debridement despite extensive soft tissue damage/loss
IIIB	High energy	Inadequate soft tissue cover with bone exposed. Requires soft tissue cover
IIIC	High energy	Disruption of the circulation – any fracture associated with an arterial injury that requires repair

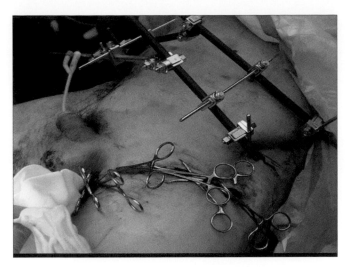

Figure 11.2 Early application of an external pelvic fixator.

Damage to pelvic organs

Damage to pelvic organs and the urinary tract is common and often associated with pelvic injury. Such injury should be looked for using the following signs: blood at the external urethral meatus, perineal haematoma or displacement of the prostate on rectal examination. In such cases, urethral catheterisation should not be attempted. Instead, an urgent retrograde urethrogram should be done; if injury is ruled out, a urethral catheter can be gently passed. In cases of injury to the urinary system, an urgent urological opinion should be sought. The same algorithm applies if a single attempt at urethral catheterisation is unsuccessful (see Chapter 10).

Damage to abdominal organs

Abdominal examination may be equivocal if there is a major pelvic injury. Diagnostic peritoneal lavage (DPL) with 10 mL/kg body-weight of normal saline can be irrigated throughout the peritoneal cavity and the effluent collected. A supraumbilical approach is best with a suspected pelvic injury to minimise the risk of a false positive related to blood entering the peritoneal cavity from a retroperitoneal haematoma. If the returned fluid is not frank blood, the red cell count in the fluid should be measured with an FBC machine (see Chapter 9). The result should be interpreted with caution. A negative result indicates no necessity for a laparotomy, but a positive peritoneal lavage does not necessarily mean that there is peritoneal organ damage

The use of focused assessment with sonography for trauma (FAST) ultrasonography (pericardial, perihepatic, perisplenic, pelvic) in the emergency department by an experienced person is a more sensitive and specific test for free fluid in the peritoneum. This can be further refined with the use of computed tomography provided the patient is stable.

Emergency laparotomy without good reason can do more harm than good as the abdominal wall contributes significantly to the tamponade of bleeding within the pelvis. Continuous monitoring of the haemoglobin concentration is essential as blood loss may be immense.

Dislocations of joints

Urgent reduction of a dislocated joint is essential to correct or prevent neurovascular compromise and to prevent late complications. Open dislocations should be treated with the same protocol as open fractures. The most common joint that presents with dislocation is the shoulder joint which usually results from low-energy injury. Reduction is usually straightforward using well-recognised methods.

Due to the inherent stability of the hip joint, a dislocation must be a result of high-energy trauma. Reduction should be performed as soon as possible in the operating theatre to minimise injury to the sciatic nerve, avascular necrosis of the femoral head and subsequent hip joint arthritis. There is commonly an associated acetabular fracture that may require later surgery.

Dislocation of the knee may be difficult to detect on plain radiographs as the position seen in the emergency department often does not reflect the position at the time of injury. A high index of suspicion is needed in patients presenting with high-energy injuries to the knee. Emergency reduction with an assessment of the vascular status of the limb is essential. Postreduction angiography must be performed to rule out an injury to the vascular tree. These injuries are also commonly associated with complex ligament disruptions requiring reconstruction and prolonged rehabilitation.

Radiology

Only when the multiply injured patient is resuscitated and the primary survey completed should radiographs of the limbs and additional pelvic and acetabular studies be considered. The standard two projections at right angles to one another are appropriate and must include the whole bone suspected of being fractured and the adjacent joints. Radiographs must be scrutinised for joint dislocations and subluxations that may be associated with fractures.

Two further pelvic views are indicated in pelvic fractures (the inlet and outlet views) (Figure 11.3) and in acetabular fractures and hip dislocations (the Judet views: 45° obliques) (Figure 11.4). In suspected shoulder pathology, an axial view should be performed in addition to the standard anteroposterior view. Oblique views should also be requested for fractures of the proximal tibia.

If computed tomography (CT) is used to study head, neck, spine, chest and/or abdomen, and a pelvic or acetabular fracture is present, 5 mm cuts through the pelvis should be requested. Five mm image CT cuts are also useful in planning the management of tibial plateau and pilon fractures, and specialised cuts are required for os calcis fractures. With the advent of spiral CT, the time for scanning patients has reduced significantly and therefore this modality will be used more frequently for early imaging of the multiply injured patient. Magnetic resonance imaging (MRI) is primarily used for imaging the central and peripheral nervous system, and soft tissue structures.

In the awake patient, the whole spine can be cleared clinically with a lateral radiograph of the cervical spine alone. In the unconscious patient, rapid spinal clearance can prevent complications such as pressure sores and help nursing staff with day-to-day care. The bony components of the spine can be assessed with radiographs (AP, lateral and peg views) and a CT scan. However, the

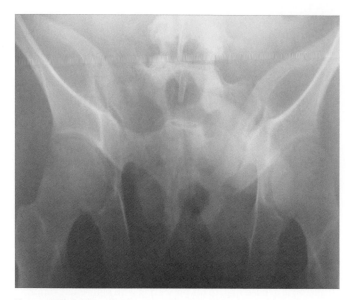

Figure 11.3 Pelvic outlet view.

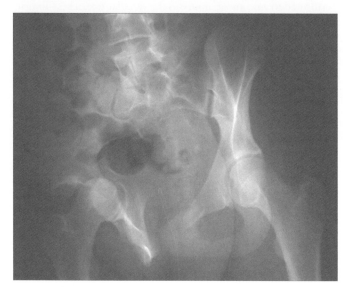

Figure 11.4 Pelvic judet view.

important ligaments that contribute to cervical stability are poorly assessed. Dynamic X-ray screening of the neck by trauma surgeons is performed in some units to look for evidence of ligamentous instability; the use of spiral CT is also gaining popularity. The thoracic and lumbar spines can be cleared with two-view radiographs and CT reconstructions.

Splintage

Correct use of splintage will afford considerable pain relief, avert further soft tissue damage and facilitate transport. To be effective, the splint must immobilise the joint above and below the fracture and include the bone on either side of a dislocation.

The arm is best supported by a simple sling and bandaged to the body. The forearm and wrist are immobilised on padded splints

or pillows. The hand should be splinted in a functional position: that is, over a bandage roll with the fingers straight. Femoral shaft fractures may be adequately controlled only by using fixed traction splints such as the Thomas splint or the modern equivalent. A traction force is applied to the leg or foot and is countered with a proximal pelvic bar.

Low-pressure (30 mmHg) inflatable double-walled polyvinyl jacket splints are commonly used to immobilise tibial, ankle and forearm fractures; they are easy to use and are effective.

Compartment syndromes

Multiply injured patients with reduced tissue perfusion and oxygenation are at high risk of developing compartment syndromes. Increasing swelling in the unyielding fascial compartments, particularly in the forearm and lower leg, as a result of tissue contusion, bleeding or ischaemia may result in autoinfarction of the compartment muscle.

Compartment syndrome is a clinical diagnosis and the first sign is increasing pain, out of proportion to that expected, which is unrelieved by strong analgesia. As the compartment syndrome evolves further, sensory deficit in the distribution of the peripheral nerves passing through that compartment, progressive swelling and tension, and pain on passive muscle stretching of the affected muscle compartment develop. The presence of peripheral pulses does not exclude an evolving compartment syndrome and is a late sign.

If signs of a compartment syndrome develop, all potentially constricting dressings, casts and splints should be released. If rapid recovery is not observed then prompt fasciotomy should be performed (Figure 11.5). A high index of suspicion must be maintained in the unconscious patient and continuous instrumented compartment pressure monitoring may be indicated. A compartment perfusion pressure of more than 30 mmHg is considered suspicious. Standard instrumentation for the measurement of compartment pressure should be available in all hospitals.

It is a fallacy that compartment syndromes do not develop in open fractures: an incidence of 15% has been reported. Even though the fascia will be disrupted at the fracture site, it may still be intact elsewhere. If the duration of a compartment syndrome has exceeded 72 h, fasciotomies should not be performed as this will expose dead

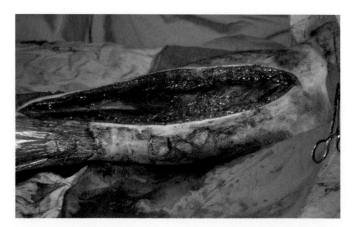

Figure 11.5 Fasciotomy.

muscle and increase the risk of infection. It is imperative that the orthopaedic surgeon is asked before any local anaesthetic blocks are used in severe limb injuries. This is because these may mask evolving compartment syndromes or ischaemic pain or both.

Traumatic amputations

Amputation is a catastrophic and life-threatening injury. Haemorrhage must be controlled as a priority. Reimplantation is possible in certain instances. In these cases the amputated part should be cleaned and wrapped in a sterile cloth that has been soaked in saline. It needs to be sealed in a sterile plastic bag, which is then immersed in a container of crushed ice and water. The part must not be placed directly on ice or allowed to freeze. Rapid transfer to a definitive care centre is essential. Amputated parts that are unsuitable for replantation may be a source of bone, skin, vessel and nerve grafts and should not be discarded.

Primary amputations

In cases of severe soft tissue damage with bone loss, primary amputation is more appropriate than an attempt to save a limb with a resultant prolonged and complicated recovery period. It is recommended that two consultant surgeons are involved when considering primary amputation. Such patients require multidisciplinary care post amputation with early referral to a limb-fitting unit.

Communication

Early communication with the appropriate specialties is essential. All open fractures will require early orthopaedic evaluation and management and most will also require the services of plastic surgery. Pelvic and acetabular fractures require prompt referral of the patient to a specialist unit with studies suggesting that best functional results are obtained when reduction and fixation are perfomed less than 11 days post injury. The appropriate inlet/outlet and/or Judet views plus CT scans should be rapidly sent for advice.

Definitive management of fractures

Closed fractures

In the multiply injured patient the conservative management of major fractures of long bones is rarely an option. The incidence, morbidity and mortality associated with adult respiratory distress syndrome, fat embolism and systemic inflammatory response syndrome may be significantly reduced if major long bone fractures are stabilised by internal or external fixation early. This is known as damage control surgery. Fixation also makes nursing of the patient easier and reduces the need for narcotic analgesia.

Open fractures

See Figure 11.6 for the management of an open fracture.

Soft tissue damage and the risk of infection are the two critical factors determining outcome in patients with serious open limb fractures. The patient's management within the first few hours can determine whether the outcome is complete recovery or lifelong disability. The infecting organisms may be the contaminating ones,

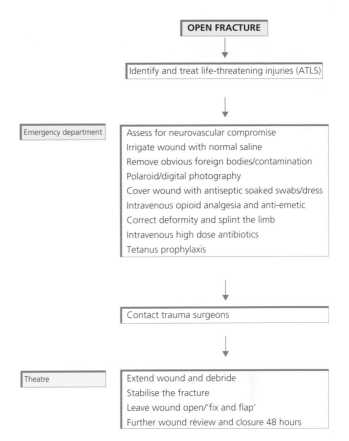

Figure 11.6 The management of an open fracture.

and samples for culture should therefore be obtained at the outset. The priorities are to clear contamination and devitalised tissue. In so doing, the amount of potential culture medium is reduced, as is the size of an infecting inoculum.

In a multiply injured patient with reduced oxygen delivery and an anticipated rise in tissue pressure, wound hypoxia and an increased susceptibility to infection are inevitable. Closure of a wound is therefore rarely indicated.

Wound debridement is often inadequately performed. The orthopaedic surgeon together with the plastic surgeon who may subsequently be required to provide tissue cover should perform debridement. Surrounding skin is shaved and the wound and surrounding area scrubbed. The wound is extended, in the long axis of the limb, as required to facilitate examination and fasciotomies performed if required. All non-viable muscle, fascia and fat are carefully but radically excised. The '4 Cs' – colour, contractility, capacity to bleed and consistency – can assess muscle viability.

Large volumes of irrigation fluid should be used, in excess of 4 L. The most commonly used irrigant is physiological saline, although Hartmann's solution and mild antiseptics can be used. There is no evidence for the use of antibiotics in the lavage fluid. It is the rate and volume of irrigant flow that are important rather than the pressure; indeed, high-flow pressure may drive contaminated tissue or foreign bodies deeper.

Skin flaps of dubious viability are best dealt with by taking a split skin graft from the flap surface. This will serve to delineate the margin of viability (the dead area will show no capillary bleeding). The harvested graft can be applied later if necrosis of the flap occurs. All loose fragments of bone should be removed.

Most open fractures are unstable. Stabilisation will promote tissue healing. This should be done using the most appropriate method for the fracture, the soft tissues, the unit in which the procedure is undertaken, and in appropriate cases following consultation with plastic surgeon. The debrided wound should initially be left open and covered with a dry dressing. Wet dressings should be avoided, except over large areas of exposed tendon or bone or both where there is no viable soft tissue that can be used to cover. The wound is ideally inspected again at 48 h. Early closure of the soft tissue wound, when it is suitable for closure, reduces the chance of infection and non-union of the fracture.

However, combined trauma and plastic surgical teams are commonly using the 'fix and flap' approach for grade IIIB fractures on day 1. Grade IIIC fractures with a vascular insult requiring repair require combined trauma/plastic and vascular teams. The trauma surgeons should stabilise the bones first, often with temporary external fixation, to provide a stable platform on which repair to the arteries, veins and nerves can proceed.

Summary

The assessment and management of limb trauma should always be secondary to resuscitation and management of life-threatening conditions.

A knowledge of the mechanism of injury and careful examination are essential if all injuries sustained by the patient are to be identified.

Assessment of the peripheral circulation is crucial to allow early detection and management of potentially limb-threatening injuries. Appropriate reduction of fractures and dislocations combined with correct splintage will reduce pain and can prevent serious complications.

A high level of suspicion is necessary in the multiply injured patient to identify nerve injuries and detect evolving compartment syndromes. Frequent reassessment and recordings of the circulation and neurological function of an injured limb are essential. The seriousness of open fractures should be appreciated and an aggressive approach to wound debridement adopted. As early as possible, there should be consultation between orthopaedic trauma surgeons and other teams, especially the plastic surgeons for open fractures, general surgeons for open pelvic fractures and vascular surgeons for suspected vascular injuries. Operative stabilisation of major long bone fractures in the first 24 h significantly reduces morbidity and mortality.

Further reading

Brinker MR. (2000) *Review of Orthopaedic Trauma*. Philadelphia: W.B. Saunders.

Bulstrode C, Buckwalter J, Carr A, *et al.* (2003) *Oxford Textbook of Orthopaedics and Trauma*. Oxford: Oxford University Press.

Duckworth T. (1995) *Lecture Notes on Orthopaedics and Fractures*. Oxford: Blackwell.

McRae R, Esser M. (2002) *Practical Fracture Treatment*, 4th edn. Edinburgh: Churchill Livingstone.

McRae R, Kinninmonth AWG. (1996) *Orthopaedics and Trauma: An Illustrated Colour Text*. Edinburgh: Churchill Livingstone.

CHAPTER 12

Eye Injuries

John Elston[1] and Andrew Gibson[2]

[1]Oxford Eye Hospital, Oxford University Hospitals NHS Trust, Oxford, UK
[2]The James Cook University Hospital, Middlesbrough, UK

OVERVIEW

- Ocular and periocular injuries can be a component of a wide range of trauma presentations and necessitate a high index of suspicion.
- Use the ocular ABCDEF protocol to identify eye injuries and prioritise referral.
- Acute visual loss due to orbital compartment syndrome may need urgent intervention in the emergency department.
- Ocular perforation may be occult; all eyelid lacerations should be evaluated and repaired by an ophthalmologist – have a low threshold for referral.
- Children with suspected eye injuries often need examination under anaesthetic.

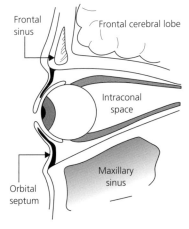

Figure 12.1 Sagittal view of the orbit and adjacent structures.

Injuries to the globe and periocular region can occur following major trauma. It is important that these injuries are identified during the secondary survey to ensure appropriate management.

Ocular injuries can occur as a result of accidents at home or work, and in sports-related injuries such as badminton and squash. Serious ocular injuries are seen following assaults and road traffic accidents. In addition, significant ocular injury can occur in connection with blast-related injuries seen in wartime and other bombings.

The mechanism of injury should alert the clinician to the possibility of ocular trauma and lead to appropriate examination. Children can present particular difficulties in assessment due to poor co-operation and may require referral to consider examination under anaesthetic.

The aim of this chapter is to outline an approach to the recognition of ocular trauma for non-ophthalmologists and then to consider some aspects of its management by ophthalmologists. During the course of the chapter, relevant anatomy will be explained and a practical method of assessing ocular injuries will be outlined followed by discussion of specific ocular injuries.

Applied anatomy

It is useful to consider the eye as a sphere situated anteriorly within the orbit. It is protected anteriorly by the bony orbital rim and the

skin of the eyelids. Superiorly, the bony walls separate the orbit from the frontal sinus and frontal lobe. Medially lie the ethmoid sinuses and inferiorly lies the maxillary sinus. The medial and inferior walls of the orbit are composed of thin bone and are the most common site of orbital blow-out fractures. Anterolaterally lies the temporal fossa, posterolaterally is the middle cranial fossa. The eyelids contain the lacrimal drainage system medially and the lacrimal gland superolaterally. The eyelid is a three-layered structure with the central cartilaginous tarsal plate giving the eyelid its strength (Figure 12.1).

The contents of the eyeball are protected by a tough collagen coat called the sclera, continuous anteriorly with the clear cornea. Overlying the sclera is the conjunctiva which is continuous with the conjuctiva of the posterior surface of the eyelids. Important structures inside the eye are the lens, the pigmented iris, the vitreous cavity and the retina.

Attached to the globe are the four rectus muscles and two oblique muscles. Leaving from the posterior aspect is the optic nerve which passes through the optic canal to the optic chiasm. The superior and inferior orbital veins lie deep within the orbit (Figure 12.2).

Assessment of ophthalmic trauma

Ophthalmic trauma can be blunt, penetrating or chemical and may involve the lids, the globe, the orbital walls and adjacent structures such as brain or sinuses. The mechanism should be ascertained from the history. Chemical injuries require urgent irrigation before

ABC of Major Trauma, Fourth Edition. Edited by David V. Skinner and Peter A. Driscoll.
© 2013 Blackwell Publishing Ltd. Published 2013 by Blackwell Publishing Ltd.

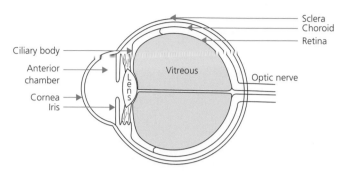

Figure 12.2 Anatomy of the eye (conjunctiva not shown).

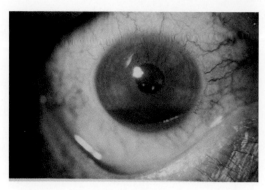

Figure 12.3 Small to moderate hyphaema.

further examination. Other important considerations in the history are the patient's past ophthalmic history, including previous surgery, and medication use. Legal considerations are particularly important if the injury is as a consequence of work or interpersonal violence. Suspect ocular injury in high-speed road traffic accidents (RTAs), injuries where glass is involved and in blast-related injuries.

Ophthalmic trauma often occurs in combination with other trauma so it is important to assess patients initially according to the standard Advanced Trauma Life Support (ATLS) guidelines. Airway, breathing and circulatory problems should be excluded before proceeding to the secondary survey when the ocular status should be assessed.

Many frontline A&E staff will have little formal ophthalmic training and so it is useful to have a robust method of assessing these patients. Initially, an inspection of the periocular region should be undertaken, looking for obvious globe rupture, globe displacement, bruising or lid laceration. Following this, a systematic assessment of ocular function should be undertaken. A useful mnemonic to remember, which is in keeping with the spirit of ATLS, is the ABCDEF of ophthalmology. Completion of this assessment will objectively assess ocular function and determine whether an ophthalmic referral is needed.

A – Acuity

The most crucial and the most likely to be omitted. If the patient is conscious and co-operative, a baseline distance visual acuity should be recorded in each eye. If no formal visual acuity chart is available then use either newsprint or some other estimate of acuity. A useful technique is to use the patient's hospital label – if this can be read at arm's length then acuity is at least 6/9 (Box 12.1).

Box 12.1 **Visual acuity measurements**	
6/6	Excellent vision – small newsprint at arm's length
6/9	Hospital label at arm's length
6/18	
6/24	
6/36	Headlines at arm's length
6/60	
CFs	Able to count fingers at arms length
HM	Hand movements
PL	Perception of light

B – Bright light examination

Use a bright light (a Mini-Maglite is ideal) to look for pupil reactions. A normal pupil responds directly when a bright light is directed into it and also consensually when the light is shone into the contralateral eye. If the direct response is less than the consensual then it suggests that a relative afferent papillary defect is present. Significant ocular trauma can lead to orbital compartment syndrome (discussed in more detail in the article by Courtney and Colucciello – see Further reading list), causing a relative afferent papillary defect requiring urgent treatment. Third nerve palsy, traumatic pupil dilation (mydriasis) and distortion of the iris are all signs of potentially serious ocular trauma and so it is necessary to assess pupil function. It is also an objective test which can be carried out in an unconscious patient, assuming opiates are not the cause of coma.

C – Cornea and conjunctiva

Use the same bright light as in B. Look for the normal corneal reflex and the visibility of intraocular contents. In significant trauma there may be iris damage causing pupil distortion. If the iris/pupil is not seen then there may be significant blood in the anterior chamber (hyphaema) (Figure 12.3). A significant subconjunctival haemorrhage raises the possibility of penetrating injury. It is useful to stain the cornea with fluorescein as this accentuates any corneal trauma.

D – Disc examination

Use a direct ophthalmoscope to examine the optic disc and macular region. Inability to see the disc suggests significant anterior or posterior segment injury, such as vitreous haemorrhage.

E – Eye movements

Eye movements test the function of the cranial nerves and the muscles. Trauma can cause mechanical limitation of eye movements such as seen in a blow-out fracture and also cause neurogenic limitation if the cranial nerves are damaged. If there is uniocular impairment of eye movement, for example due to blow-out fracture and inferior rectus entrapment, patients will complain of double vision.

F – Fields

Confrontation visual field assessment is a quick and objective test of visual function.

Whilst this ABCDEF approach may seem a little simplistic, it is a valuable tool to assist those unfamiliar with ophthalmic assessment to avoid missing a significant eye injury. It is safe to say that a patient with normal visual acuity, no relative afferent pupillary defect (RAPD), normal corneal reflex, normal disc examination with full eye movements and full visual fields is unlikely to have a significant ophthalmic injury.

Practical approach to ophthalmic trauma

The aim of the ABCDEF approach is to identify the likelihood of significant ophthalmic injury. If ophthalmic trauma is present then a simple working approach is to consider whether the ocular injury is:

- causing visual loss that is reversible with prompt treatment
- globe injury
- associated with orbital or adnexal injury
- caused by chemical injuries.

If there is concern about ocular injury, a thorough assessment by an ophthalmologist should be requested. The ophthalmologist may use additional equipment to facilitate examination such as a slit lamp and indirect ophthalmscope. Furthermore, the ophthalmologist may request additional investigations such as ultrasound or computed tomography (CT). CT is the usual first-line examination in the trauma setting as it is widely available and with the appropriate cuts can demonstrate the globe and orbit and allow anatomical location and diagnosis of most trauma or its consequence. Plain X-ray and magnetic resonance imaging examination have limited utility in most trauma settings.

Reversible visual loss

The most likely cause of acute reversible visual loss is an orbital compartment syndrome. This can occur acutely following trauma due to haemorrhage or be delayed as a consequence of secondary infection or orbital emphysema. The orbit is a contained structure so expanding mass lesions such as haemorrhage or infection inside the orbit lead to raised orbital pressure and compression of the optic nerve. If the pressure on the optic nerve is not reduced then permanent visual loss may occur. Patients with orbital compartment syndrome will have a painful eye, decreased vision and a relative afferent papillary defect. These patients require urgent treatment to reduce orbital pressure through lateral canthotomy or drainage of abscess.

To perform a lateral canthotomy, infiltrate local anaesthetic into lateral canthus and lower lateral lid. Using straight sharp scissors, cut from lateral canthus to orbital rim. Grab the lower lid and pull toward ipsilateral ear. With blades of the scissors open, slide the blades toward the nose with one blade lying in the fornix and the other underneath the skin. Advance and cut simultaneously. This movement will divide the lateral canthal tendon and release the orbital pressure (Figures 12.4–12.6).

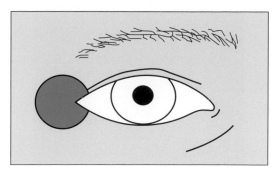

Figure 12.4 Shaded area in lateral canthus raised by bleb of local anaesthetic.

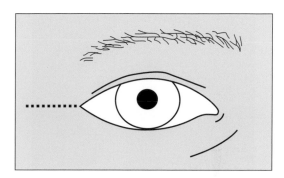

Figure 12.5 Incision line in lateral canthus.

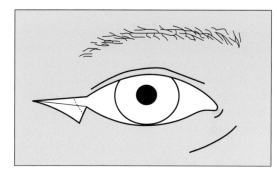

Figure 12.6 Lower cut edge of wound turned out.

The optic nerve can also be injured via penetrating injury or indirect contusion. Traumatic optic neuropathy describes the situation of decreased vision with relative afferent pupil defect without signs of significant anterior or posterior segment damage or orbital compartment syndrome. Although both high-dose intravenous steroids and optic canal decompression have been proposed to treat the condition, robust evidence to support these treatments is lacking.

Globe injury

Significant globe injury will be associated with decreased vision, usually a RAPD, loss of normal corneal reflex, inability to see the disc and abnormal field exam. The integrity of the globe may be obviously disrupted but a penetrating injury from a fine sharp fragment may leave only subtle signs such as shallow anterior chamber, distorted iris, focal cataract or wound leak (Figures 12.7

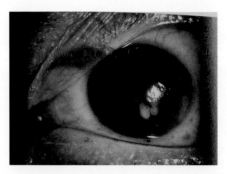

Figure 12.7 Full hyphaema with disruption of normal anterior chamber anatomy.

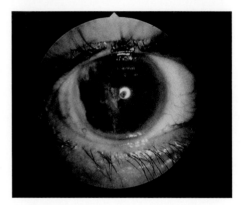

Figure 12.8 Iridodialysis in lateral half of iris.

and 12.8). In children if there is any suspicion of a penetrating eye injury then an examination under anaesthetic may be required.

Patients with globe injury require management by an ophthalmologist. A protective cartella shield should be placed over the injured eye to prevent any further pressure on the eye whilst an ophthalmology assessment is sought.

The principle of management is firstly to perform a primary repair to reinstate the integrity of the globe. Surgery to repair corneoscleral trauma requires special microsurgical equipment, particularly an operating microscope, and so may require transfer to appropriate facilities. Once the eye has settled following the trauma, further ophthalmic surgery may be required to reconstruct the anterior segment or to deal with the retinal sequelae of injury. In addition, patients with significant ocular trauma are at risk of developing a retinal detachment later on and should be informed of this risk.

Orbital and adnexal injury

Blunt trauma to the periocular region may result in injury to the bony orbit. The most common injury is the blow-out fracture which usually involves the medial wall or floor. Enophthalmos and diplopia with altered cheek sensation suggest a blow-out fracture of the orbital floor and damage to the maxillary nerve which runs in the floor. A CT scan will confirm the diagnosis. Usually it is better to delay surgery for 7–10 days to allow post-trauma swelling to settle. However, paediatric patients with a blow-out fracture with

inferior rectus entrapment can experience a significant oculocardiac reflex which leads to a profound bradycardia and mandates urgent surgery. The indications for surgical repair of blow-out fractures are not clearly defined but if there is significant enophthalmos, diplopia in primary position or significant loss of orbital floor area (over 50%), surgery should be recommended.

Penetrating orbital injuries can result in retained intraorbital foreign bodies and should be suspected from the mechanism of injury. As a general rule, posterior located inorganic foreign bodies can be left *in situ*, while organic material such as wood usually leads to orbital cellulitis and should be removed. If the foreign body is lying anteriorly and causing visual symptoms then it should be removed. See Figures 12.9 and 12.10

Lacerations to the lid margin are usually obvious as the action of orbicularis oculi tends to pull the lid apart. The presence of a lid laceration increases the chance of a globe rupture and requires formal ophthalmic assessment to exclude a more significant injury. If there are signs of medial lid trauma it is important to consider

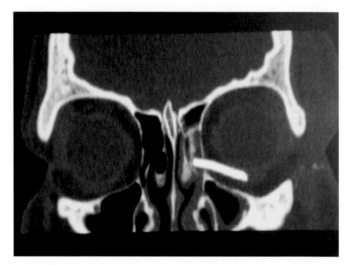

Figure 12.9 Foreign body on CT.

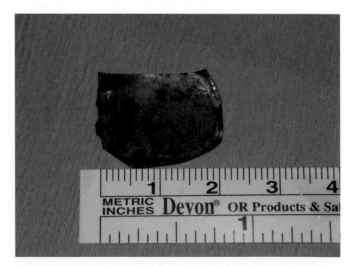

Figure 12.10 Foreign body on removal.

damage to the lacrimal drainage apparatus. Medial to the puncta lies the canaliculus which drains tears from the lid to the lacrimal sac and then into the nose. If canalicular trauma is not repaired correctly then patients will be left with symptomatic watering. Dog bites to the face and nose are often associated with medial lacerations involving the canaliculus.

Injury to the levator muscle which lifts the eyelid can occur following trauma. Although in many cases function recovers, in some cases formal ptosis surgery is needed. See Figures 12.11–12.13.

Patients with lid lacerations should be referred to the ophthalmologist for reconstruction.

Chemical trauma

Chemical trauma to the eye can cause significant ocular morbidity. Both acid and alkali may be responsible for significant ocular injury. Alkalis, however, penetrate ocular tissues rapidly, leading to internal and external eye damage and require management by an ophthalmologist once the initial vigorous irrigation has taken place. Significant chemical injuries will result in a significant drop

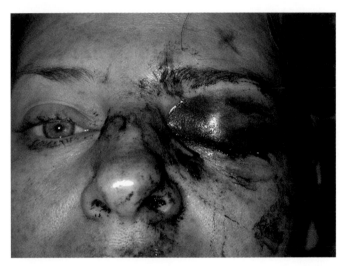

Figure 12.11 Bomb blast injury to left eye.

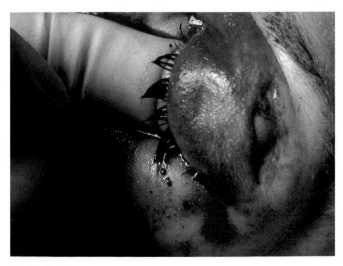

Figure 12.12 Upper lid laceration

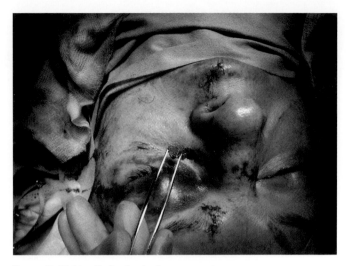

Figure 12.13 Metallic foreign body on removal.

in vision and loss of corneal clarity. The mainstay of acute treatment is irrigation to remove the irritant and neutralise the pH. Topical and systemic ascorbate can be used to promote recovery and a short course of topical steroids is sometimes used along with topical antibiotics.

Summary

It is important to consider ocular injury following major trauma. By carrying out the appropriate assessment during the secondary survey, the possibility of ocular injury should be identified. The ABCDEF is a useful mnemonic to help non-ophthalmologists to perform a thorough assessment of ocular function and identify the likelihood of injury. If there is visual loss associated with the injury, consider whether it is due to orbital compartment syndrome and consider appropriate urgent action.

Further reading

Courtney DM, Colucciello SA. (2002) Eye trauma. In: Cameron P (ed) *Pediatric Emergency Medicine*, 2nd edn. Dallas, TX: American College of Emergency Physicians, pp. 126–32. A straightforward practical guide to the assessment and management of this important subgroup. Available online emj.bmj.com.

Guly CM, Guly HR, Bouamra O, Gray RH, Lecky FE. (2006) Ocular injuries in patients with major trauma. Emerg Med J 23: 915–17. A large retrospective analysis of the Trauma Audit Research Network (TARN) database over 15 years. Serious eye injuries were rare: major risk factors were RTA, male gender and presence of facial fractures.

Mazzoli RA, Ainbinder DJ, Hansen EA. (2003) Orbital trauma. In: Thach AB (ed) *Ophthalmic Care of the Combat Casualty*. Washington, DC: Storming Media, pp. 335–83. This very detailed and well-illustrated chapter is also available online www.bordeninstitute.army.mil/published/ophthalmic.

Poon A, McLuskey PJ, Hill DA. (1999) Eye injuries in patients with major trauma. J Trauma 46: 494–9. Emphasises the association of RTA, skull base/facial fracture and potentially vision-threatening eye injuries.

Rodriguez JO, Lavina AM, Agarwal A. (2003) Prevention and treatment of common eye injuries in sports. Am Fam Physician 67: 1481–8. Available online with excellent photos illustrating eye injuries and practical tips on investigation and management www.aafp.org.

CHAPTER 13

Medical Problems in Trauma Patients

Tom Hughes

John Radcliffe Hospital, Oxford, UK

OVERVIEW

Medical problems:

- are a cause of preventable mortality and morbidity in trauma
- may cause trauma
- may be caused by trauma
- need early identification and a team approach.

Why are medical problems important?

Deaths from trauma have been declining in most developed countries over the last 10 years. Despite the large cost of trauma to the community, estimated to be £750,000 per life in 1993, collection of high-quality data about trauma is limited.

Research in California in the 1970s suggested that trauma-related deaths characteristically occurred in one of three distinct periods (Figure 13.1).

- Immediate – within the first hour (50%)
- Early – within the first 1–4 hours (30%)
- Late – after the first 4 hours (20%)

Causes of the first peak include unsurvivable injury and untreated major causes of airway and breathing problems, such as tension pneumothorax. These deaths usually occur out of hospital. Injury prevention and safety measures such as better road and car design, seatbelts and airbags have reduced the first peak, as well as much improved prehospital care.

Deaths in the second peak may be caused by uncontrolled haemorrhage or multiorgan/multisystem damage that overwhelms the body's compensatory mechanisms. These deaths are likely to occur in the resuscitation room or operating theatre. Better trauma management systems, education and standards of care such as the Advanced Trauma Life Support course are credited with reducing the second peak.

Medical causes are commonly implicated in the third peak: adult respiratory distress syndrome (ARDS), multiorgan dysfunction

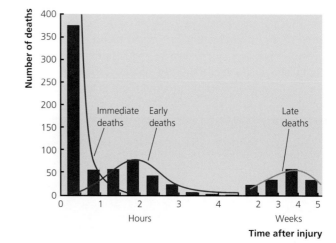

Figure 13.1 Trimodal death distribution.

syndrome (MODS), coagulopathy and thromboembolism, cerebral injury, sepsis and co-morbid conditions. Increasingly sophisticated emergency department (ED) and intensive care unit (ICU) care and better understanding of the pathophysiology of trauma have reduced the third peak, yet some of these deaths may still be preventable.

In countries with low rates of penetrating trauma such as the UK, the 'three peaks' model is a 'two peaks' model, with deaths in the middle third being minimal, giving an 80%/20% distribution.

Therefore once a patient has survived to hospital, medical problems are an important cause of morbidity and mortality in trauma patients.

Avoidable mortality and morbidity

A multidisciplinary review of Australian trauma patients defined specific problem areas that were found to contribute to poor outcomes in trauma patients (Table 13.1, Figure 13.2).

Medical problems as they affect trauma are considered below in the following categories:

- medical problems *causing* trauma
- medical problems *caused* by trauma
- medical problems *complicating* trauma.

ABC of Major Trauma, Fourth Edition. Edited by David V. Skinner and Peter A. Driscoll.

Table 13.1 Common system errors in trauma management.

Prehospital	Emergency department	ICU/HDU/ward
No paramedic	Inappropriately junior staff	Inadequate fluids
Too long at scene	Delayed consultant attendance	Inadequate blood transfusion
No 'scoop and run'	Delayed consultant surgeon	Inadequate coagulation factors
Inadequate documentation	Delayed neurosurgical consultation	No CVP monitoring
Delayed airway management	Inadequate documentation	Inadequate respiratory support
Inadequate respiratory support	Delayed respiratory support	Inadequate chest injury management
Inadequate IV access/fluids	Inadequate IV fluid/blood	Inadequate analgesia
Failed intubation/IV access	Inadequate bleeding control	No surgical/neurosurgical consultation
Delayed chest compressions	Delayed CT scan	Delayed repeat CT
	Delayed investigations	Inadequate brain perfusion
	Inadequate monitoring	No DVT prophylaxis

CT, computed tomography; CVP, central venous pressure; DVT, deep vein thrombosis; HDU, high-dependency unit; ICU, intensive care unit; IV, intravenous.

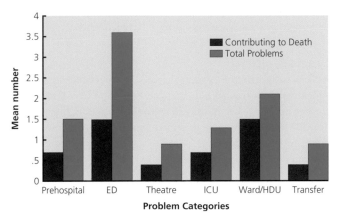

Figure 13.2 Problems in trauma by area.

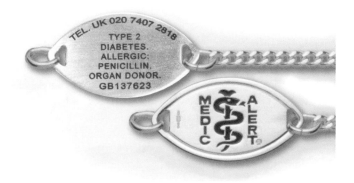

Figure 13.3 Medic-Alert bracelet. (Reproduced with permission from medic-alert.org.uk)

Medical problems that cause trauma

Trauma history: AMPLE mnemonic

The key points of the medical history relevant to trauma can be remembered easily using the mnemonic AMPLE, and should be taken from the patient as soon as is practicable (Box 13.1).

Box 13.1 **AMPLE**

A – Allergies
M – Medications
P – Previous medical history
L – Last ate/drank
E – Event/environment

- *Allergies*: it is important to differentiate true allergy (e.g. blotchy, itchy rash or anaphylactoid reaction) from a mild or predictable adverse effect, e.g. nausea.
- *Medication*: a list of medicines is a valuable guide to previous medical history, particularly in a patient who is unable to give a history. A Medic-Alert bracelet or locket is an important clue in this situation (Figure 13.3).
- *Previous medical history*: awareness of medical/surgical/anaesthetic problems can minimise the risk of complications.

- *Last ate/drank*: a full stomach increases the risk of aspiration during anaesthetic procedures.
- *Event/environment*: this includes the events that lead up to trauma, and any exposure to heat/cold or hazardous materials.

Collapse

The most useful tool in trying to ascertain a cause for collapse is a careful history, taken as soon as possible after the event, corroborated where possible by witnesses.

Key questions to ask

Is the patient known to have diabetes/ epilepsy/ heart failure?

- Epileptic seizures or hypoglycaemia may cause unconsciousness.
- Heart failure predisposes to ventricular arrhythmias.

What was the patient doing at the time?

- Posture/ occurred on standing/looking up/micturition.

Can the patient remember passing out/falling?

- A period of feeling dizzy and 'the room spinning' may indicate a vasovagal episode or abnormally slow heart rate.
- Patients with seizures or who have sudden ventricular arrhythmias will have minimal warning.

Did the patient lose consciousness? For how long?
When consciousness was regained, was it full consciousness?

- A witness account is very helpful.
- A seizure is usually followed by a period of confusion.

Was amnesia present?

- Retrograde amnesia – inability to remember events before injury.
- Anterograde amnesia – inability to remember events after injury.

Action

A full medical history and examination, including cardiovascular and neurological systems, are necessary in cases of syncope. A chest radiograph and an electrocardiogram (ECG) are indicated in most cases. Medical referral as appropriate.

Cardiovascular causes of collapse

The classic 'faint' which occurs when the heart is slowed by the parasympathetic outflow of the vagus nerve is a 'vasovagal' episode. Many factors may play a part in this, including strong emotion, vagal hypersensitivity and fatigue.

A true faint needs to be differentiated from other causes, such as orthostatic (or postural) hypotension, which is hypotension present only when the patient is vertical. When moving from lying to standing, a patient's blood pressure should increase. A common cause of orthostatic hypotension is intravascular volume depletion, often caused by diuretics or dehydration, but also reduced autonomic sensitivity, e.g. β-blockers or autonomic neuropathy.

Any history of heart failure or any ECG abnormality in combination with a history of collapse should be reviewed by an Emergency Physician.

Action

Lying and standing blood pressure should be measured.

If the history is consistent with that of a single vasovagal episode with full recovery, no further action may be necessary. Patients with repeated episodes of 'faints' should be referred for investigation.

Seizures

A witness is particularly valuable in establishing the diagnosis, but post 'seizure' confusion, lateral tongue biting and incontinence are strongly suggestive of epileptiform seizures.

Seizures occurring in patients not known to be epileptic or seizures in known epileptics that are outside the 'normal' pattern for the patient may need further investigation, particularly if there is objective evidence of neurological dysfunction.

Common factors precipitating seizures are lack of sleep and sub-therapeutic doses of antiepileptic drugs. Drug (e.g. benzodiazepine) and alcohol withdrawal also cause seizures, which may occur despite significant levels of alcohol/drug being present. What matters is the relative amount of the drug compared to the usual level.

A vasovagal collapse may be followed by a few seizure-like 'jerks' but then rapid recovery, whereas a true 'grand mal' seizure is followed by a period of post-ictal confusion.

Action

Seizures occurring in a patient known to have epilepsy, when occurring in their normal pattern or as a result of non-compliance,

rarely need further investigation if the patient recovers fully after the seizure.

Patients with a history consistent with a seizure who recover fully but who are not known to be epileptic should have a computed tomography (CT) scan of their brain. This scan should be performed on their first admission if they have objective neurological signs. Otherwise, the patient should be discharged with plans for CT and electroencephalogram (EEG) prior to outpatient review in 4–6 weeks.

Patients who have suffered a seizure should always be advised not to drive pending formal neurological review, and such advice must be recorded in the medical notes. The patient's understanding and intention to comply with the advice should also be recorded; if the patient shows intention of rejecting the advice, the doctor usually has a duty to notify the licensing authorities. Patients should also be advised against swimming alone, climbing ladders or activities that might be dangerous were they to have a further seizure.

Drugs and alcohol

Alcohol is known to be a common factor in street violence, domestic violence and fatal road crashes. Since 2005, blood samples after road crashes may be taken in the UK without consent if the patient is not able to give consent, e.g. is unconscious. Other countries have mandatory testing for alcohol and drugs after road crashes and/or random breath testing; these appear to be effective policies.

Medical problems caused by trauma

Acute respiratory distress syndrome

Acute respiratory distress syndrome (ARDS) is the presence of interstitial fluid in the lungs despite normal pulmonary arterial and venous pressures. It is common after significant blunt trauma affecting the thorax, but can occur as a result of major trauma elsewhere in the body. Usually presenting within 48 h of injury, leakage of fluid into the alveoli results in a stiff lung that does not exchange gas well, resulting in hypoxia.

Action

Treat in the intensive care unit. Patients usually need intubation and ventilation.

Massive transfusion

Patients with uncontrolled bleeding from major trauma may lose many times their blood volume (normally 5 L in an adult). Aside from the challenge of physically replacing the fluid, transfusing large amounts of cold fluid in an exposed patient risks hypothermia and coagulopathy.

Action

Bleeding should be controlled as soon as possible, as well as specific therapy for coagulopathy and hypothermia.

Coagulopathy

Coagulopathy may occur after major trauma, with or without massive transfusion, and is often under-recognised and therefore undertreated.

The clotting cascade is impaired in the cold, acidotic, hypoperfused patient, and therefore laboratory measures (at 37°C) of clotting factors may give false reassurance about the 'real-life' situation.

Action

The mainstay of treatment is surgical control of bleeding together with correction of acidosis, hypotension and hypothermia. Early haematological advice should be sought to guide the replacement of clotting factors.

Hypothermia

Prolonged exposure to cold conditions prior to hospital or transfusion of large volumes of cold fluid can cause hypothermia. Although hypothermia appears to have a neuroprotective effect, this must be balanced against the fact that the body's enzymes are significantly impaired below 34°C which will result in coagulopathy.

Action

Patient temperature should be kept above 34°C. Warm air blankets (e.g. Bair Hugger) and warm humidified oxygen are the most effective means of warming patients with mild to moderate hypothermia. Intravenous fluids should be warmed.

Multiple organ dysfunction syndrome

Multiple organ dysfunction syndrome (MODS), previously known as multiorgan failure, occurs when two or more of liver, heart, kidney and lungs are significantly impaired. The organ damage is probably mediated by a series of inflammatory mediators similar to those in severe sepsis. In the absence of sepsis, this is known as the systemic inflammatory response syndrome (SIRS) and mortality is 30% or above.

Action

Treatment is largely supportive, usually on the intensive care unit, and aims to optimise the body's pathophysiological response to trauma.

Fat embolism

Fat is a normal part of the bone marrow and is released into the venous circulation from fractures. The fat embolises to the pulmonary and then systemic circulations, and can also precipitate disseminated intravascular coagulation. Approximately 24–48 h after the injury, fat emboli provoke an inflammatory reaction; in the skin this is a widespread petechial rash, also seen on the conjunctiva and retina. A similar inflammatory reaction is seen in all internal organs: emboli to the lungs may result in ARDS, emboli to the brain cause oedema that may cause headache, confusion and seizures.

Action

Fat embolism may be prevented by early fixation of large fractures, particularly long bone fractures, which appear responsible for the most severe cases of fat embolism.

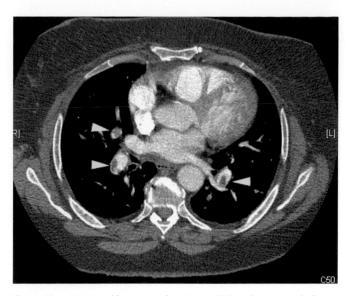

Figure 13.4 CT scan with contrast showing multiple pulmonary emboli (arrowed).

Thromboembolism: pulmonary embolism and deep venous thrombosis

Thromboembolism is relatively common and is difficult to diagnose, as symptoms are non-specific and there is no one test that is sensitive, specific and cheap. D-dimer is a fibrin degradation product and therefore likely to be raised by trauma alone. Changes in chest radiographs, electrocardiographs or arterial blood gases may suggest pulmonary embolus, but none can reliably exclude it.

The preferred investigations for thromboembolism are currently Doppler ultrasound scanning of leg veins for deep venous thrombosis (DVT) and high-resolution CT pulmonary angiography for pulmonary embolism (Figure 13.4).

Action

Optimum prophylaxis in blunt trauma patients is achieved by a combination of early mechanical prophylaxis using pulsatile foot pumps and low molecular weight heparin started once bleeding has been controlled, usually 12–24 h after admission.

Medical problems that may complicate trauma

Principles

While trauma is generally a condition of the young, older patients with significant pre-existing medical diseases need specific management in the context of trauma. Major trauma should be treated with a team-based approach, involving clinicians from medical and critical care teams as appropriate. Patients with a long-term medical condition such as renal failure are usually well known to their medical teams, who appreciate early contact regarding their management, as this enables complications to be predicted and avoided.

Diabetes

Diabetes is common and increasing in prevalence. Patients with diabetes with critical illness have improved outcomes when their blood glucose is well controlled. Patients with diabetes are more prone to infection, and osteomyelitis is a particular danger in lower limbs with co-existent vascular disease. Neuropathy in patients with long-standing diabetes can mask trauma, as gross disruption of joints may occur with no pain – the neuropathic (Charcot) joint. Neuropathy may also obscure other disease processes; autonomic neuropathy may blunt the body's normal response to hypovolaemia or ischaemia, e.g. the silent myocardial infarction, compartment syndrome.

Action

Patients with diabetes with major trauma should be managed with a sliding scale insulin regime until stable. Scrupulous debridement of wounds and a low threshold for antibiotic use are advisable. Patients with neuropathy are at high risk of pressure sores.

Heart failure

Heart failure is the inability of the body's pump to maintain an adequate supply of oxygen to the tissues. In physiological terms, the Frank–Starling curve is reduced at all levels, meaning that the heart is less tolerant of under- or overfilling and has reduced ability to increase output in the face of physiological stress (Figure 13.5).

In the context of trauma, both hypovolaemia and overtransfusion can reduce cardiac output. Patients with severe heart failure (ejection fraction of less than 30% or breathless on walking less than 50 meters) are particularly likely to have problems.

Action

Patients known to have heart failure should have careful monitoring of fluid balance. Patients with severe heart failure and significant trauma are likely to benefit from a central venous line and an early medical/critical care opinion.

Ischaemic heart disease

Ischaemic heart disease is rare in men below 40 years and women below 50 years of age.

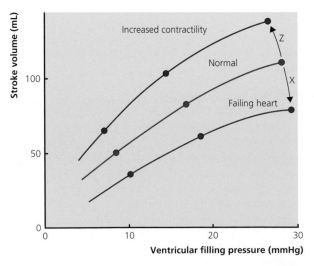

Figure 13.5 Frank–Starling curve.

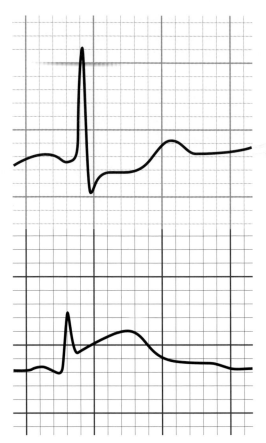

Figure 13.6 Comparing single QRS complex with ischaemic (ST down) and infarcted (ST up) complexes.

Cardiac ischaemia may occur in trauma, particularly in hypovolaemia as the increased heart rate increases myocardial oxygen demand (Figure 13.6).

Body Mass Index

People with high (>30) or low (<20) Body Mass Index are at increased risk of complications and mortality following major trauma. Obesity can result in immobility, hypoventilation and pressure sores. Very thin people are at risk from pressure sores and the catabolic state following trauma.

Action

Scrupulous care of pressure areas and nutritional care are particularly important in these patients. Good analgesia in patients with chest injuries prevents hypoventilation and chest infections.

HIV/AIDS

Treatment modification is rarely necessary unless the patient has very low immunological function. The regime of drugs for HIV is tightly specified and may be difficult to maintain in the acute phases of the injury; there is no evidence that this impairs long-term prognosis.

Renal failure

Patients with chronic renal failure may be at increased risk of fractures due to renal bone disease. The physiological stress of major trauma is tolerated less well by patients with renal failure, as the ability of the body to manage acid–base disturbance is impaired.

Acute renal failure may be precipitated by prolonged hypovolaemia and/or precipitation of myoglobin in the renal tubules, the myoglobin being released from damaged muscle.

Action

Very close monitoring of fluid balance and early consultation with a renal physician are advisable.

Drugs that impair renal function should be avoided, and modified doses used for those which are renally excreted.

Adrenal suppression

Patients on long-term oral steroids or powerful inhaled steroids, such as fluticasone, lose the ability to increase their endogenous steroid production appropriately in response to stress, resulting in hypoadrenalism. Hypoadrenalism may also occur as a result of trauma, systemic illness or drugs such as etomodate.

Hypoadrenalism affects a host of neuroendocrine functions, and will cause hypotension that will not correct with normal measures. Patients on long-term exogenous steroids are immunosuppressed and normal signs of infection may not occur.

Action

Hydrocortisone 50–100 mg four times daily while the patient is unwell. The dose should be weaned as the patient improves.

The risk of infection, which may not be clinically obvious, is high in these patients, so medical staff must be extremely vigilant.

Chronic lung disease

Trauma patients with chronic lung disease such as chronic obstructive pulmonary disease (COPD) are at high risk of lung infections. Patients with type II respiratory failure, who rely on a degree of hypoxia to drive their respiration, are particularly vulnerable.

Action

Close monitoring using oxygen saturation and blood gas measurement. Early consultation with intensive care is advisable if ventilation is compromised.

Adequate analgesia reduces hypoventilation and the risk of chest infections; this may include intercostal nerve blocks or thoracic epidural infusions.

Drug and alcohol withdrawal

Patients who are dependent on alcohol or drugs will undergo withdrawal while in hospital. These patients often use more than one group of alcohol, benzodiazepines, opiates and street drugs.

Severe benzodiazepine and alcohol withdrawal commonly cause agitation and tremors and may cause seizures.

Opiate withdrawal should be suspected in any agitated patient with visual hallucinations, particularly if these involve insects crawling on the skin.

Action

Large doses of benzodiazepines may be necessary to control withdrawal symptoms in alcohol- and benzodiazepine-dependent patients, e.g. diazepam 10–20 mg PO every hour until symptoms are controlled. The long half-life of diazepam and its metabolites results in a gradual withdrawal and prevention of seizures. An alternative is a tapering dose schedule of chlordiazepoxide.

Opiate withdrawal symptoms may benefit from non-steroidal anti-inflammatory drugs (NSAIDs) and clonidine in addition to benzodiazepines; seek specialist advice.

Chronic alcoholics tend to be deficient in thiamine, risking neurological and cardiac disease. This is easily preventable by administration of a multivitamin preparation (including vitamins B,C and thiamine) to all patients dependent on alcohol on admission. This should be repeated for such patients who are in hospital for a long period.

The future

Research into manipulating the body's response to trauma is in its infancy, and the prospect of a 'magic bullet' for trauma-related organ dysfunction remains as far off as ever. The current range of treatments for trauma is a relatively blunt tool, and recent research has caused clinicians to question many of the assumed benefits of trauma treatments, e.g. intravenous fluids.

The heterogeneous nature of trauma and poor data collection make it difficult and expensive to perform good-quality research in this area. Much research in the management of critically ill patients relates to severe sepsis, and the validity of extrapolating these data to trauma patients is questionable. Research from trauma populations with high rates of penetrating trauma such as in the USA is often not applicable to the UK and similar countries where most trauma is blunt.

Haemorrhage

Control of haemorrhage in blunt trauma is rarely as urgent as is the case in penetrating trauma. There are some data to suggest that activated factor VII is effective in controlling ongoing bleeding in trauma patients, and trials are in progress to evaluate this.

Early goal-directed therapy

'Goal-directed therapy' tailors therapy to maximise the body's oxygen extraction; this is commonly achieved by measuring the oxygen saturation of mixed venous blood and comparing with that of arterial blood. Other surrogate measures of efficient oxygen usage that have been used are the lactate level, cardiac output, pulse waveform analysis, oesophageal Doppler and gastric tonometry.

Use of goal-directed therapy in the emergency department has been shown to be beneficial in severe sepsis, but there is not yet good evidence to demonstrate benefit in trauma.

Molecular biology

Molecular biology offers the prospect of targeted manipulation of the inflammatory cascade that results in ARDS and MODS. To date, there has been little success; anti-tumour necrosis factor (TNF) proved ineffective. Activated protein C is licensed for use in severe sepsis, and research into a possible role in trauma patients is ongoing.

Further reading

Department of Human Services. (1999) *Review of Trauma and Emergency Services*. Victoria, Australia: Department of Human Services. www.health.vic.gov.au/trauma/review99/

Trauma: Who Cares? (2007) National Confidential Enquiry into Patient Outcome and Death. http://www.ncepod.org.uk/2007t.htm

CHAPTER 14

Radiological Assessment

James Rankine,[1] *David Nicholson,*[2] *Peter A. Driscoll*[2] *and Dominic Barron*[1]

[1]Leeds General Infirmary, Leeds, UK
[2]Hope Hospital, Salford, UK

OVERVIEW

- In many centres, the lateral cervical radiograph, chest and pelvic radiographs remain important first-line imaging investigations in the resuscitation room, though practices are changing with the advent of multislice computed tomography.

- Multislice computed tomography technological advances have revolutionised the imaging of the polytrauma patient, allowing imaging from the head to pubis in as little as 30 sec.

- The computed tomography scan is performed with intravenous contrast, allowing detection of vascular injury, and this has largely replaced diagnostic angiography.

- Oral contrast is no longer required for the detection of intestinal injury on computed tomography, reducing previous delays waiting for contrast to enter the small bowel.

- Multiplanar reformats are very useful for the detection of bony injury and have largely replaced the need for thoracic and lumbar spine radiographs.

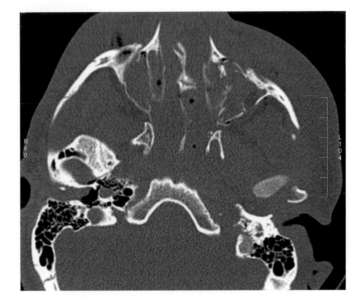

Figure 14.1 Axial CT showing Le Fort 3 injury.

Until recently, trauma imaging was limited to the use of plain radiographs in the resuscitation room with additional imaging restricted to head computed tomography (CT) and bedside ultrasound. The development and widespread availability of multislice CT scanners have, however, revolutionised imaging of the trauma patient with the ability to perform rapid whole-body scanning. It is now widely accepted that a polytrauma CT scan should cover the head, cervical spine, chest, abdomen and pelvis.

These scanners use multiple detectors to acquire information, vastly increasing the amount of data that can be acquired in a single scan. A scan covering the vertex to the pubis can be done in approximately 30 sec. These data are then further processed to provide diagnostic images of the bony pelvis, thoracic and lumbar spine. Approximately 1000 images for interpretation are generated in these cases.

Head

It is now well recognised that skull radiographs are of little value in head trauma as it is the intracranial injuries that matter. CT is the

imaging modality of choice for this. It clearly demonstrates bleeds, intracranial air and fluid levels as well as providing indirect evidence of raised intracranial pressure. If there is a significant associated facial fracture then a dedicated fine detail scan of the face may be helpful (Figure 14.1).

This importance of CT in head trauma is recognised in the National Institute of Health and Clinical Excellence (NICE) guidelines which advocate that all significant head injuries should have CT (see Further reading). Although this is good practice, the financial and logistical implications for radiology departments remain an ongoing problem yet to be resolved nationally.

Cervical spine

In the multiply injured patient, there is a high incidence of cervical fracture and the ready availability of CT is replacing the full series of cervical radiographs as a means of clearing the C-spine. A single lateral radiograph is taken initially to check for major injuries and then a detailed CT of the whole cervical spine is performed, covering down to at least the bottom of T1 and preferably the bottom of T4.

ABC of Major Trauma, Fourth Edition. Edited by David V. Skinner and Peter A. Driscoll.
© 2013 Blackwell Publishing Ltd. Published 2013 by Blackwell Publishing Ltd.

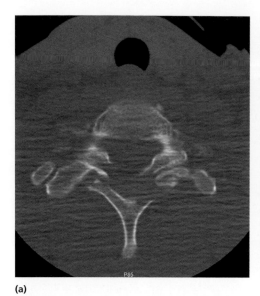

(a)

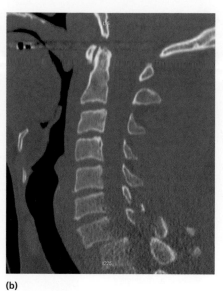

(b)

Figure 14.2 (a) Axial CT with disruption of the facets and posterior elements. (b) The sagittal reformat highlights the 50% translation of C7 relative to T1 consistent with a bifacet fracture dislocation.

Sagittal and coronal reformats are mandatory as axial fractures may be difficult to appreciate on the axial images alone (Figure 14.2).

There remains considerable debate as to whether the C-spine can be cleared after a normal CT. Most centres have the patient reassessed by a senior clinician after a normal CT and where there remains strong clinical concern, then further imaging by magnetic resonance imaging (MRI) is undertaken (Figure 14.3). MRI is now routinely used for the investigation of patients with abnormal neurological symptoms and signs following trauma. The ability of MRI to image the soft tissues is an advantage over CT. Spinal cord injury and ligamentous disruption can be demonstrated.

Chest

Injuries to this area are common, can be rapidly life threatening and are often initially clinically occult. The initial screening anteroposterior (AP) radiograph remains necessary to look for unsuspected pneumothoraces and mediastinal injuries. CT with vascular contrast enhancement is used to look for major vessel injuries and has largely replaced the invasive investigation of thoracic angiography. It is also far more sensitive than the chest radiograph for pneumomediastinum and small pneumothoraces (Figure 14.4).

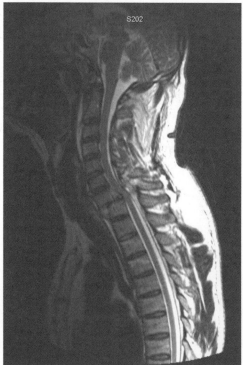

Figure 14.3 This is a sagittal T2-weighted MRI from the same patient as in Figure 14.2. This shows stripping of both the anterior and posterior longitudinal ligaments, cord compression and disruption to the posterior elements.

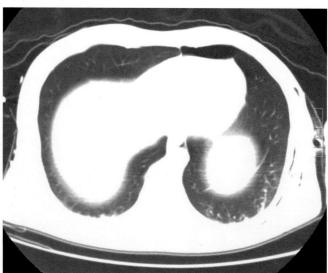

Figure 14.4 Axial CT showing a small left pneumothorax.

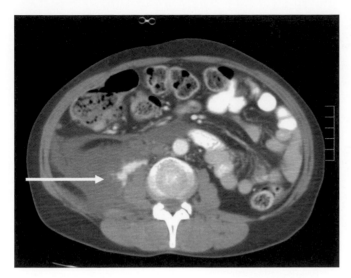

Figure 14.5 Axial CT demonstrating active bleed (*arrow*) in the right retroperitoneum with large associated haematoma.

Abdomen

The scan is then carried straight on to cover the abdomen. Only vascular contrast enhancement is now used. Prior to the advent of multislice scanners, oral contrast was routinely used to look for duodenal rupture. The superior image quality now available with high-quality coronal reformats means that this is no longer necessary. This change in practice means that patients can now be brought for a trauma scan as soon as the patient is ready rather than waiting for oral contrast to go through, as used to be the case.

Where bladder injuries are suspected then a CT cystogram can be performed at the end of the standard scan. This technique is extremely accurate and quick to perform.

There are many advocates of using ultrasound instead of CT. However, although ultrasound is good at assessing for free fluid, it does not necessarily show the source of the injury. CT not only shows free fluid and air but will usually show the origin of the fluid, and characterise the severity of the injuries in the solid organs (Figure 14.5). Ultrasound, except in very skilled hands, can frequently underestimate or miss these solid organ injuries.

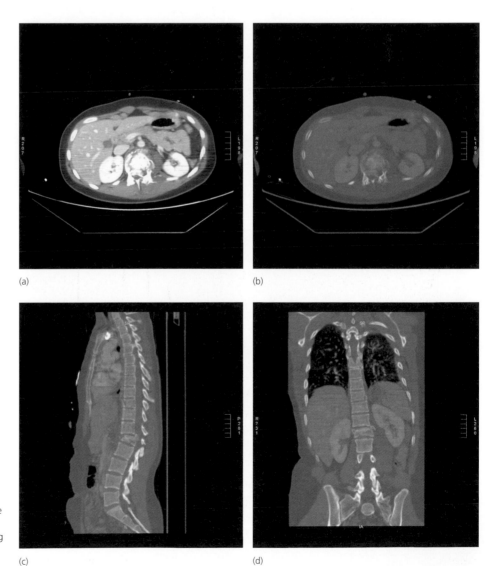

(a)

(b)

(c)

(d)

Figure 14.6 (a) Axial image of the abdomen showing fracture of the spine with associated haematoma. (b) The same image on bone windows shows better delineation of the same fracture. (c,d) These are the sagittal and coronal reformats of the same dataset showing the fracture dislocation of L1 as well as a further fracture at T10.

There is, however, a definite move to introduce ultrasound in prehospital care. Hand-held ultrasound devices are now freely available and there is great value in a paramedic calling in to say that the patient they are bringing in has free intraperitoneal fluid.

Post processing

Once the torso scan has been completed, modern CT techniques allow the data to be reprocessed and diagnostic data regarding the bony pelvis, lumbar and thoracic spines can be obtained (Figure 14.6).

Ultrasound

Focused assessment with sonography for trauma (FAST) is popular in emergency departments as it is fast, can be done at the bedside and involves no ionising radiation. There is no doubt that it is of value when looking for free fluid but it should be borne in mind that up to 34% of trauma patients with visceral trauma have no free fluid. Furthermore, accurate assessment of the solid organs is very user dependent.

Pathways

The key to optimising these facilities is well-developed trauma care pathways. It is essential that imaging is considered as soon as the patient is known about in the emergency department. In a polytrauma patient, CT should be informed as soon as possible. It is possible to carry out the above 'pan scan' and have the patient back to the emergency department within 20 min. The main delay is now the availability of a 24/7 immediate CT service. This certainly represents best practice but clear funding streams are difficult to identify.

Further reading

National Institute for Health and Clinical Excellence. (2003) *Head Injury: Triage, Assessment, Investigation and Early Management of Head Injury in Infants, Children and Adults*. London: National Institute for Health and Clinical Excellence.

CHAPTER 15

Role of the Trauma Nurse

Jill Hill

John Radcliffe Hospital, Oxford, UK

> **OVERVIEW**
>
> - How to prepare for managing a major trauma.
> - Providing a team approach.
> - Caring for a trauma patient.
> - Special circumstances and equipment.
> - Patient advocacy and safety.

Major trauma can cause death within a very short time, with survivors facing impending death in the subsequent hours (ATNC 2003). It is therefore essential to provide structured, efficient multidisciplinary care, paying particular attention to the 'golden hour' detailed by the Advanced Trauma Life Support (ATLS) programme.

Each member of the trauma team plays a key role in providing support to the patient, his friends and relatives and, importantly, to their own colleagues within the team. An effective team involves a group of individuals who share a common goal with the knowledge, skills and dedication to achieve an agreed outcome. Nurses play a pivotal role within this team, contributing a 360° degree perspective. This includes familiarity with the environment, time to provide explanation to the patient or relatives and the ability to use expanded skills. The nurse can also provide crowd control, as although a trauma incident may be an excellent learning environment, there may have to be limits to the numbers of learners so as not to compromise patient care.

Effective teams function optimally with clear communication, co-ordination of skills and knowledge, circumstantial decisions and the direction of a good leader. Absence of any part of this can result in an uninformed, chaotic and potentially dangerous situation putting the safety and well-being of not only the patient but also members of the team at risk. Therefore it is essential that roles are clearly identified and each team member is sure of their own and their colleagues' responsibilities.

There will be local variation regarding the composition of the trauma team and it is essential that the team approach extends beyond the 'golden hour'. The role of the trauma nurse is key to the multidisciplinary approach promoted through ATLS and beyond to provide excellence in patient care.

Preparation

When receiving a patient who has suffered traumatic injury, it is common to be given advanced warning of the patient's arrival. This can include a courtesy call from ambulance control reporting progress from the scene, information regarding the arrival of an air ambulance, as well as a mobile phone call or radio phone patch from the ambulance transporting the patient.

Local preference will determine what information is provided by the crew but it is important that vital aspects concerning the patient's condition are included. Initially the time of the call should be noted so that the correct expected time of arrival (ETA) is accurate. The crew should then state the approximate age and sex of the patient and outline the mechanism and the injuries sustained. They will then relay the patient's vital signs including conscious level, any interventions they have made such as intubation, intravenous (IV) access and state their ETA. Finally, the above should be repeated back to the crew and any further relevant questions asked.

Depending on the severity of the injuries, asking for advance notice to activate a major haemorrhage protocol could prove very helpful. Major haemorrhage protocols consider the overall outcome for the patient. Although the protocol may vary according to the size and scale of the hospital, O negative blood is sent in an insulated box so it is there for the arrival of the patient. The lab is also ready to receive a blood sample from the patient at the earliest opportunity, and along with type and cross matching blood, they also prepare additional clotting products such as fresh frozen plasma (FFP).

When the call has ended preparation for the patient's arrival is made. This includes nominating an appropriate area, usually the resuscitation or designated trauma room, informing colleagues within the unit so they can provide additional support and calling together the trauma team. The structure of the trauma team will vary according to local policy; ideally there will be a consultant level, ATLS trained clinician as team leader. He/she will be joined by an anaesthetist, two further doctors such as registrar or senior house officers (SHO), three ED nurses, a radiographer and a porter. Dependent on the type of trauma, a general surgeon may also be required.

ABC of Major Trauma, Fourth Edition. Edited by David V. Skinner and Peter A. Driscoll.
© 2013 Blackwell Publishing Ltd. Published 2013 by Blackwell Publishing Ltd.

The role of the nurse is diverse and interchangeable but in order for the team to function, each member must be aware of their responsibilities. Nurse 1 is in charge of the airway and communication with the patient. However, in many circumstances this job is taken by the anaesthetist. This leaves nurse 1 to assist with procedures, communicate with the patient and their relatives and usually direct the other nurses. Nurse 2's primary role is charting, involving documenting at 3–5-min intervals the patient's vital signs, Glasgow Coma Score (GCS), fluids and drugs administered and injuries sustained. Nurse 2 may also be responsible for attaching the monitoring equipment as the patient arrives. Nurse 3 acts as a runner which involves exposing the patient on arrival, drawing up medication such as analgesia or antibiotics and preparing dressings. Nurse 3 may also prime warmed fluids, prepare cannulation equipment and prepare chest drain bottles if it is likely they will be required to save vital minutes when the patient arrives.

Protective clothing such as full-length aprons, gloves and goggles should be worn by all members along with lead aprons to enable an uninterrupted X-ray series.

On arrival

When the patient arrives, in most cases they will be immobilised with a cervical collar and head bolsters and will have been transported on a spinal board. As the patient is moved onto the trolley, silence is maintained for the team to receive handover from the ambulance crew. The primary role of the nurse is to remove the patient's clothing in order to fully expose all possible injuries; this usually involves cutting the clothing. Monitoring equipment including non-invasive blood pressure (BP), three-lead electrocardiogram (ECG) and oxygen saturation probe is attached immediately and BP should be monitored at least every 3–5 min. A respiratory rate trend is also vital as an increase or decrease is one of the earliest signs of deterioration in the patient's condition. The GCS is obtained from nurse 1 or the anaesthetist along with pupil size and reaction. Nurse 2 should document this on the designated trauma chart along with any medication or fluids given at the scene of the accident or en route to hospital. While the senior doctor completes the primary survey, the SHOs may be inserting cannulae and taking blood. The nurse may be able to complete this task if they have the skills but not at the expense of the other vital elements mentioned above.

It is essential to remove the patient from the spinal board at the earliest opportunity and dependent upon the patient's GCS, they may be able to verbalise any pain, discomfort or loss of sensation in their limbs. However, although an unconscious patient will be unable to express pain, they should still be removed from the spinal board to prevent pressure sores developing. The log roll at the end of the primary survey enables the spine board to be removed safely whilst maintaining the spine in line.

It is important to continue communication with the patient at all times. Telling the patient your name, explaining what is happening and why, asking if there are friends or relatives to be contacted will help to reduce their anxiety. This is an important aspect of the trauma nurse's role as it can be so easily omitted within the technological diagnostics and high-stress environment of the resuscitation room. Maintaining good communication with the patient will in turn allow the rest of the trauma team to be directed towards any discreet injuries. The nurse can assume advocacy for the patient by voicing particular concerns and, importantly, assessing their levels of pain.

Pain

A conscious patient may be able to express pain by screaming or vocalising where the pain is and factors that exacerbate it. Various methods of accurately scoring the levels and intensity of pain are available, such as the Likert scale or for children the Wong–Baker Faces Rating Scale. Using a pain ladder, asking the patient to score their pain between 0 and 10 with 0 being no pain and 10 the worst pain they have ever experienced, will give a subjective opinion of their pain. As people differ in their tolerance to pain, this may be the most appropriate way to assess the patient and their injuries individually.

Analgesia and antiemetic drugs can be administered at the earliest opportunity as prescribed by the doctor. Commonly, opiates such as morphine sulphate given intravenously and titrated to pain are a quick, safe and effective form of analgesia.

If the patient has a significantly reduced GCS due to injury or anaesthesia it is still crucial that pain relief is considered. Closely monitoring vital signs may reveal a tachycardia which may be triggered by pain; this may settle with analgesia although should not be considered as a sole cause.

Investigations

After the doctor has completed the primary survey, X-rays of the cervical spine, chest and pelvis are usually taken. Although the radiation risk lies with the radiographer, there are other factors that require consideration. If the patient is female and of childbearing age, a pregnancy test may be required. However, this should not delay essential investigation or treatment which could put the patient's and any potential baby's lives at risk. If the patient is conscious this may need to be explained and justified and the appropriate measures taken to minimise the risks, such as placement of lead aprons. The nurse may also need to explain to relatives the need to leave the room temporarily whilst radiographs are taken along with the assurance that they will be brought back in as soon as possible.

The log roll is usually combined with the rectal examination. Many units now have access to portable ultrasound equipment so that trained members of the trauma team can identify signs of internal bleeding. As an alternative, conventional methods such as diagnostic peritoneal lavage (DPL) may require preparation. In most circumstances, more comprehensive imaging such as computed tomography (CT) scanning is required as a matter of urgency. In most hospitals the CT scanner is located in the X-ray department which means moving the critically injured patient out of the relative safety of the ED into an area with little or no resuscitation equipment.

Computed tomography

When transferring the patient out of the ED to the X-ray department, careful consideration of potential complications is vital to ensure emergency equipment and medications are immediately available. Some units have specific transfer packs which carry most emergency supplies such as airway and cannulation equipment, anaesthetic drugs and fluids, etc. However, it is important not to overstock or tightly pack the equipment as in an emergency situation finding specific items may prove difficult. Local policy and the geography of the department will vary and this will dictate what procedures should be followed in the case of an emergency. Notwithstanding, the basic rules of ATLS following the ABCDE approach should be a priority.

A common-sense approach when transferring the patient should minimise any potential problems. Ensure that the patient is attached to a portable monitor and that observations are continued at regular intervals whilst the patient is being scanned. Be sure that there is a full tank of oxygen available prior to transfer, particularly if piped oxygen is unavailable in the X-ray department. A portable suction device is essential to quickly alleviate any airway obstruction whilst away from the ED. Attempt to have a clear path to the CT scanner which may involve a specified person, perhaps a porter, walking slightly ahead of the patient and clearing the way which will in turn promote a safer environment for other patients. Ensure there are enough people available on arrival to safely transfer the patient onto the CT table. Throughout any transfer, continued communication with the patient is essential, particularly if the patient is conscious. In order to obtain adequate scan pictures, the patient needs to remain as still as possible to reduce any artefact which is more likely if the patient understands what is going to happen.

What next?

Some patients with life-threatening injuries may require urgent surgery and need immediate transfer to theatre from the CT scanner. However, dependent upon circumstances, even the critically injured patient may need to wait for surgery. Patients who have less severe injuries and do not need further immediate intervention are transferred back to the ED. It is at this stage that further management plans are made or additional interventions performed. If not performed already, the senior doctor will carry out a secondary survey to identify any further injuries.

Injuries such as limb fractures, wounds and so on can now be dealt with. Experienced nurses with the appropriate training play a pivotal role in cleaning, closing and dressing wounds along with immobilising fractures with the appropriate cast or splint. Observing for changes in neurovascular status of a limb is an equally important task.

During this period other interventions may be undertaken such as inserting a urinary catheter or assisting the anaesthetist to insert an arterial cannula for invasive monitoring. These additional adjuncts are not necessarily vital to the survival of the patient but enable closer monitoring which in turn can identify an early deterioration in their condition.

Transfer

When planning to transfer the patient to definitive care, whether this is to theatre, a ward or another hospital, preparation is required.

Documenting and securing patients' property is an important part of the nurse's role. In an increasingly litigious society, nurses can safeguard themselves and their colleagues by documenting all items removed from the patient, including cut or soiled clothing, labelling it and securing it in a bag. Valuable items such as mobile phones, money, jewellery, etc., should be logged separately and placed in a safe or locked area until they can be safely returned to the patient or their family. Any property taken by the family or by the police, who may require it for forensic evidence or to gain information for next of kin, should be documented in the patient's notes.

When the receiving area is identified, telephoning ahead to ensure they are ready will prevent any unnecessary delay on arrival. Taking the same precautions as transferring to the X-ray department will promote a safer relocation from the ED. Continued communication with the patient and their relatives is essential to minimise anxiety and confusion.

Special circumstances

The role of the nurse is varied and ever changing. Therefore it is necessary to adapt to any situation and judge each circumstance as it arises. Treating a gravely ill patient may require the need to 'pull out all the stops' where individual tasks may be less defined.

When needing to infuse fluids or blood at a very fast rate, the use of a rapid infuser can aid the process. Models will vary but generally they provide the ability to infuse and warm fluid very quickly and to deliver more than one bag at a time. Because of the speed involved, it requires one nurse to continually work the machine, interchanging bags, checking blood products and observing cannulae or lines. As the use of the rapid infuser may be sporadic, regular checking of the equipment and a good working knowledge of how it operates is essential.

Other situations such as thoracotomy, burr holes or surgical airways can result in even the experienced nurse feeling overwhelmed and unprepared. In these situations, tensions run high and stress levels increase, causing a feeling of apprehension. Debriefing using hindsight when the situation is over and talking through aspects of the events can help to reconcile any concerns or questions that may have arisen. It is advisable to endeavour to meet soon after the event and this is likely to be within the following week. It should not be viewed as an opportunity to apportion blame or criticism, but to give a balanced overall account of the events in an environment where people feel comfortable asking and answering relevant questions.

Debriefing may not be helpful for all situations or all individuals but offering it as an option aids the continued support of the team.

Summary

The trauma nurse is an experienced adaptable team player with a variety of skills and attributes to make a positive contribution to the trauma team and in turn the trauma patient. Clear communication skills are vital in every aspect of the trauma nurse's role. Good communication within the team will promote a well-bonded and efficient service where members can anticipate change and address it together. Honest communication with the patient, their family and friends will help to decrease their anxiety and encourage confidence.

Unlike the medical role in a trauma team, the varied nature of the trauma nurse's role requires many skills and the ability to adapt and interchange these skills according to the situation. Switching from one task to another is expected and essential to keep the team progressing.

With an ATLS focus on the 'golden hour', there is little time for error and patient safety is not an aspect for compromise. Therefore preparation, anticipation and planning are essential. The role of the trauma nurse provides a 360° perspective of the trauma patient's care. With the potential for high mortality soon after injury, it is vital that a multidisciplinary approach is embraced to promote the best possible outcome for the patient.

Further reading

Advanced Trauma Nursing Course Manual. (2003)

American College of Surgeons Committee on Trauma. (2004) *Advanced Trauma Lift Support Course for Physicians*, 7th edn. Chicago: American College of Surgeons.

Christie J, Langstaff D. (2000) *Trauma Care: A Team Approach*. Oxford: Butterworth Heinemann.

Wong D, Baker C. (1988) Pain in children: comparison of assessment scales. Pediatr Nurs 14(1): 9–17.

CHAPTER 16

Scoring Systems for Trauma

Maralyn Woodford

University of Manchester, Manchester, UK

OVERVIEW

- Trauma scoring systems include measurements of host vulnerability (age, gender), anatomical severity and physiological derangement.
- In Europe, the TRISS methodology has been superseded.
- Any assessment of the effectiveness of a trauma system should be based on casemix standardised outcomes.
- Process measures are equally important in evaluating trauma systems.

Trauma care systems deal with patients who have an almost infinite variety of injuries requiring complex treatment. The assessment of such systems is a major challenge in clinical measurement and audit. Which systems are most effective in delivering best outcomes? Implementing recommendations for improved procedures will often incur additional costs: will the expense be worthwhile? Clearly, casemix-adjusted outcome analysis must replace anecdote and dogma. Outcome prediction in trauma is a developing science which enables the assessment of trauma system effectiveness. An improvement in trauma care is essential; audit is one of the tools that can be used.

The effects of injury can be defined in terms of input (an anatomical component and the physiological response) and outcome (mortality and morbidity) (Box 16.1). These must be coded numerically before we can comment with confidence on treatment or process of care. Elderly people survive trauma less well than others, so age must be taken into account and the association between gender and age is also considered to be important. Most recent work has been concerned with measurement of injury severity and its relation to mortality. Assessment of morbidity has been largely neglected, yet for every person who dies as a result of trauma, there are two seriously disabled survivors.

Input measures

Injury is assessed through the anatomical component and the physiological response. These two elements are separately scored.

Box 16.1 **Analysis of trauma care**

Input

- Anatomical injury
- Physiological derangement
- Age
- Gender

Process

- Variations in the system of care
- Variations in patient care

Outcome

- Survival: alive or dead at 30 days
- Disability:
  - temporary or permanent
  - neurological
  - musculoskeletal

Examples: Glasgow Outcome Score, SF12, EU5D

Anatomical scoring system

The Abbreviated Injury Scale (AIS), first published in 1969, is anatomically based. There is a single AIS score for each injury a patient may sustain. Scores range from 1 (minor) to 6 (incompatible with life) (Association for the Advancement of Automotive Medicine 1990). Table 16.1 shows examples of injuries scored using the AIS.

Table 16.1 Examples of injuries scored by the Abbreviated Injury Scale (AIS 2005).

Injury	Score
Shoulder pain (no injury specified)	0
Wrist sprain	1 (minor)
Closed undisplaced tibial fracture	2 (moderate)
Basal skull fracture	3 (serious)
Incomplete transection of the thoracic aorta	4 (severe)
Complex liver laceration	5 (critical)
Laceration of the brainstem	6 (incompatible with life)

ABC of Major Trauma, Fourth Edition. Edited by David V. Skinner and Peter A. Driscoll.
© 2013 Blackwell Publishing Ltd. Published 2013 by Blackwell Publishing Ltd.

There are more than 2000 injuries listed in the AIS 2005 dictionary, which is in its fifth edition. Intervals between the scores are not always consistent; for example, the difference between AIS3 and AIS4 is not necessarily the same as that between AIS1 and AIS2. (Copies of the booklet are available from www.carcrash.org.)

Patients with multiple injuries are scored by adding together the squares of the three highest AIS scores in three predetermined regions of the body. This is the Injury Severity Score (ISS) (Box 16.2). Scores of 7 and 15 are unattainable because these figures cannot be obtained from summing squares. The maximum score is 75 ($5^2 + 5^2 + 5^2$). By convention, a patient with an AIS6 in one body region is given an ISS of 75. The ISS is non-linear and there is pronounced variation in the frequency of different scores; 9 and 16 are common, 14 and 22 unusual (Baker & O'Neill 1976).

Box 16.2 **Injury Severity Score (ISS)**

To obtain this:

- use the AIS90 dictionary to score every injury
- identify the highest AIS score in each of the following six areas of the body:
  1 head and neck
  2 face
  3 chest and thoracic spine
  4 abdomen, lumbar spine and pelvic contents
  5 bony pelvis and limbs
  6 body surface
- add together the squares of the highest scores in three body areas.

An example of an ISS and associated calculation is shown in Box 16.3.

Box 16.3 **Case study**

A man is injured in a fall at work. He complains of pain in his neck, jaw, and left wrist and has difficulty breathing. There are abrasions around the left shoulder, left side of the chest, and left knee. Examination of the cervical spine (with radiography) suggests no abnormality. There is a displaced fracture of the body of the mandible. There are also fractures of the left wrist and left ribs (4–9), with a flail segment.

Injury	AIS score
Fracture of body of mandible	2
Fracture of lower end of radius(not further specified*)	2
Fracture of ribs L4–9 with flail segment	4
Abrasions (all sites)	1
Neck pain†	0

*If fracture of radius was known to be displaced or open the AIS would be 3. If not specified, the lower score is used.
†Symptoms are not scored if there is no demonstrable anatomical injury.
ISS = $2^2 + 2^2 + 4^2 = 24$

For the purpose of the analysis described here, the ISS should be calculated only from operative findings, appropriate investigations or necropsy reports. The overall ISS of a group of patients should be identified by the median value and the range, not the mean value. Non-parametric statistics should be used for analysis.

Physiological scoring systems

Historically, the physiological responses of an injured patient have been assessed by the Revised Trauma Score (RTS). The physiological parameters that make up the RTS are respiratory rate, systolic blood pressure and Glasgow Coma Scale (GCS) (Tables 16.2 and 16.3). The RTS was developed following statistical analysis of a large North American database to determine the most predictive independent outcome variables. Selection of variables was also influenced by their ease of measurement and clinical opinion. In practice, the RTS is a complex calculation, combining coded measurements of the three physiological values. To calculate the RTS, the coded value for each variable is multiplied by a weighting factor derived from regression analysis of the database.

After injury, the patient's physiological response is constantly changing but for the purposes of injury scoring, and by convention, the first measurements, when the patient arrives at hospital, are used. If the patient is intubated before arrival, an RTS cannot be measured.

Current practice

The latest European research has shown the GCS to be the most valuable physiological predictor (Bouamra *et al.* 2006). If the

Table 16.2 Glasgow Coma Scale.

Component	Response	Score
Eye opening	Spontaneous	4
	To speech	3
	To pain	2
	None	1
Best verbal response	Orientated	5
	Confused	4
	Inappropriate words	3
	Incomprehensible sounds	2
	None	1
Best motor response	Obeys commands	6
	Localises to pain	5
	Withdraws from pain	4
	Flexion to pain	3
	Extension to pain	2
	None	1

Table 16.3 Modification of Glasgow Coma Scale for children.

Component	Response	Score
Best verbal response	Appropriate words or social smiles, fixes on and follows objects	5
	Cries but is consolable	4
	Persistently irritable	3
	Restless, agitated	2
	Silent	1
Eye and motor response		Scored as for adults

patient is intubated before arrival, a GCS measured at the scene of the incident can be used.

The GCS is the accepted international standard for measuring neurological state. The state may be represented as a single figure (for example, GCS = 15) or as the responses in each of the three sections of the scale (for example, eyes = 4, verbal response = 5, motor response = 6). Coma is defined as a GCS of <9. Various modifications of the scale have been suggested for use in small children. Some doctors reduce the maximum score to that which is consistent with neurological maturation. A more useful clinical device, which ensures more accurate communication and simplifies epidemiological research, is to retain the maximum score of 15 but redefine the descriptions.

Trauma outcome prediction methodology

The degree of physiological derangement and the extent of anatomical injury are measures of the threat to life. Mortality will also be affected by the age and gender of the patient.

Traditionally the 'TRISS' methodology combined four elements – the RTS, the ISS, the patient's age, and whether the injury was blunt or penetrating – to provide a measure of the probability of survival (Ps). The acronym was tortuously developed from **Tr**auma score and **I**njury **S**everity **S**core (Champion *et al.* 1990).

From the database of the Trauma Audit and Research Network (TARN; www.tarn.ac.uk), the outcome prediction model has been updated to reflect the characteristics of the European trauma population when calculating the survival probability. Specifically:

- outcome (survival or death) is measured at 30 days reflecting outcomes from the injuries rather than any pre-existing diseases
- using the GCS as the only physiological marker improves the logistic regression model and increases the number of cases that can be included in outcome predictions by 20% without sacrificing the integrity of the model.
- an improved second-order model for ISS over the original linear functional form used in TRISS, fitting significantly better than a first-order model
- patients who are transferred to another hospital for further care, intubated at scene and those with burns injuries can now be included in the core data set that defines one model for all cases
- injured children are now included and regression coefficients created for ages 0–5, 6–10 and 11–15 years
- one outcome predictor model is now used for both blunt and penetrating injured patients
- analysis of the data set shows that increases in mortality with age are more pronounced for males and that there is an age/gender interaction that must be taken into account in the new outcome prediction model.

In order to achieve the best statistical model, there must be a balance between good prediction and accuracy rates and clinical 'face validity'. The data used for the model's development also must reflect 'real-world' data. The recent statistical modelling work at TARN reflects these concerns. Finally, the predictions of any model will only be valid if the data set includes the great majority of index cases.

The probability of survival (Ps) of each injured patient is calculated using:

· Age · Gender · Glasgow Coma Scale · Injury Severity Score

It is important to realise that Ps is merely a mathematical calculation; it is not an absolute measure of mortality but only an indication of the probability of survival. If a patient with a Ps of 80% dies, the outcome is unexpected because four out of five patients with such a Ps would be expected to survive. However, the fifth would be expected to die and this could be the patient under study. The Ps is used as a filter for highlighting patients for study in multidisciplinary trauma audit.

Full calculations are shown at www.tarn.ac.uk/resources.

Comparing systems of care

Comparison of the probabilities of survival of all patients seen at a particular hospital with the observed outcome can be used as an index of overall performance. Probabilities of survival are combined in the 'standardised W statistic' (Ws) to assess a group of patients (Hollis *et al.* 1995).

Standardised W statistic

The Ws provides a measure of the number of additional survivors, or deaths, for every 100 patients treated at each hospital accounting for different mixes of injury severity. The 'standardised Z statistic' (Zs) provides a measure of its statistical significance.

A high positive Ws is desirable as this indicates that more patients are surviving than would be predicted from the TRISS methodology. Conversely, a negative Ws signifies that the system of trauma care has fewer survivors than expected from the TRISS predictions. Consequently, poorly performing trusts have the opportunity to evaluate their trauma care systems through comparative national audit and improve the care provided. Trusts performing better should continue to monitor their healthcare system for injured patients.

Comparisons have become more relevant to clinicians after extensive work was undertaken to base the regression analysis on statistics derived from the TARN database. The Ws can be shown graphically with 95% confidence intervals to illustrate clinical differences between hospitals (Figure 16.1).

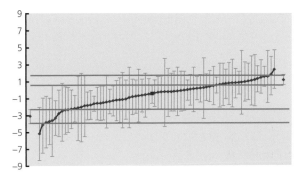

Figure 16.1 Comparative outcome. Summary Ws scores with 95% confidence intervals.

Trauma Audit and Research Network

The method used in the Trauma Audit and Research Network for England, Wales (Lecky *et al.* 2000) and throughout Europe and Australia to audit the effectiveness of systems of trauma care and the management of individual patients was first developed in North America. The Ps12 methodology is applied in all patients with trauma who are admitted to hospital for more than 3 days, managed in an intensive care area or referred for specialist care, or who die in hospital. Additional information is sought on the process and timing of care interventions and length of stay.

The TARN provides a valuable method of comparing patterns of care in different parts of the country. It is reliant on careful collection of data in a consistent format to allow collation and comparison of results. This is integral to the new electronic system of data collection and reporting and to the training provided by TARN staff. Deaths caused by trauma are too varied, too complicated and too important to be discussed in isolation in individual hospitals.

The wider perspective of TARN is increasingly recognised as the only valid approach to trauma audit and is being taken up by regional and national bodies for this purpose. Identification of deficiencies is valuable only if a mechanism exists to correct them. Local audit meetings and national comparisons must be used to stimulate appropriate changes in systems of trauma care.

The development of the TRISS and Ps methodologies has been a major advance in the measurement of injury severity. The detailed structure of the scales and the method of developing a single number to represent threat to life are, however, under constant review (Bouamra *et al.* 2006).

An alternative method of measuring anatomical injury has been described which uses the root sum squares of the AIS scores for the head and trunk (anatomical profile). It has been incorporated into a system for the characterisation of trauma (ASCOT), using different weightings for the AIS scores of a patient's most severe injuries regardless of body region (Champion *et al.* 1996). These developments may lead to even more accurate scoring systems.

European trauma registries are now collaborating within the EuroTARN initiative (http://eurotarn.man.ac.uk/) to compare crude outcomes (% mortality) in similar groups of patients. As there is large trauma system variation across Europe, it is hoped this collaboration will help identify the true role and benefits of 'trauma centres' and other system characteristics which have yet to be determined.

Measurement of outcome in terms of survival or death is, however, a crude yardstick. Further progress is required in measuring disability after injury (Box 16.4). Most life-threatening visceral injuries leave the patient with little disability. In contrast, the many more patients who sustain musculoskeletal sequelae are largely ignored in the statistics. Much effort will be required to develop outcomes measures based on disability; these are essential if the treatment of the multiply injured patient is to be based on sound scientific principles.

Further details of TARN can be obtained from www.tarn.ac.uk.

Box 16.4 **Definition of impairment, disability and handicap**

- *Impairment* has an anatomical or physiological basis and is usually a consequence of musculoskeletal or cerebral injury (e.g. an amputated finger). It is easy to measure but variably related to the patient's activity.
- *Disability* is a functional consequence of an impairment that affects the patient's ability to perform the activities of daily life. Its measurement is relevant to the patient's needs but it is influenced by the environment.
- *Handicap* refers to the disability within an individual's social and professional role. It may reflect a change in lifestyle, which is influenced by society. Handicap is difficult to relate to specific injury and difficult to measure.

References

Association for the Advancement of Automotive Medicine, Committee on Injury Scaling. (1990) *The Abbreviated Injury Scale – 1990 Revision.* Des Plains, IL: Association for the Advancement of Automotive Medicine.

Baker SP, O'Neill B. (1976) The injury severity score: an update. *J Trauma* 16: 882–5.

Bouamra O, Wrotchford AS, Hollis S, Vail A, Woodford M, Lecky FE. (2006) A new approach to outcome prediction in trauma: a comparison with the TRISS model. *J Trauma* 61(3): 701–10.

Champion H, Sacco WJ, Copes WS, Gann DS, Gennarelli TA, Flanagan ME. (1989) A revision of the Trauma Score. *J Trauma* 29: 623–9.

Champion H, Copes WS, Sacco WJ, *et al.* (1990) The Major Trauma Outcome Study: establishing national norms for trauma care. *J Trauma* 30: 1356–65

Champion H, Copes WS, Sacco WJ, *et al.* (1996) Improved predictions from A Severity Characterization of Trauma (ASCOT) over Trauma and Injury Severity Score (TRISS): results of an independent evaluation. *J Trauma* 40: 42–9.

Hollis S, Yates DW, Woodford M, Foster P. (1995) Standardized comparison of performance indicators in trauma: a new approach to case-mix variation. *J Trauma* 38: 763–6.

Lecky F, Woodford M, Yates DW. (2000) Trends in trauma care in England and Wales 1989–97. *UK Trauma Audit and Research Network. Lancet* 355: 1771–5.

CHAPTER 17

Handling Distressed Relatives and Breaking Bad News

Chris A. J. McLauchlan

Royal Devon and Exeter Hospital, Exeter, UK

OVERVIEW

- Initial contact, reception and the vigil.
- Breaking the news.
- Facing reality, including witnessing resuscitation.
- Actions and a checklist after a death including legal, cultural, spiritual issues and tissue donation.
- Providing information and follow-up.
- Staff support.

Coping with major trauma is stressful for both staff and relatives. Handling distressed relatives is still underemphasised but the training of such issues at medical school is improving, although junior staff may have little experience. It is a time that the relative will always remember and, if handled badly, will leave lasting scars. Alternatively, skilled early handling of the bereaved will enable them to make a smoother journey through grief and improve the long-term outlook.

Giving bad news is never easy but it can be especially difficult in cases of major trauma when there is physical damage to the loved one (Box 17.1). The nature of the patient's problem and the bad news can be varied. The management of the relatives may begin before they arrive at hospital and carry on until well after death or discharge of the patient. The principles of management apply to the emergency department as well as the intensive treatment unit or admitting ward. Providing genuine care and support for relatives is the key to their management.

Box 17.1 Problems associated with breaking bad news in cases of trauma

- Death or severe injury is sudden and unexpected.
- The victim is often young.
- The prognosis is often unsure.
- Staff are often very busy.
- Relatives may already have been notified in an unskilled manner.
- The victim may have committed suicide.
- Alcohol or drug intoxication may have been a contributing factor.

ABC of Major Trauma, Fourth Edition. Edited by David V. Skinner and Peter A. Driscoll.
© 2013 Blackwell Publishing Ltd. Published 2013 by Blackwell Publishing Ltd.

Initial contact

When a victim of major trauma arrives in the emergency room the priority is immediate resuscitation. Once identified, the closest relatives or friends should be notified.

Communication with the emergency services can provide important information that is useful when handling the relatives. The ambulance crew and police, as well as giving details about the incident, may have already seen the relatives or know of their whereabouts. It is usually better for a sympathetic police officer to make the initial contact in person rather than for a telephone call to be made from the hospital, but local knowledge may be important. The police may also be able to help with transport.

If the telephone is used, information should be given by an experienced nurse or doctor and a lone relative advised strongly against driving to hospital alone. Mentioning that the victim is unconscious often helps to impart a certain severity to the lay person, although the full severity of death is usually best explained in person at the hospital (Boxes 17.2 and 17.3). If relatives are not told of the victim's death, however, they may blame themselves for not arriving at the hospital before death. It is important to dispel any self-recrimination by giving the relatives the exact information, including the time of death, when they attend.

If the relatives have to travel great distances or from overseas, the full details, including death, may have to be explained over the telephone. Find out if the relative is alone and, if so, suggest that he or she seeks support locally. Offer to telephone for support.

Arrival of relatives at the hospital

Anxious relatives should be met by a named link nurse and not be kept waiting around in reception. It is important that the nursing sister co-ordinates the information so that the staff, in particular those at reception, know that potentially distressed relatives are expected (Figure 17.1). They should be welcomed and not made to feel in the way. Staff should remember that it is not only the victim's relatives who may be distressed: in some instances, it may be a close friend or partner of either sex.

There should be a private room or office where relatives and friends can wait and be seen by medical staff. Ideally, this room should be solely for relatives and friends, have a homely décor, yet be nearby and private but not isolated. An outside view is desirable

Box 17.2 **Various outcomes of major trauma**

- Death.
- Serious head injury.
- Multiple injuries.
- Spinal injury.
- Major burns.
- Loss of a limb.
- Loss of sight.

Box 17.3 **Handling the initial contact with relatives**

- It may be preferable for a police officer to make contact in person.
- Information conveyed by telephone should be given by an experienced nurse or doctor.
- Relatives should not drive to hospital alone.
- The full severity of injuries or death may be best explained at the hospital.

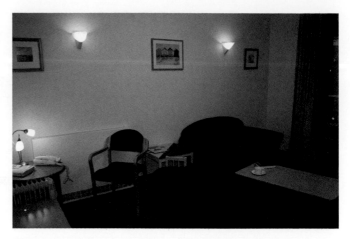

Figure 17.2 Relatives' room.

or at least a controlled view of a corridor. It is a myth that such details are not remembered by distressed relatives.

Distressed relatives should be given privacy and not be kept waiting in reception areas, which may be impersonal and busy (Box 17.4, Figure 17.2).

Box 17.4 **Essential features of a relatives' room**

- Privacy.
- Telephone, preferably direct dial.
- Hand basin.
- Mirror.
- Appropriate décor and furniture.
- Advice and information leaflets (out of sight).
- Tea cups and drink facilities.
- Toys for children.

Breaking the news

Remember to ask relatives for the medical history of the patient. This history may be vital if the patient is receiving certain drugs such as steroids or anticoagulants, and an idea of the quality of life may be useful in elderly victims or those with disease. Providing a history can also make relatives feel that they are doing something useful.

During attempted resuscitation, if not already involved, relatives should be given early warning of the patient's critical condition. Regular updates by the same person (usually the link nurse) are also appreciated and may help to break the bad news in stages. It also allows relationships to form, which will help in providing the support that may be needed later.

The link nurses should introduce a doctor, preferably a senior one, to the relatives as soon as possible to provide further information. There are no firm rules as to who should break the news, but ideally it should be someone senior with the time, warmth and communication skills. Relatives will expect to see a doctor for medical information and an idea of the prognosis: 'Will he be all right, doctor?'.

Advice for the doctor (or other breaker of news)

Breaking bad news has to be tailored to the situation and the particular relatives, but the following principles generally apply.

- On leaving the emergency area, you may be stressed, so take a moment to compose yourself and think about what you are going to say while you take a few deep breaths. Also remove evidence of blood stains, etc., so that you are physically and mentally prepared.
- Take an experienced nurse with you. The link nurse can be a great support and can carry on where you leave off.
- Confirm that you are speaking to the correct relatives. Briefly ascertain what information they already have.
- Enter the relatives' room, introduce yourself and sit down near the patient's closest relatives at eye level. Do not stand holding

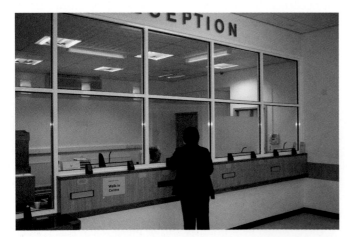

Figure 17.1 Reception area.

the door handle like a bus conductor ready to jump out. Giving the impression that you have time to talk and listen is important.

- Look at the person you are talking to, be honest and direct and keep it simple. Be prepared to emphasise the main points. Avoid too much technical information at this stage (although if a patient has multiple injuries there may be much going on). If death is probable, say so; do not beat around the bush.
- After breaking bad news, allow time and silence while the facts sink in.
- If the seriousness of the situation does not seem to have been accepted, re-emphasise the facts and consider showing them the patient or deceased person immediately.
- Be prepared for a variety of emotional responses or reactions (Box 17.5). Some people stick at one reaction, whereas others go through several reactions. These reactions are not your fault – rather, they imply that you have got the message across.
- Allow and encourage reactions such as crying. Provide tissues and facilities for relatives to make themselves presentable to the world again.
- Although it is upsetting, close relatives appreciate the truth and your honest empathy.
- At this stage there is no substitute for genuine care and support. A sensitive nurse is a great asset.
- Tea usually appears, and this is another sign that the relatives' distress is appreciated.
- During the interview it is a helpful and natural comfort for staff to touch and/or hold the hand of the relative. Various social and cultural factors may influence the appropriateness of touching, but generally if it feels right, then it is probably right.
- Likewise, during the interview it may be natural for the staff to have sad feelings, and these need not be completely hidden. Some sign of emotion may help distressed or bereaved people to realise that the staff do have some understanding and it is not just another 'case'.
- Avoid platitudes; for example, after a death, comments such as 'You've still got your other son' are not helpful, as it is the dead person whom the relatives want back. Also avoid false sympathy, as in 'I know what it's like', but rather empathise, as in 'It must be hard for you ...' or 'It must feel very unreal and a shock for you ....', etc, reflecting back their emotions.

Box 17.5 Some immediate grief reactions

- Numbness – that is, acceptance but no feeling.
- Disbelief.
- Acute distress.
- Anger, including against the medical professions.
- Blaming themselves, others or even the deceased.
- Guilt.
- Acceptance.

A sensitive nurse is a great asset after bad news has been broken (Figure 17.3).

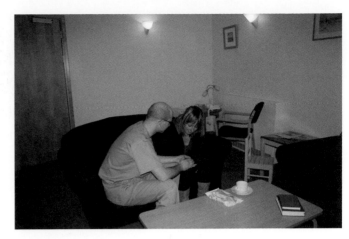

Figure 17.3 Sensitive nurse.

Encourage and be prepared for questions to be asked during the interview. They may disclose any misunderstandings and present a chance to re-emphasise the message. The question of pain and suffering is common and should be discussed routinely, with reassurance as appropriate. The prognosis may be unknown initially, and you should say so. If death or serious disability is possible, however, then it is only fair to be honest and warn the relatives. It will be a worse shock later if they have been protected from this knowledge.

Do not be afraid to say that you do not know the answers to medical or philosophical questions such as 'Why me?'. Other difficult questions may arise from feelings of guilt or when a relative was involved in but not injured in the same accident. Special problems may arise if the relative feels directly responsible – for example, as the driver in an accident. Other complications may include a recent squabble before the accident, with subsequent self-recrimination. The 'If only ...' rumination can be a type of guilt response that is fruitless and should be understood but discouraged at the outset. Just listening may be all that is needed.

If death has already occurred, the same principles as above apply. It is important to use the word 'death' or 'dead' early and avoid euphemisms such as 'passed on' or 'lost', which can be misinterpreted. The news is usually hard to accept and so it must be as clear as possible, abrupt as it may seem. People usually need an explanation as to the cause of death of a loved one. It may be helpful to explain the inevitability in the light of the known injuries and that 'everything possible was done'. Worries about their own first aid at the scene of the accident may need talking through.

Children should not be excluded from the proceedings in the mistaken belief that they need protection. They will be afraid and may have fantasies and feelings of guilt, and need more information and listening to rather than less. Parents and carers may need support and explanation about a child's or teenager's reaction.

Staff actions during the interview with the bereaved are summarised in Box 17.6.

Box 17.6 Staff actions during the interview with the bereaved

Allow:

• time
• the bereaved to react
• silence
• touching
• questions

Avoid:

• rushing
• 'protecting' from the truth
• platitudes
• false sympathy
• euphemisms
• talking instead of listening

Whenever possible, relatives should be given a clear explanation of the cause of death. Children should not be excluded from the proceedings – they need more information and listening to, rather than less. Reality is preferable to fantasy, so allow relatives to see even critically ill patients, albeit briefly.

Management of relatives

Seeing the patient

It should be possible, as well as beneficial, for close relatives to see the patient briefly before he or she is rushed off to theatre, the intensive treatment unit or even another hospital (Box 17.7). Although distressing, reality is usually preferable to fantasy, and this brief contact window may also be beneficial to the conscious patient. Otherwise, it may be some hours or the patient may die before the relatives see them. Relatives may ask to enter or remain in the resuscitation area during emergency treatment, especially of infants and children.

Box 17.7 Seeing the patient

• Staff should respond promptly to allow and encourage early contact with the patient.
• Allowing relatives in the resuscitation room is now accepted practice and has advantages for all parties.

Relatives in the resuscitation room

Should relatives enter the resuscitation room? It is now accepted practice for relatives to be offered this opportunity, and evidence suggests that it can be beneficial if certain safeguards are in place (Boxes 17.8 and 17.9) (Department of Health 2005, Merlevede 2004). These include constant support and explanation from an experienced member of staff and a free choice to stay or leave – although, of course, if their presence in any way impedes the resuscitation effort, the team leader must be aware that they can be taken out. By being present, even briefly, a relative may better appreciate the seriousness of the situation and the vigour of

resuscitation efforts (Resuscitation Council 1996). In major trauma particularly, the level of invasive procedures can increase rapidly, and careful explanation and the opportunity (or encouragement) for the relatives to leave must be provided by the support nurse.

Initially some staff are apprehensive about the presence of relatives but the concept should be gently introduced with reminders of the safeguards and benefits. Experience and feedback from relatives and published evidence certainly support the concept, with only occasional problems. The offer to relatives to enter the resuscitation area should be reconsidered if it is felt that it may not be in the best interests of the patient – for example, if there is overt aggression, especially with alcohol intoxication.

Box 17.8 Relatives in the resuscitation room: key safeguards

• Offer the opportunity but without duress.
• Prepare the relative first.
• Support and accompany the relative throughout.
• Generally restrict to one or two people.
• Ensure the team leader and team are aware.
• The patient remains the priority.
• Provide time for questions afterwards.

Box 17.9 Allowing relatives in the resuscitation room: potential benefits

• Helps relative accept reality and avoid denial.
• Relative feels involved.
• Relative sees that 'all was done'.
• Avoids painful separation and feeling of having let down their loved one if not present.
• Relative able to speak to and touch loved one.
• Allows autonomy for relatives.
• Breaking the bad news is easier for staff.

Seeing the body after death

The opportunity to see the dead person should always be offered and gently encouraged if there is any doubt (Box 17.10). Well-meaning friends may try and discourage this act, which is an important part of accepting reality, and relatives may also like to see the place of death.

The imagination by relatives of the extent of injuries is usually far worse than the reality. The actions and words of staff when relatives are with the body should give 'permission' for relatives to touch, hold, kiss or say goodbye to their loved one. Staff will often carefully prepare a body before viewing in the clinical area or chapel. Ideally, there should be a private cubicle near the resuscitation area, made as non-clinical as possible, to allow relatives time with the deceased person. There should also be a non-religious 'chapel of rest' for later opportunities for visiting, usually at the hospital mortuary. Religious insignia can be added as appropriate. The relative may also like to be left alone with the body and must be given permission to stay as long as they wish or is practically possible. Hospitals should ensure that there is a system in place to allow key relatives to visit the mortuary in emergencies, out of hours, including weekends.

Box 17.10 **Seeing the body**

- Seeing the dead person is an important part of accepting reality and relatives may also like to see the place of death.
- If a relative wishes to be left alone with the body, he or she must be given permission to stay as long as they wish or is practically possible.

Other actions (Box 17.11)

Although they are stunned by events, it is often small touches of care that relatives appreciate and remember, such as being given a lock of hair from their dead child (or adult relative) by a thoughtful nurse.

Box 17.11 **Checklist of actions in the event of a patient's death**

- Notify the general practitioner, other relatives and friends, and the coroner's officer.
- Ensure that the minister or chaplain has been called if the relatives wish and any religious or ethnic issues considered.
- Give an information or help leaflet to the relatives.
- Notify the social worker if he or she is available.
- Give useful telephone numbers and contact addresses (and your name) to the relatives.
- Remember to check the donor register and ask about any wishes regarding tissue donation.

Always ask if there is anyone else whom the relatives would like to be contacted – for example, a close friend or a minister. The relatives or appropriate minister should be consulted about any religious or ethnic issues and the correct procedures. Staff should be aware of the main minority ethnic groups in their area. The hospital chaplains can be a source of great support to both relatives and busy staff.

The wishes that the deceased may have had regarding tissue donation should be raised sensitively with the relative. (Organ donation will not normally be viable after cardiac arrest.) Staff may find it difficult, but relatives should have the choice and may later regret not being able to fulfil their loved one's wishes. For some, it can also be something of a consolation to know someone else has benefited. The finding of an organ/tissue donation card provides a good opening and the patient's name can also now be checked with the national donation registry. It is generally best to decouple this question from breaking the bad news, so perhaps return to the relatives after half an hour and say something like: 'Do you know if _____ had any wishes regarding their (organs and) tissues after death?' or 'Had you talked about donation with _____?'.

Corneas can be donated up to 24 h after death and heart valves up to 48 h. In some areas, it may also be able to donate skin and bone,

but check with your local donation co-ordinator. The co-ordinator for your area can then answer questions, provide advice on consent, and then take over the situation. Referring the death to the coroner is not a contraindication. It is known that many more people could benefit from donation if more staff feel able to ask.

If a mechanism of counselling and follow-up exists locally, consider borrowing their expertise in appropriate cases of trauma.

Sedation may be requested for relatives, usually by a third party, but it is generally inappropriate as it dulls reality and may delay acceptance. Grieving cannot be avoided so easily.

Information and follow-up

Long-term management and bereavement counselling are not within the scope of this chapter, but arrangements for follow-up may need to be initiated at the outset. If the nurse or doctor concerned in the emergency department feels able, he or she can offer to be available for any questions later. Some departments have a social worker who can provide practical help and co-ordinate follow-up. If death occurs, it is helpful to have a routine checklist, which includes notifying the general practitioner. An open invitation can be posted to the relatives, offering an interview with a consultant so that questions on the events or necropsy findings can be answered. Many take up this offer, sometimes months later, to fill in gaps in their information which helps them to make some sense of what happened.

An up-to-date leaflet explaining official procedures slipped into a relative's pocket is useful for later perusal (for example, leaflet D49, *What to Do after Death*, published by the Department of Health) (Figure 17.4). Participation by the coroner's officer, who may be a policeman, should be explained. Warning relatives of the possibility that they may develop symptoms of post-traumatic stress disorder is appropriate in certain cases. Such symptoms include depression, anxiety and flashbacks, with a wide range of severity. Also, a necessary part of follow-up may be to warn them about the possibility of avoiding or unhelpful actions by neighbours.

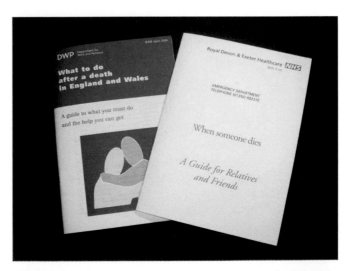

Figure 17.4 Booklets explaining bereavement, the local arrangements and official procedures after a death.

A local leaflet explaining possible reactions, and local information on the coroner, registration of a death and arranging the funeral should also be provided. Details of any support organisations such as CRUSE, RoadPeace or any local groups should be included (Box 17.12).

Box 17.12 National contact addresses

CRUSE Bereavement Care
crusebereavementcare.org.uk
Email: helpline@cruse.org.uk
Helpline: 0844 477 9400 daytime

The Compassionate Friends (for bereaved parents)
www.rcf.org.uk
Helpline: 08451 232304

Foundation for the Study of Infant Deaths
fsid.org.uk
Tel: 0808 802 6868
Email: helpline@fsid.org.uk

NHS National Organ Donor Register
www.organdsonation.nhs.uk
Tel: 0300 123 2323

National Blood Service
www.blood.co.uk
Tel: 0300 123 2323

RoadPeace (information and support after deaths on the road)
www.roadpeace.org
Helpline: 0845 4500 355

Samaritans (for the despairing)
www.samaritans.org
PO Box 9090, Stirling FK8 2SA
Helpline: 08457 909090

Sudden Death Support Association (support for families after accidental or traumatic deaths)
Dolphin House, Part Lane, Swallowfield, Reading, Berkshire RG7 1TB
Tel: 0118 988 9797

TACT: Trauma After-Care Trust (support for bereaved people experiencing post-traumatic stress disorder)
www.tacthq.demon.co.uk
Butfield, 1 The Farthings, Withington, Gloucestershire GL54 4DF
Tel: 01242 890306
Email: tact@tacthq-demon.co.uk

Staff support

Lastly, do not forget the carers. Staff do not recognise their own needs, and encouragement and 'permission' are needed for them to express their feelings. Senior staff should be responsible for facilitating this, and for recognising that some staff may need further support or even professional counselling. There are many different reactions, the most common of which are sadness, anger and guilt (Parris *et al.* 2007). Staff, including the ambulance crew, may identify with particular people or situations. For example, the death of a child will be particularly upsetting, especially for members of staff with children of the same age. Part of the debriefing on major trauma must include an opportunity for members of staff to express their feelings. After a major trauma (or any emotive incident), staff should be allowed a short break to recover and perhaps discuss the incident before returning to more mundane duties.

After a critical incident (that is, any incident causing an unusually strong emotional reaction), staff should be given an opportunity to defuse. This is done by compulsorily calling together all staff involved and providing key facts; then, with the leader keeping a low profile, the group should be allowed to freely discuss the incident and their roles. The beginning of nurse report or handover may also be an opportunity to defuse. The meeting is best terminated, once all is said, by the leader expressing thanks and noting the team's strengths, and that distress is normal after such events; for example, 'It was the event that was abnormal, not you . . .'.

After a large-scale or major incident, staff should be demobilised at the end of the incident or shift. As with defusing, everyone who took part should attend; however, demobilisation has a time limit (10–15 min) and is characterised by clear leadership and limited participation by staff. The leader provides a factual overview of the incident, the casualties and their progress, and reassures the staff that they did a good job. The meeting should finish in the same way as a defusing session, with the additional offer of further support if necessary.

Occasionally, staff may request or need critical incident stress debriefing. This is a more formal procedure, where the staff member sees a trained counsellor over several sessions. There is probably no advantage in providing such debriefing routinely, but staff should have access to a local facility.

The purpose of informal or formal support is to allow staff to return to normal function, acknowledge distress, and show them that someone cares. Senior staff must not be forgotten, and should support one another. Facilitating such support presents a challenge in busy, often understaffed departments, but meeting the challenge is rewarded by a reduction in staff stress and related problems.

Summary

The suddenness and severity of major trauma make it especially difficult to cope with, for relatives and staff. However bad the news is, relatives need direct, honest information and genuine care and support. Many doctors find this important part of their work difficult. Reasons have been suggested for this (Robinson *et al* 1998). Awareness may help the situation, and lead to more emphasis during training on acquiring the appropriate skills.

The principles of dealing with distressed relatives can be summarised as follows.

- Empathise; sit, listen and reflect back relatives' reactions rather than making assumptions or categorising them.
- Enable relatives to accept the reality and pain by being honest and allowing them easy access to their loved one.
- Encourage them, by suggesting 'You will be able to cope' (with help if needed).
- Encounter your own feelings and express them later, perhaps as part of a debriefing or defusing session.

Acknowledgement

I thank Sister Susan Judge, Reverend Bob Irving, Dr Sheila Cassidy and the staff of the emergency department, Derriford Hospital, Plymouth, for ideas and advice; Jackie Eccleson for typing the manuscript; and the photographic department. I also thank the relatives whose actions, comments and questions have formed the basis of this chapter.

Further reading

Department of Health. (2005) *When a Patient Dies*. www.dh.gov.uk /policyandguidance/healthandsocialcare/bereavement/fs/en

Merlevede E, Spooren D, Henderick H, *et al.* (2004) Perceptions, needs and mourning reactions of bereaved relatives confronted with a sudden unexpected death. Resuscitation 61: 341–8.

Parris RJ, Schlosenberg J, Stanley C, *et al.* (2007) Emergency department follow-up of bereaved relatives: an audit of one particular service. Emerg Med J 24: 339–42.

Resuscitation Council (UK). (1996) *Should Relatives Witness Resuscitation?* London: Resuscitation Council (UK).

Robinson S, MacKenzie-Ross S, Campbell Hewson G, Egleston C, Prevost A. (1998) Psychological effect of witnessed resuscitation on bereaved relatives. Lancet 352: 614–17.

Wright B. (1996) *Sudden Death*, 2nd edn. Edinburgh: Churchill Livingstone.

CHAPTER 18

Trauma in Pregnancy

Rebecca S. Black and Deborah J. Harrington

John Radcliffe Hospital, Oxford, UK

OVERVIEW

- Pregnant women must be managed on a tilt.
- The primary survey is identical to that for the non-pregnant patient.
- Adequate resuscitation of the mother is the best way to resuscitate the fetus.
- Blood loss is frequently underestimated.
- Cardiac arrest in pregnancy requires caesarean section to improve the chances of maternal survival.

In pregnancy, the aims of resuscitation and treatment are the same as in the non-pregnant patient with the addition of maintenance of the uteroplacental unit. However, anatomical and physiological changes must be taken into consideration from the primary survey onwards. Assessment of the fetus takes place after the primary survey.

Airway and breathing

The airway may be difficult in pregnancy. Intubation can be made more hazardous by oedema of the face and neck (especially in pre-eclampsia) and by increased breast size. Pregnant patients are more likely to regurgitate and aspirate because of delayed gastric emptying and increased reflux. Continuous cricoid pressure should be applied during positive pressure ventilation of any pregnant woman.

Circulation

The fetus is an end-organ and fetal distress can be an early sign of maternal hypovolaemia. This is because the mother will decrease blood flow to the fetoplacental unit to compensate for hypovolaemia before there are any obvious clinical signs. A pregnant woman can lose 35% of her circulating blood volume before signs of hypovolaemia develop. Blood pressure in particular is

unreliable. Mothers become tachycardic long before they develop hypotension.

In heavily pregnant (i.e. third trimester) women, lying supine causes aortocaval compression. Pregnant women, with a uterus palpable above the umbilicus, must be managed on a tilt, and tilted to the left hand side (Box 18.1).

Box 18.1 **Key treatment point**

To prevent aortocaval compression, **pregnant women MUST be placed on a TILT**.

Primary survey

As in the non-pregnant patient, the primary survey starts with the airway with cervical spine control, but in addition the patient must be tilted. This can be achieved on an extrication board, aiming for a tilt of at least 15° and up to 30°. Alternatively the uterus can be displaced manually to the left.

High-flow oxygen is always indicated in pregnant trauma victims. Intravenous fluid is required with two large-bore cannulae. Blood should be sent for testing (Box 18.2). Most patients in the UK carry their own 'hand-held' obstetric notes (Box 18.3) which should provide information about relevant issues. If the blood group is known then group-specific blood can be requested.

Physiological changes in pregnancy are shown in Box 18.4.

Box 18.2 **Blood tests in pregnant trauma patients**

Full blood count.
  Urea and electrolytes.
  Cross-match.
  Clotting.
  Amylase.
  Glucose.
  Pregnancy test.*

*A pregnancy test should be sent early in gestation or if any doubt about pregnancy status exists.

ABC of Major Trauma, Fourth Edition. Edited by David V. Skinner and Peter A. Driscoll.
© 2013 Blackwell Publishing Ltd. Published 2013 by Blackwell Publishing Ltd.

Box 18.3 **Obstetric 'hand-held' notes**

Notes should contain information on:

- Blood group.
- Rhesus status.
- Serological status (hepatitis B, HIV).
- Recent haemoglobin level.
- Known allergies.
- Current pregnancy:
  - Gestation
  - Number of fetuses
  - Placental site
  - Current medication
  - Pregnancy complications (e.g. pre-eclampsia, diabetes).
- Previous pregnancies:
  - Number of previous pregnancies
  - Previous pregnancy complications (e.g. caesarean section, postpartum haemorrhage).
- Past medical history.

Box 18.4 **Pregnancy changes**

- Cardiac output increased by 40% from first trimester.
- Pulse rate increased by 10%.
- Blood pressure falls from the first trimester, rising back towards pre-pregnancy levels during the third trimester.
- Plasma volume increases by 50%.
- There is a physiological anaemia and iron deficiency is common (normal range for pregnancy 11–14 g/dL).

Assessment of the fetus can be performed according to the contents of Box 18.5.

Secondary survey

Assessment of the mother is similar to the non-pregnant patient. X-rays should not be withheld if indicated in trauma. The radiographer should be made aware and the fetus shielded wherever possible.

Fetomaternal haemorrhage

A Kleihauer test should always be sent (usually an EDTA tube of blood sent to haematology). This test determines the amount of fetal blood in the maternal circulation.

Women who are Rhesus negative should be given an intramuscular injection of anti-D. The anti-D prevents the mother developing Rhesus antibodies. A dose of 500 IU of anti-D immunoglobulin is sufficient for a fetomaternal haemorrhage of up to 4 mL. The Kleihauer test result will indicate if the fetomaternal haemorrhage has been greater than this and therefore if any further anti-D is required.

Anti-D should be administered as soon as possible after the sensitising event and always within 72 h. If pregnant women delay

Box 18.5 **Assessment of the fetus**

Check hand-held obstetric notes if possible.

History

- Fetal movements.
- Uterine pain/tenderness/tightenings/contractions.
- Vaginal loss.

Examination

- Symphysiofundal height.
- Uterine tenderness/irritability/contraction.
- Speculum to look for blood/liquor.
- Digital examination to assess cervical dilation/effacement.

Investigation

- Ultrasound can be used to assess:
  - fetal heart: presence and rate
  - fetal movements
  - fetal position
  - placental site
  - amniotic fluid volume
  - *retroplacental clot
  - **uterine rupture
- Cardiotocography: to monitor fetal heart rate pattern.

*Placental abruption (separation of the placenta from the wall of the uterus) leads to formation of a retroplacental clot. A retroplacental clot may be seen on ultrasound but the diagnosis of abruption is usually clinically obvious. An abruption large enough to be seen on scan will have clinical symptoms and signs. These include uterine pain, tenderness and hardness (classically the uterus is 'woody hard'). There is often vaginal bleeding but some or all of the blood may be concealed, in which case the woman will show a level of shock out of proportion to the revealed blood loss. Fetuses tolerate abruption poorly and with a large abruption may well be dead. There may be a coagulopathy, particularly if the abruption is large enough to cause fetal death.

**An abnormal fetal position with free fluid in the abdomen may suggest uterine rupture. If the fetus is free in the abdomen it will probably be dead (Box 18.6).

Box 18.6 **Indications for caesarean section**

- Access required at caesarean section to adequately assess abdominal organs.
- Penetrating abdominal trauma.
- Uterine rupture.
- Unstable pelvic/lumbosacral fracture with woman in labour.
- Fetal distress with a viable fetus.
- Maternal cardiac arrest.

in presenting then there is still evidence of some benefit up to 10 days after the sensitising event so anti-D should still be given in these circumstances.

In the case of Rhesus-positive women, no anti-D is required but if the Kleihauer shows that a significant fetomaternal haemorrhage has occurred then the fetus warrants further monitoring and surveillance.

Blunt trauma

Blunt trauma is caused by road traffic crashes, assaults and falls. It commonly causes placental abruption. Blood loss is frequently underestimated. In placental abruption, caesarean section is not necessarily indicated, especially if the fetus is dead. Delivery following abruption whether abdominally or vaginally is likely to lead to postpartum haemorrhage (PPH). Disseminated intravascular coagulation (DIC) can further exacerbate blood loss.

Uterine rupture is rare but fetal mortality is high if it does occur. Caesarean section is indicated and caesarean hysterectomy is sometime required. Again, the risk of PPH is high.

All pregnant women should be advised on the correct use of seatbelts in pregnancy. Three-point seatbelts should be worn with the lap strap placed as low as possible beneath the 'bump', lying across the thighs with the diagonal strap above the bump lying between the breasts – 'above and below the bump, not over it'.

Domestic violence is common in pregnancy and should not be forgotten as a cause of trauma.

Penetrating trauma

The uterus is vulnerable to penetrating trauma, particularly in late pregnancy. Fetal survival is poor but maternal survival is better. The uterus provides some degree of protection to maternal organs such as the bowel.

Cardiac arrest

This is rare in pregnancy. The reversible causes occurring in pregnancy are:

- hypoxia
- hypovolaemia
- hyperkalaemia and other metabolic disorders
- hypotension
- thromboembolism
- toxicity
- tension pneumothorax
- cardiac tamponade
- eclampsia.

It is difficult to perform effective cardiopulmonary resuscitation (CPR) in a pregnant woman. Pregnant women become hypoxic more quickly because of increased oxygen consumption and a reduced functional residual capacity. Delivery of the fetus reverses these effects and therefore improves the chances of maternal survival.

Chest compression should be slightly above the centre of the sternum to adjust for elevation of the diaphragm and abdominal contents caused by the gravid uterus. If the woman is on a firm surface she should be tilted. If not, the uterus should be manually displaced.

Defibrillation, if appropriate, is performed using standard defibrillation doses. There is no evidence of adverse fetal effects from a direct current defibrillator.

If after 4 minutes of effective CPR there has been no return of spontaneous circulation, a caesarean section should be instigated. It is for the benefit of the mother and not the fetus. CPR must

be continued during the procedure. Delivery is achievable in less than 1 min. A midline laparotomy incision has the advantage of being quick and relatively bloodless and allows access to the other internal organs (and possibly internal cardiac massage). If, however, the operator is more comfortable with a low transverse abdominal incision then this is considered acceptable. A scalpel and two clamps for the umbilical cord are the only equipment required.

Although the aim of the perimortem caesarean section is to improve the mother's chances of successful resuscitation, neonatal survival has been reported and is related to gestation. In the most recent triennial report into maternal deaths in the UK (2006–08), there was a 47% survival in fetuses delivered after 36 weeks' gestation.

The 2000–2002 report commented on postmortem (Box 18.7) caesarean section: 'In this and all previous triennia, no baby has survived a postmortem caesarean section . . . These findings underscore the futility of attempting a postmortem section'.

Box 18.7 **Types of caesarean section**

Perimortem

Carried out *in extremis* while the mother is undergoing active resuscitation.

Postmortem

Carried out after the death of the mother in order to save the fetus.

Burns

The outcome for the mother with burns is unaffected by pregnancy. The fetal outcome depends on the extent of the burn and on gestation. If the fetus is more than 32 weeks' gestation then delivery is advised if the burns are extensive.

Further reading

CEMACH. (2003) *Why Mothers Die 2000–2002. Report on Confidential Enquiries into Maternal Deaths in the United Kingdom.* London: CEMACH.

CEMACH. (2006) *Saving Mothers' Lives 2003–2005 – The 7th Report of the Confidential Enquiries into Maternal Deaths in the United Kingdom.* London: CEMACH.

Centre for Maternal and Child Enquiries (CMACE). (2011) Saving Mothers' Lives: reviewing maternal deaths to make motherhood safer: 2006–08. The Eighth Report on Confidential Enquiries into Maternal Deaths in the United Kingdom. BJOG 118(Suppl. 1):1–203.

Cox C, Grady K. (1999) *Managing Obstetric Emergencies.* Oxford: BIOS Scientific Publishers.

Grady K, Howell C, Cox C (eds). (2007) *Managing Obstetric Emergencies and Trauma: The MOET Course Manual,* 2nd edn. London: RCOG Press.

Nelson-Piercy N. (2010) *Handbook of Obstetric Medicine,* 4th edn. Oxford: Informa.

Royal College of Obstetrics and Gynaecologists. The use of anti-D immunoglobulin for Rhesus prophylaxis. Green Top Guideline no.22, March 2011. www.rcog.org.uk.

Vanden Hoek TL, Morrison LJ, Shuster M, *et al.* (2010) Part 12: Cardiac Arrest in Special Situations: 2010 American Heart Association Guidelines for Cardiopulmonary Resuscitation and Emergency Cardiovascular Care. Circulation1;22:S829–S861.

CHAPTER 19

Paediatric Trauma

John J. M. Black

John Radcliffe Hospital, Oxford, UK

OVERVIEW

- Paediatric major trauma systematic assessment.
- Trauma team activation.
- Primary and secondary survey.
- Prehospital and emergency department initial management.
- Complex injury assessment.

Trauma remains the most common cause of death in childhood; road traffic accidents and falls account for more than 80% of significant injuries (Box 19.1).

Box 19.1 **Causes of childhood trauma**

- *Age 0–1 years*: choking/suffocation, burns, drowning, falls.
- *Age 1–4 years*: road traffic accidents (as vehicle occupant), burns, drowning, falls.
- *Age 5–14 years*: road traffic accidents (as vehicle occupant or pedestrian), bicycle injuries, burns, drowning.

The response of children to injury is quite different from that of adults, physically, physiologically and emotionally. The more frightened the child, the less will he or she be able to contribute to management. All symptoms may be denied.

Because children are small, blunt mechanisms of injury often result in multisystem injury. An injured child must therefore be assumed to have multiple injuries until proven otherwise. Life-threatening injuries found in the primary survey must be treated as soon as they are identified; treatment must not be delayed while evaluation of the child is completed.

Although injured children present several specific problems, the approach for their initial management is similar to that adopted for adults. Physiologically compromised children must be assessed and treated simultaneously by a well-lead and experienced trauma team.

ABC of Major Trauma, Fourth Edition. Edited by David V. Skinner and Peter A. Driscoll.
© 2013 Blackwell Publishing Ltd. Published 2013 by Blackwell Publishing Ltd.

A structured approach is essential to ensure correct identification and prioritisation of injuries.

Which hospital?

Ideally, seriously injured children should be transported directly from the scene of injury to an emergency department (ED) with appropriate paediatric, surgical and critical care support on site that can manage the child's entire injury pattern. Hospitals that manage high volumes of major trauma have better patient outcomes. The need to undertake interhospital transfer invariably significantly delays time to definitive surgical care which in itself can also impact significantly on subsequent morbidity and mortality. In the UK, recent audits have demonstrated that it takes an average of 2 h for well-run district general hospitals to assess, initially manage and then package patients for transfer. Until regional major trauma centres ('National Trauma Service') are set up and supported by integrated ambulance transport and critical care networks throughout the UK, children will continue to be transported to the nearest hospital's emergency department, irrespective of its surgical resources. Regional trauma network roll out is due to be completed in England during 2012 (see Chapter 21).

Trauma team activation

A trauma team, with predetermined roles and responsibilities, should be assembled at the time of a request from the ambulance service through a dedicated phone line into the emergency department control room. Criteria should be agreed locally but should factor in high-energy injury mechanism, physiological compromise or signs of severe injury to more than one body region (Box 19.2). A reduced level of consciousness is one of the most useful single clinical predictors for major trauma.

Failure to assemble a trauma team prior to patient's arrival in the emergency department will seriously compromise the quality of patient handover and there is a very real risk that the patient's management may stall upon arrival at hospital. The handover to the trauma team should be undertaken in a standardised manner once the patient has been transferred onto a resuscitation room trolley and the airway has been handed over to an identified clinician (see Box 19.2). This should not take longer than 1–2 min at the most (see Chapter 21).

Box 19.2 Trauma team activation

Mechanism

- Fall from significant height (first floor or above).
- Ejection from vehicle.
- Penetrating injury to neck or torso.
- Death of same vehicle occupant.
- Near drowning.

Examination findings

- Airway obstruction.
- Hypoxia, respiratory distress or ventilatory failure.
- Signs of shock.
- Reduced level of consciousness (AVPU score of V or less).
- Serious injury to more than one body region.

ATMIST handover

- Age.
- Time of incident.
- Mechanism of Injury.
- Injuries identified top to toe
- Treatment.
- Summary and immediate needs.

Primary survey and resuscitation

After handover, the patient should undergo a prompt systematic primary survey and any immediately life-threatening injuries should be treated as they are identified (Box 19.3). This is best done by an experienced clinician who should verbalise their findings for the team leader who should remain 'hands off' and focus on team direction. If relatives of the child have accompanied him or her to hospital, a team member should obtain an 'AMPLE' history (Box 19.4).

Box 19.3 Structured approach to the injured child

- Primary survey and resuscitation.
  - Airway and cervical spine control
  - Breathing and ventilation
  - Circulation and haemorrhage control
  - Dysfunction of the central nervous system
  - Exposure and environment
- Secondary survey.
- Definitive care.

Box 19.4 AMPLE history

- Allergies
- Medication
- Past medical history
- Last ate and drank
- Environment – accident details

With an estimate of the weight of the child, it is possible to predict appropriate volume replacement and drug doses. An approximate weight can be derived from nomograms based on head-to-toe length (Broselowe/Sandell tape or the Oakley Paediatric Resuscitation Chart; see Figure 19.1). Alternatively, for children aged 1–10 years the following formula can be used to estimate body weight:

$$\text{Body weight (kg)} = \{\text{Age (years)} + 4\} \times 2$$

The appropriate sizes and indications for use of paediatric equipment according to age (approximate weight) of the child are shown in Table 19.1. Normal values for paediatric vital signs in patients not crying are shown in Table 19.2.

Airway management with cervical spine control

After control of catastrophic but compressible external haemorrhage by prehospital personnel, maintenance of airway patency is the most critical part of the initial assessment and management of the injured child. A child with noisy breathing has partial airway obstruction that requires immediate assessment and appropriate intervention.

Children have specific anatomical differences from adults that can hinder airway maintenance and may complicate definitive airway management.

- Relatively large occiput, which causes flexion of the head on the neck when the child lies on a firm surface, e.g. a spinal board; this may cause complete upper airway obstruction.
- Small oral cavity with a relatively large tongue.
- A compressible floor of the mouth.
- Hypertrophy of the tonsils and adenoids (common in preschool children), more likely to bleed if traumatised.
- A large, horseshoe-shaped, floppy epiglottis which, with its more acute angle with the laryngeal opening, makes access to the relatively cephalad and anterior larynx difficult.
- Short (in infants, non-existent) cricothyroid membrane makes needle cricothyroidotomy difficult; surgical cricothyroidotomy is impossible in infants.
- Cricoid ring is the narrowest part of the upper airway.
- Short trachea; this increases the risk of mainstem bronchus intubation.
- Symmetry of the carina in the infant, which may result in inadvertent intubation of either main bronchus.

All injured children must receive supplemental oxygen via a well fitting and moulded Hudson (non-rebreathing) reservoir mask, which will deliver an inspired oxygen concentration of approximately 85%. Fogging of the inside of the mask will confirm airway patency and spontaneous ventilation and can give an indication of respiratory rate. If the child appears to be apnoeic, the head should be placed in the neutral position. If this alone is not adequate to open the airway, a jaw thrust will passively bring the tongue anteriorly and thus potentially relieve airway obstruction within the oropharynx. A jaw thrust is less likely than a chin lift to compromise an unstable cervical spine injury. Take care to place the fingers accurately under the mandible to avoid precipitating airway obstruction (Figure 19.2).

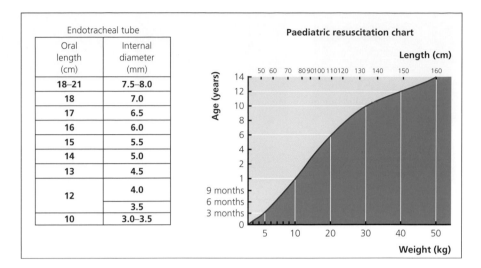

Figure 19.1 Paediatric resuscitation chart.

Table 19.1 Appropriate sizes and indications for use of paediatric equipment according to the age (approximate weight) of the child.

Equipment	0–6 months (1–6 kg)	6–12 months (4–9 kg)	1–3 years (10–15 kg)	4–7 years (16–20 kg)	8–11 years (22–33 kg)
Airway/breathing:					
Oxygen facepiece	0	0/1	1	1/2	2/3 (Adult)
Oral airways	000/00	0/1	0/1	1/2	2
Resuscitator	Baby	Baby	Baby/adult	Adult	Adult
Breathing system	"T" piece	"T" piece	"T" piece	"T" piece	Coaxial
Tracheal tubes (uncuffed; mm diameter)	2.5–3.5	3.5–4.0	4.0–5.0	5.0–6.0	5.5–7.0
Stylet	Small	Small	Small/medium	Medium	Medium
Suction catheter (FG)	6	8	10–12	14	14
Circulation:					
Intravenous cannula (G)	24/22	22	22/18	20/16	18/14
Central venous pressure cannula (G)	20	20	18	18	16
Arterial cannula (G)	24/22	22	22	22	20
Ancillary equipment:					
Nasogastric tube (FG)	8	10	10–12	12	12–14
Chest drain (FG)	10–4	12–18	14–20	14–24	16–30
Urinary catheter (FG)	5 Feeding tube	5 Feeding tube/Foley (8)	Foley (8)	Foley (10)	Foley (10–12)

Exact measurements in children are extremely important. Endotracheal tubes are measured in mm outside diameter (OD). Catheters, naosgastric tubes and chest drains are measured in French Gauge (FG) or Charrière (CH) (the same) which is the circumference in mm. ΠD is the formula for a circumference, so divide by Π (roughly 3) for the diameter in mm. G is short for SWG (standard wire gauge), which is an entirely different method of measuring needles.

Table 19.2 Normal values for paediatric vital signs in patients not crying.

Age	Heart rate (beats/min)	Blood pressure (systolic) (mm Hg)	Respiratory rate (breaths/min)	Blood volume (ml/kg)
<1 year	120–140	70–90	30–40	90
2–5 years	100–120	80–90	20–30	80
5–12 years	80–100	90–110	15–20	80

Gurgling when the child starts to breathe may indicate blood or secretions in the upper airway, which should be cleared by judicious use of suction under direct vision.

Grunting or snoring indicates upper airway obstruction by the tongue. If a jaw thrust relieves this, an oropharyngeal airway of appropriate size is likely to be needed to maintain airway patency.

A nasopharyngeal airway may be better tolerated in a less obtunded child but particular care must be taken when inserting these devices because of the vascularity of the nasal mucosa. Suspicion of an anterior base of skull fracture is a relative but not an absolute contraindication to nasal airway use.

Stridor in an injured child implies upper airway obstruction at laryngeal level and the need for a definitive airway at the earliest opportunity (e.g. inhalation burn).

Children who require regular upper airway suctioning and who tolerate an oral airway are likely to require early definitive airway management in the context of major trauma, as will children who remain hypoxic despite high-flow oxygen.

In any child with significant injury above the level of the clavicles, an unstable cervical spine injury must be assumed until excluded, accepting that this is a rare injury in children. Restore the child's

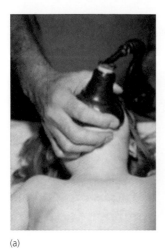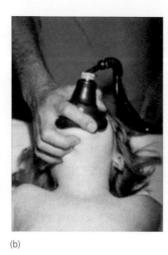

(a)   (b)

Figure 19.2 Maintaining a clear airway. (a) WRONG – supporting fingers placed in the submental triangle causing posterior displacement of the tongue and airway obstruction. (b) CORRECT – placement of the hand and jaw lift.

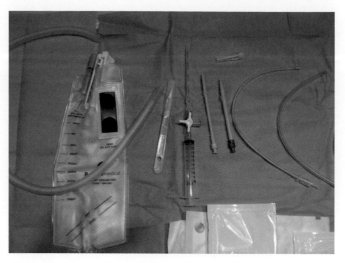

Figure 19.3 A percutaneous seldinger chest drain set designed for use in small children. This set has been specifically designed for prehospital use in a major incident.

head and neck to the neutral position and hold manually with inline mobilisation in the first instance. Hold the head thus until a suitable semi-rigid collar or sand bags and tape have been applied. The child will usually have been placed onto a long board to facilitate vehicular extrication and placed in an orthopaedic scoop stretcher by prehospital personnel to facilitate spinal packaging for onward transport to hospital. The child should be removed from any spinal packaging device at the earliest opportunity to reduce pain and the risk of decubitus ulceration of the skin, and to facilitate radiographic imaging. Unless the patient is being transported directly to the operating theatre, this should be done by the end of the primary survey. Modern resuscitation room trolleys provide perfectly adequate thoracolumbar support.

Breathing

If opening and clearance of the child's airway do not result in spontaneous ventilation, then assisted ventilation via a bag-valve-mask (BVM) with a reservoir attached will be required to deliver 100% oxygen. Placing an oropharyngeal airway before starting assisted ventilation may improve airway patency and also reduce gastric distension and thus the risk of aspiration. The BVM must have a blow-off valve set at 30–40 cm of water to reduce the risk of causing pulmonary barotrauma and life-threatening gastric dilation. It may be necessary to obstruct (with caution) the BVM blow-off valve in the face of low pulmonary compliance to achieve satisfactory ventilation.

An alternative strategy to using airway adjunct and BVM is the use of an appropriate sized laryngeal mask airway which may in non-anaesthetic hands achieve more effective ventilation.

Children who develop tension pneumothorax will require prompt pleural decompression (needle thoracocentesis or finger thoracostomy) and subsequent tube thoracostomy. Large simple pneumothoraces associated with hypoxia are also likely to require tube thoracostomy (Figure 19.3), especially if positive pressure ventilation will be required (e.g. for emergency surgery).

Tracheal intubation

Indications for tracheal intubation in an injured child are:

- failure to maintain or protect the airway
- failure of ventilation or oxygenation
- the anticipated clinical course.

Failure to anticipate upper airway obstruction after an inhalation burn or penetrating wound to the anterior neck may be catastrophic, because distortion of the upper airway anatomy may make later intubation extremely difficult. Non-alert head-injured children with or without focal neurological signs should be considered for early endotracheal intubation for safe transfer to the computed tomography (CT) suite. Unstable children who will require early definitive surgery or transfer to a tertiary centre should be intubated before leaving the emergency department. The hazards of transfer, even to a nearby radiology department, cannot be overstated.

Laryngoscopes with straight blades are widely used in infants. Traditionally curved blades have been used in older children, and the 'adult method' adopted for laryngoscopy (blade inserted into the vallecula). However, with airway trauma and a distorted upper anatomy, the straight Miller blade can be extremely valuable if inserted into the proximal oesophagus and then slowly withdrawn; the tip is used to control the epiglottis directly, thus providing optimal exposure of the glottis. This is particularly helpful when inline immobilisation has left the glottis in an unfavourable position. Any semi-rigid cervical collar should be loosened or removed before laryngoscopy to prevent needless restriction of mandibular movement.

Immediate management of critically ill children is greatly enhanced by storing airway, breathing and circulation equipment in colour-coded resuscitation cart drawers using the Broselow type system. Cuffed endotracheal tubes may be useful when pulmonary compliance is low in the context of severe injury. Should endotracheal intubation be required in the field, use of armoured (reinforced) endotracheal (ET) tubes introduced using a stylet may be particularly helpful in small children in whom ET tube kinking can become a problem when they are being packaged and transported to hospital. See Box 19.5.

Endotracheal tubes must be well secured; they are easily displaced, especially in small children. The use of Elastoplast tape using a 'split-trouser' technique is very effective in achieving this.

Box 19.5 **Endotracheal tube sizing**

Uncuffed ET tubes should be used until puberty. The correct size can be derived from the formulae:

- ET tube length (cm) = {age (years)/2} + 12
- ET tube diameter (mm) = {age (years)/4} + 4

Cricothryoidotomy

The indication to perform a needle cricothyroidotomy is the 'cannot oxygenate, cannot ventilate' scenario. Surgical cricothyroidotomy should be avoided in children under 12 years old, because of the high risk of damage and late stenosis to the narrowest part of the paediatric airway – the cricoid ring. If a surgical airway is needed formal tracheostomy should be undertaken. The technique for needle cricothyroidotomy is shown in Figure 19.4.

Gastric drainage

An orogastric tube must be passed as soon as the airway has been secured, to prevent gastric distension, diaphragmatic splinting and compression of inferior vena cava, which has the potential to compromise oxygenation and cardiac output. This is a priority in any child that has been resuscitated using a bag valve mask when gastric distension is a common complication of this technique.

Circulation and haemorrhage control

Catastrophic external (compressible) haemorrhage control – <C>ABC – is now the first priority for first responders at the scene of injury and can usually be controlled by direct pressure using elasticated compression bandages. Tourniquets may be required to control life-threatening extremity haemorrhage following limb mangling, proximal amputation, blast or ballistic injury. Ideally, pelvic and long bone fractures should be stabilised and restored to length at the earliest opportunity to achieve early haemorrhage control (see Chapter 21). Vital signs and central capillary refill should be recorded and peripheral skin colour and temperature should be noted. Central capillary refill provides a better guide to adequacy of perfusion in the field setting: in the author's experience the gums are the most suitable location to do this as this assessment is not compromised by ambient environmental temperature. Gum capillary refill may also be particularly useful in both adults and children in the context of major burns.

Normal values for vital signs vary with age. A child's normal systolic blood pressure can be estimated by using the formula:

$$\text{Systolic BP (mmHg)} = 80 + (2 \times \text{age in years}).$$

The physiological reserve of a child's circulation is greater than that of an adult, so vital signs may be only slightly abnormal despite considerable blood loss. Therefore the early diagnosis of impending shock in children is based on the appearance of the skin, the temperature of the extremities, the capillary refill time (normal less than 2 sec) and altered sensorium. The degree of shock, and hence blood loss, can be estimated from the classification of shock (Table 19.3). A resting tachycardia may be the result of fright, pain or hypovolaemia. Hypotension is a late, preterminal sign of hypovolaemic shock.

Circulatory access

Venous access in hypovolaemic children with collapsed veins is difficult, especially in those under 6 years of age.

If there is any difficulty in gaining peripheral intravenous access in unconscious children, immediate intraosseous access should be established. The usual sites are the medial upper tibia, distal to the proximal epiphysis, or the distal third of the femur, proximal to the lateral femoral condyle. Alternative sites include the proximal humerus or calcaneum. Intraosseous (IO) access enables vascular

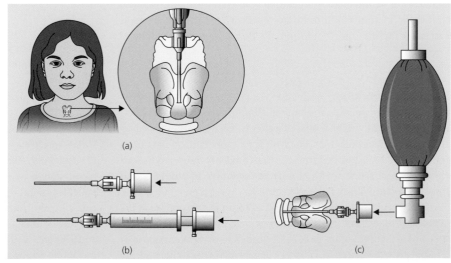

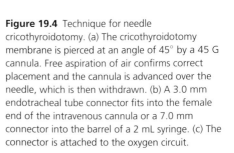

Figure 19.4 Technique for needle cricothyroidotomy. (a) The cricothyroidotomy membrane is pierced at an angle of 45° by a 45 G cannula. Free aspiration of air confirms correct placement and the cannula is advanced over the needle, which is then withdrawn. (b) A 3.0 mm endotracheal tube connector fits into the female end of the intravenous cannula or a 7.0 mm connector into the barrel of a 2 mL syringe. (c) The connector is attached to the oxygen circuit.

(a)

(b)

(c)

Table 19.3 Advanced Trauma Life Support classification of shock in children.

	Class I <15%	Class II 15–25%	Class III 25–40%	Class IV >40%
Cardiovascular system (heart rate in beats/min)	Heart rate ↑ 10–20% Blood pressure normal	Tachycardia (>150) Systolic blood pressure ↓ Pulse pressure ↓	Tachycardia (>150) Systolic blood pressure ↓↓ Pulse pressure ↓↓	Tachycardia/bradycardia Severe hypotension Peripheral pulses absent
Respiratory rate (breaths/min)	Normal	Tachypnoea (35–40)	Tachypnoea	Respiratory rate falls
Skin	Normal	Cool, peripheries cool and clammy	Cold, clammy, cyanotic	Pale, cold
Central nervous system	Normal	Irritable, confused, aggressive	Lethargic	Comatose
Capillary refill time	Normal	Prolonged	Very prolonged	

access to be readily established in less than a minute suitable for drug and fluid administration. All intravenous fluids (crystalloid or blood) must be actively injected into the marrow, usually with a 50 mL syringe. There are now new commercially IO systems suitable for use in larger children and adults (for example, EZ IO) (see Chapter 21).

Alternative sites of venous access include the external jugular or femoral veins. Internal jugular access is hazardous to attempt in a child with a potential cervical spinal injury. The widespread adoption of early IO access has made venous cutdown a procedure rarely performed in critically ill children.

Cellulitis, osteomyelitis or extravasation of intravenous fluids fluids producing a compartment syndrome are potential but rare complications; the IO needle should be removed as soon as adequate venous access has been obtained.

As soon as venous access has been established, blood should be drawn for group and cross-matching and blood glucose estimation, and also for a full blood count and baseline biochemistry. A full cross-match will take about 45 min if the child has not been previously transfused. Type-specific blood can usually be obtained in 15 min and O rhesus-negative blood should be stored in every resuscitation room. Arterial access should be obtained in unstable children, but attempts to achieve it should not delay transfer of the child to an operating theatre or to CT, but it will optimise close monitoring of the child's circulation, gas exchange and response to therapy. A transfixion technique as illustrated in Figure 19.5 is easiest in infants, and should initially be attempted in peripheral arteries.

Fluid administration

The early use of colloids and human albumin in the initial resuscitation of critically ill and injured patients has been questioned by the Cochrane investigators. Until we have more clinical data from much needed randomised trials, current advice is to use crystalloid (physiological saline) in the initial resuscitation of children who have been injured. See Figure 19.6.

All intravenous fluids should be warmed. In prehospital care, the current guidance for older children is that they should receive a bolus of crystalloid of up to 250 mL titrated to presence/absence of a radial pulse and presence/absence of central pulses in penetrating

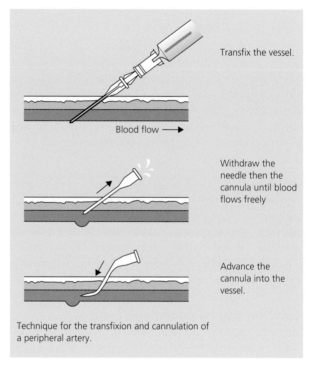

Transfix the vessel.

Blood flow ⟶

Withdraw the needle then the cannula until blood flows freely

Advance the cannula into the vessel.

Technique for the transfixion and cannulation of a peripheral artery.

Figure 19.5 Technique for the transfixion and cannulation of a peripheral artery.

trauma. There is not enough evidence of consensus on what volumes to give infants or young children. However, there is consensus that attempts to administer fluids should not delay transport of patients to hospital.

Current advice in hospitals remains that children should receive an initial bolus of crystalloid 20 mL/kg which should be given rapidly and the cardiovascular response must be dynamically determined. Unless cardiovascular stability is achieved, a second 20 mL/kg bolus of crystalloid should be given. If stability is still not obtained, blood should be given and surgical advice promptly obtained. If patients present with the features of class III or IV shock, blood and clotting factors (tranexamic acid and FFP) should be transfused early as trauma associated coagulopathy (TAC) develops quickly, and a surgical opinion urgently sought. The presence of significant metabolic acidosis (lactate >4 or BE <−5.0) is a useful predicator

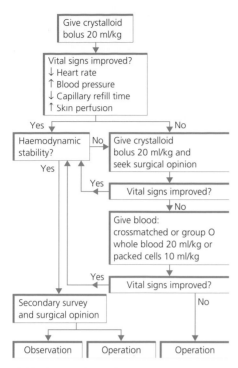

Figure 19.6 Fluid administration pathway.

Table 19.4 Glasgow Coma Scale.

Component	Response	Score
Eye opening	Spontaneous	4
	To speech	3
	To pain	2
	None	1
Best verbal response	Orientated	5
	Confused	4
	Inappropriate words	3
	Incomprehensible sounds	2
	None	1
Best motor response	Obeys commands	6
	Localises to pain	5
	Withdraws from pain	4
	Flexion to pain	3
	Extension to pain	2
	None	1

Table 19.5 Modification of Glasgow Coma Scale for children.

Component	Response	Score
Best verbal response	Appropriate words or social smiles, fixes on and follows objects	5
	Cries but is consolable	4
	Persistently irritable	3
	Restless, agitated	2
	Silent	1
Eye and motor response		Scored as for adults

Neurological dysfunction

The major determinants for survival following a severe head injury are oxygenation and cerebral perfusion. There is therefore little to be gained by focusing on assessment of the head and possible spinal injury until the airway and breathing have been secured and cardiovascular stability obtained. In practice, an initial brief mini neurological examination is performed to assess level of consciousness and papillary reaction. Initially, the AVPU score is sufficient and later a modified Glasgow Coma Scale (GCS) should be determined (Box 19.6; Tables 19.4 and 19.5) during the secondary survey.

Box 19.6 AVPU scoring for level of consciousness

- **A**: **a**lert
- **V**: responds to **v**oice
- **P**: responds to **p**ain
- **U**: **u**nresponsive

Exposure

Removal of all clothing is essential to allow a complete physical examination and facilitate practical procedures. Until the patient has been 'log rolled' and the back examined, up to 50% of the patient has not been adequately checked. Children, especially infants, lose heat rapidly as a result of their high ratio of surface area to weight, thin skin and lack of subcutaneous tissue.

Considerable heat loss may have occurred at the site of injury and during transportation to hospital. Monitoring and maintenance of core temperature is a vital component of initial assessment. A fall in body temperature causes a rise in oxygen consumption as endogenous processes begin to increase heat production, with peripheral vasoconstriction and consequent metabolic acidosis and associated coagulopathy. The ambient temperature of the resuscitation room should be raised and overhead heaters and warming blankets used. Children do not respond well to being exposed in unfamiliar environments and covering the child will also help to preserve dignity.

Trauma X-ray series

Radiographs of the chest and then the pelvis must be taken at the earliest opportunity towards the end of the primary survey; that is, within the first 15 min of admission in major trauma cases. Cervical spine radiographs are not an immediate priority, as injured children should always be treated and handled as if they had an unstable injury of the cervical spine, accepting that this is a rare event. Radiographs should be delayed until cardiorespiratory stability has been obtained. Better quality films will be obtained in the radiology department, where they may be combined with CT if necessary (Figure 19.7).

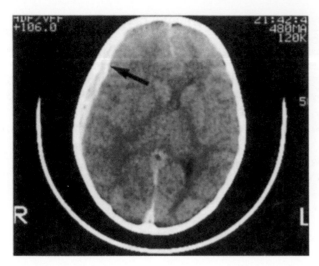

Figure 19.7 Computed tomogram showing right subdural haematoma.

Secondary survey

The principles for the secondary survey are shown in Box 19.7.

Box 19.7 Principles for the secondary survey

- Assess the child systematically, from head to toe, front and back.
- Finding an injury should not stop the remainder of the evaluation.
- Log roll the child to prevent secondary injury to the spinal cord.
- Be gentle and explain clearly to the child any procedure to be performed.
- Record vital signs repeatedly and assess response to therapy.

Head and neck

Fully examine the head for lacerations, the skull for fractures, the eyes for injury (also remember penetrating injury) and pupillary function, the ears and nose for leakage of cerebrospinal fluid, the face for fractures and lacerations, the mouth for loose teeth and finally, the neck for cervical vertebral displacement. Frequent assessment of the GCS is essential. In the infant, palpation of the open fontanelle may give a direct assessment of intracranial pressure.

The initial management of severe head injury is shown in Box 19.8. Primary brain damage that occurs at the time of the injury cannot be reversed. Secondary brain damage occurs as a result of cerebral hypoxia or hypercarbia or profound hypotension and can be minimised by ensuring full oxygenation, optimising ventilation and maintaining adequate cerebral perfusion pressure (Box 19.9).

A child's brain is vulnerable to accelerative, decelerative and shear forces that result in focal intracranial mass lesions (cerebral contusions, lacerations and haemorrhages) and cerebral oedema. Raised intracranial pressure secondary to diffuse cerebral swelling and axonal injury is the most common cause of death in children with head injuries.

Acute subdural haematomas are often bilateral; there is a high incidence of an associated primary brain injury and seizures, and a low incidence of skull fractures.

Box 19.8 Initial management of severe head injury

- Adequate oxygenation (but avoid hyperoxia).
- Trachael intubation.
- Controlled ventilation (maintain ET $PaCO_2$ 4.5–5.0 kPa).
- Restoration of mean arterial pressure (>70 mmHg) and early haemorrhage control.
- Prompt neurosurgical referral.
- Administration of mannitol 0.5–1.0 g/kg (following neurosurgical advice only).
- Timely and safe transfer to a neurosurgical unit or neuro-intensive care unit.

Box 19.9 Causes of secondary brain injury

- Hypoxia.
- Hypercarbia.
- Cerebral ischaemia:
  - Systemic hypotension
  - Fall in cerebral perfusion secondary to raised intracranial pressure from cerebral oedema or an intracranial mass lesion.

If there is no history of appreciable trauma, consider the possibility of non-accidental injury.

Extradural haematomas are most often unilateral and associated with a high incidence of skull fractures and a low incidence of seizures. The biphasic presentation of extradural haematomas ('lucid interval') is less common in children.

About 75% of skull fractures are linear, but they may be depressed, compound or basal, and in children younger than 3 years, the cranial sutures can undergo traumatic separation (diasteal fractures).

The clinical manifestations of raised intracranial pressure or skull fractures are the same in children as in adults. Infants with open fontanelles and mobile sutures, however, are more tolerant to an expanding intracranial mass, although when decompensation does occur it is rapid and often irrecoverable. A bulging fontanelle or suture diastases in an infant imply serious cerebral trauma.

The indications in hospital for establishing a definitive airway in children with head injury are coma (GCS <9, i.e. not obeying, speaking or opening eyes), loss of protective laryngeal reflexes, ventilatory insufficiency (PaO_2 <9 kPa on air or <13 kPa on oxygen; $PaCO_2$ >6 kPa), spontaneous hyperventilation ($PaCO_2$ <3.5 kPa) or respiratory arrhythmia. The aim should be to initially achieve a PaO_2 >15 kPa on supplemental oxygen and a $PaCO_2$ of 4.0–4.5 kPa.

Restoration of systemic blood pressure by judicious volume replacement is vital and should not be limited by concerns about the potential for aggravating cerebral oedema. For serious head injuries, a neurosurgical opinion should be sought early and a brain CT scan performed as soon as the patient is haemodynamically stable. There is increasing evidence that therapy directed at lowering intracranial pressure (ICP), guided by direct ICP monitoring, improves neurological outcome. Early decompressive craniectomy may have a role in selected patients with medically refactory intracranial hypertension.

In children, head injury alone does not usually produce shock and hypotension as a result of hypovolaemia; most bleeding usually occurs elsewhere in the body. Extensive scalp lacerations, however, may bleed sufficiently to cause hypovolaemic shock in small children. In small infants intracranial haemorrhage alone may be sufficient to cause hypovolaemia.

After head injury vomiting and seizures are more common in children than in adults. Both symptoms tend to be self-limiting, but if either persists a serious head injury should be suspected. Repeated seizures cause an increase in intracranial pressure by increasing cerebral blood flow, and anticonvulsants should be given. Intravenous diazepam 0.15–0.25 mg/kg is the drug of first choice; this may cause respiratory depression and may precipitate the need for ventilation. Phenytoin 15–20 mg/kg by slow intravenous injection (1–2 mg/kg/min) may subsequently be necessary with continuous electrocardiogram monitoring.

Minor head injury is extremely common in children and vomiting is a poor predictor of intracranial injury. Selective plain radiography of the skull may have a place if reserved for children who are well enough to be discharged from hospital (full level of consciousness, no neurological symptoms and no neurological signs) but have local signs within the scalp consistent with a vault fracture. The identification of a skull fracture by X-ray increases the likelihood of intracranial haemorrhage 10-fold in this context. CT is now readily accessible in all UK emergency departments and thresholds for CT should be low if there is any clinical suspicion of intracranial injury, witnessed loss of consciousness, or if a vault fracture has been identified on plain films (Box 19.10). Children with minor head injury should be observed in the ED or admitted until they are fully conscious and systemically asymptomatic.

Box 19.10 **Criteria for immediate request for CT scan of the head in children (NICE)**

- Loss of consciousness lasting more than 5 min (witnessed).
- Amnesia (antegrade or retrograde) lasting more than 5 min.
- Abnormal drowsiness.
- Three or more discrete episodes of vomiting.
- Clinical suspicion of non-accidental injury.
- Post-traumatic seizure but no history of epilepsy.
- GCS less than 14, or for a baby under 1 year GCS (paediatric) less than 15, on assessment in the emergency department.
- Suspicion of open or depressed skull injury or tense fontanelle.
- Any sign of basal skull fracture (haemotympanum, 'panda' eyes, cerebrospinal fluid leakage from the ear or nose, Battle's sign).
- Focal neurological deficit.
- If under 1 year, presence of bruise, swelling or laceration of more than 5 cm on the head.
- Dangerous mechanism of injury (high-speed road traffic accident either as pedestrian, cyclist or vehicle occupant, fall from a height of greater than 3 m, high-speed injury from a projectile or an object).

GCS, Glasgow Coma Scale.

Spinal injury

Spinal cord injuries are rare in children, constituting only 5% of all spinal cord trauma. Nevertheless, there should be a high index of suspicion in any child with major trauma, especially if he or she has an appreciable head injury and a reduced level of consciousness.

Careful clinical and radiological examination should be undertaken (see Chapter 8). Assessing paralysis and altered sensation, however, can be very difficult, especially in infants. Mass flexion withdrawal in response to stimulation may be indistinguishable from normal withdrawal in this age group. Furthermore, 50% of children with serious spinal injuries have normal radiographs, and radiological normality should not deter a clinical diagnosis of spinal injury. Conversely, the presence of epiphyses in immature spine may lead to erroneous diagnosis of spinal injury by clinicians (Boxes 19.11, 19.12 and 19.13). The thoracolumbar spine can usually be cleared using plain X-rays, supplemented by CT when necessary.

Box 19.11 **Confusing radiological features of the cervical spine in children**

Growth centres resemble fractures

- Cartilaginous plate at the base of the odontoid (closes at 3–5 years).
- Secondary ossification centre at apex of odontoid (present from 2–12 years).
- Secondary ossification centre at tip of spinous processes.

Pseudosubluxation

- Anterior displacement of C2 on C3 (30% of children under 7 years). Much less commonly C3 on C4.

Hypermobility

- Increased distance between dens and anterior arch of C1 (15% of children under 5 years).

Clearing the cervical spine in unconscious children is potentially problematic and spinal cord injury may occur in the absence of a spinal fracture. There is now good evidence that the cervical spine can be safely cleared in unconscious children using modern multislice CT alone.

Children under 10 years should receive anterior/posterior and lateral plain films without an anterior/posterior peg view.

In children under 10 years, because of the increased risks associated with irradiation, particularly to the thyroid gland, and the generally lower risk of significant spinal injury, CT of the cervical spine should be used only in cases where patients have a severe head injury (GCS $\leq$ 8), or where there is a strong clinical suspicion of injury despite normal plain films (for example, focal neurological signs or paraesthesia in the extremities), or where plain films are technically difficult or inadequate (NICE).

Early removal of tightly fitting cervical collars dramatically reduces the risk of decubitus ulceration, simplifies nursing care, and helps significantly reduce elevated intracranial pressure in head-injured patients, especially when nursed head up.

It is essential that all children are removed from spinal immobilisation devices at the earliest opportunity after arrival in the ED to prevent unnecessary discomfort. A common misconception is that ED patient trolleys do not provide adequate thoracolumbar support.

Thorax

Blunt chest trauma is common in children, whereas penetrating injury is rare. The approach to diagnosis and management is the same as in adults. About 15–20% of children with major injuries have chest trauma that requires immediate management. Early diagnosis is essential: of the children who die of chest injury, more than 90% die in the first few hours after the accident. Most thoracic injuries (85–90%) can be managed by standard, non-operative techniques.

More than 50% of patients with thoracic trauma have associated injuries, most commonly of the head, abdomen or an extremity.

The chest wall should be examined for bruising, wounds and asymmetry of movement, and surgical emphysema. The high compliance of a child's chest wall, however, allows ready transfer of energy to intrathoracic structures, and appreciable organ damage may be present with minimal evidence of chest wall injury (Box 19.14).

If a *pneumothorax* (indicated by inequality of air entry) is under tension it requires immediate decompression (Figure 19.8). Classically this should be by needle thoracocentesis before placement of an intrapleural drain. The site *must* be lateral to the midclavicular line if the anterior approach is used, because of risk of injury to the great vessels and heart in the presence of significant mediastinal shift. In the older child, in experienced hands, the chest can be rapidly vented through a stab incision used for intercostal drain placement in the fifth intercostal space anterior axillary line. Percutaneous chest drainage sets are useful for chest drainage in smaller children and occasionally in prehospital care (see Figure 19.3).

The threshold for draining simple traumatic pneumothoraces should be low, especially if it is anticipated that the child will be ventilated, because of the potential risk of tension, unless the patient can be very closely observed (HDU/PICU).

Open pneumothorax is unusual in children. It is initially managed by giving high-flow oxygen, covering the wound on three sides with an airtight dressing, thus creating a one-way outlet valve on the chest wall, and insertion of an intercostal drain.

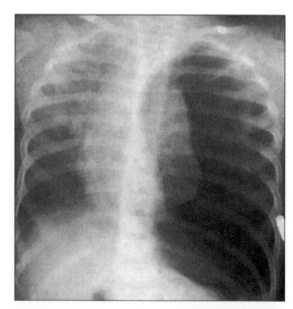

Figure 19.8 Radiograph of left tension pneumothorax causing deviation of the mediastinum to the right.

Flail segments are also uncommon in children but may require early treatment with chest drainage, intermittent positive pressure ventilation and positive end-expiratory pressure, as these injuries are usually associated with a severe pulmonary contusion. Gas exchange predictably deteriorates for 24–48 h after injury associated with an increase in the work of breathing. Haemoptysis, subcutaneous emphysema, and a persistent air leak after drainage of a pneumothorax all suggest significant underlying lung injury.

Patients with *pulmonary contusion* present with tachypnoea, breathlessness and hypoxia. The symptoms are often exacerbated by inhalation of gastric contents, especially if the abdomen has been compressed. If the child has undergone a garroting type injury, tracheal rupture should be suspected, especially if there is cervical subcutaneous emphysema and laryngeal crepitus. Noisy breathing and a persistent (massive) leak through the chest drain with failure to re-expand the lung suggest a tracheal or major proximal bronchial tear.

As in adults, *diaphragmatic rupture*, most commonly on the left side, is often missed clinically, especially in ventilated children, but should be suspected if the left side of the diaphragm is not clearly visualised on the chest radiograph.

Myocardial contusion is rare in children but is suggested by arrhythmias in a child who has sustained significant blunt trauma to the anterior chest wall. Continuous three-lead ECG monitoring is essential for 24 h. Baseline echocardiography should be performed to rule out structural cardiac injury (free wall, valve or septal injury or rupture). See Boxes 19.15 and 19.16.

Box 19.15 **Indications for cardiothoracic surgical referral**

- Large air leak or persistent haemorrhage following chest drain insertion.
- Cardiac tamponade.
- Major vascular disruption (also consider interventional radiology if available).

Box 19.16 **Factors that suggest aortic rupture**

- A deceleration injury.
- A widened mediastinum.
- Fractures of the first or second ribs.
- Obliteration of the aortic knuckle in the chest radiograph.
- Displacement to the right of a nasogastric tube.

Although mediastinal mobility in children means that there is a lower incidence of rupture of the great vessels than in adults, aortic transection (which most commonly occurs close to the origin of the left subclavian artery) is suggested by a deceleration injury, widened mediastinum, fractures of the first or second ribs, and obliteration of the aortic knuckle in the chest radiograph. Displacement of a nasogastric tube to the right is also suggestive of this injury.

Abdomen

The basic principle governing the evaluation of a child with a possible abdominal injury is to determine whether an operation is necessary, either for an acute abdomen or for controlling haemorrhage. As in thoracic injuries, blunt trauma is most common. Penetrating wounds are rare but, when present, may require exploration. Emergency laparotomy for haemorrhage control is a relatively rare requirement, even in severely multiply injured children.

Early passage of a nasogastric tube of appropriate size is essential in children. Careful and gentle clinical examination of the conscious child may produce evidence of significant abdominal injury, although free blood in the peritoneal cavity may be clinically silent as it is a physiological solution, at least initially. Any sign of direct injury to the abdominal wall, in the context of a high-energy injury mechanism, may signify occult but significant abdominal visceral injury. The pattern and methods of clinical examination are the same as in adults.

As in adults, the spleen and liver are the solid organs most commonly injured; a conservative approach is usually initially adopted as haemorrhage is usually self-limiting in children. Splenectomy has significant long-term health implications, leaving a child with lifelong vulnerability to pneumococcal sepsis.

Rapid deceleration forces may cause abdominal compression and result in other injuries (Box 19.17). Bowel perforation detected clinically or by CT is an indication for immediate laparotomy. Pancreatic injury is usually treated conservatively unless it is complicated by late pseudocyst formation.

Box 19.17 **Abdominal injuries caused by rapid deceleration forces**

Duodenal

- Perforation
- Obstructing haematoma

Pancreatic

Rupture of the hollow viscera

- At the ligament of Treitz
- Near the ileocaecal valve

Mesenteric avulsion

Renal

- Vascular
- Parenchymal
- Collecting system

Bladder rupture

A renal injury should be suspected in every child with tenderness of the flank and haematuria. This injury can be well defined on a CT scan and again is usually managed conservatively unless there is uncontrolled haemorrhage. The lumbar spine, ribs and pelvis are also commonly injured (Figure 19.9).

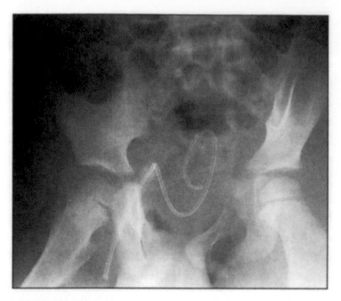

Figure 19.9 Radiograph showing fractured pelvis caused by a crush injury. A suprapubic catheter is *in situ*.

A full bladder is readily ruptured because of its intra-abdominal location in a child. Management is usually conservative with urethral drainage. Any clinical suspicion of urethral rupture should be confirmed by urethrography. Initial management is with a fine silastic Foley catheter passed ideally by an experienced urologist.

Clinical assessment of the abdomen is limited in an unconscious child. Major trauma centres are increasingly using serial abdominal ultrasound examinations in the ED resuscitation room, to look for free intraperitoneal fluid in children with persistent haemodynamic instability. This has helped to expedite the early transfer to theatre of children with uncontrolled intra-abdominal haemorrhage. Stable but multiply injured children should undergo early contrast-enhanced CT to exclude occult intrathoracic or intra-abdominal injury.

Diagnostic peritoneal lavage is now rarely performed in the UK unless there is no access to (or time to use) CT. The consultant surgeon responsible for the child's inpatient care should undertake it.

Soft tissue and skeletal injuries

The principles of management of skeletal and soft tissue damage in children are the same as those for adults. In children the history of the injury is important. The radiological diagnosis of skeletal injury around the joints is more difficult in children because of the growth plate and lack of mineralisation of the epiphysis.

The pattern of fractures is different in children. They may involve the growth plate (Salter–Harris classification types I–V) (Figure 19.10), greenstick (through only one cortex of a long bone) or buckle (bony angulation without a fracture). Because of potential arresting of growth, malalignment of joints and traumatic arthritis, it is essential to recognise any fractures involving the epiphysis and joint articular surfaces.

Supracondylar fractures at the elbow have a high incidence of associated vascular injury. The proportional blood loss after pelvic or long bone fractures in children is greater than in adults and may be an important cause of initial haemodynamic instability. These fractures must be effectively splinted. A number of commercially available splints enable this to be readily achieved in the field as well as the ED. See Chapter 21.

The presence of multiple old healed fractures should alert the medical team to the possibility of non-accidental injury.

Burns

Scalds from hot water are the most common cause of burns in children, and management does not differ appreciably from that of adult patients (see Chapter 22).

The change in body proportions as children grow means that calculation of the percentage total body surface area burnt cannot be based on the adult 'rule of nines'. An accurate estimation of the percentage of the total body surface area burnt (partial and full thickness) requires the use of detailed charts (Lund & Browder) (Figure 19.11). The surface of a child's palm approximates to 1% of the body surface area.

Crystalloid fluid replacement (in addition to maintenance fluid requirements) required in the first 24 hours can be calculated using the Baxter–Parkland formula:

$$4 \text{ mL/kg} \times \% \text{ burn}$$

The child should be given half of this requirement in the first 8 h after the time of the burn. The adequacy of fluid replacement is monitored by ensuring a urine output of at least 1 mL/kg/h in children over 1 year of age and 2 mL/kg/h in infants.

The indications for transfer to a regional burns unit include:

- 10% partial- and/or full-thickness burns
- 5% full-thickness burns
- burns to special areas (face, hands and genitalia).

If a burnt child presents with signs of hypovolaemic shock, then an additional source for blood loss should be urgently sought.

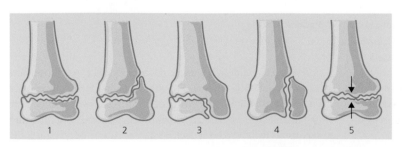

Figure 19.10 The Salter–Harris classification of epiphyseal fractures.

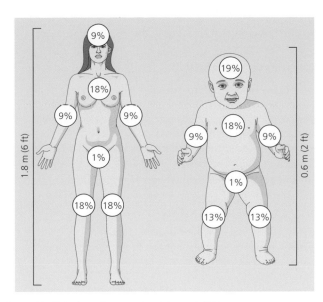

Figure 19.11 Body surface area in adults and children.

Clingfilm is an ideal emergency dressing for extensive burns and provides effective pain relief (protection from draughts). Topical sulphadiazine should be avoided in the first instance because it complicates the assessment of depth of partial-thickness burns at 48 h (by staining the burn).

Pain relief in children

Adequate control of pain is humane and will improve a child's co-operation with diagnosis, investigation and management. It is important to quantify pain scores at the time of initial assessment and the observational Alder Hey triage pain scoring system is being used increasingly widely to determine this in UK EDs. Intravenous morphine should be titrated to effect in the conscious older child in severe pain (Box 19.18).

> Box 19.18 **Control of pain**
>
> - After resuscitation, give a bolus of morphine 50 μg/kg intravenously.
> - Titrate further doses of 25 μg/kg against the patient's response.
> - Oramorph and intranasal diamorphine are useful alternatives in young children.

In younger children with isolated extremity fractures, Oramorph at a dose of 200–400 μg/kg in combination with splinting of the fracture in a back slab cast will often produce rapid and satisfactory analgesia without the initial trauma of gaining intravenous access. In children too distressed to take anything orally, intranasal diamorphine works extremely rapidly and produces excellent analgesia, especially in children under 5. This is now being increasingly used in many UK emergency departments as first-line analgesia for young children with fractures or significant injury.

Throughout the secondary survey, the child's response to resuscitation and general condition should be constantly reassessed. Subsequent management depends on the expertise and facilities of the receiving hospital. If the anaesthetic, surgical and intensive care services are not suited to the care of children, a protocol for transfer to a designated paediatric centre should be an important part of the initial evaluation and management.

Non-accidental injury

A wide variety of injuries can be caused by physical child abuse (Figure 19.12). Inconsistencies in the mechanism of injury and physical findings, certain specific injury patterns, delays in presentation to the ED or a background of domestic violence should alert the clinical team to the possibility of intentional injury. The diagnostic criteria for non-accidental injury are shown in Box 19.19.

Initial resuscitation and management of the battered child are the prime responsibilities of the ED medical team, but it is essential that multidisciplinary assessment teams are involved at the outset of the child's management. Thresholds should be low for admitting such children for detailed assessment in suspicious cases.

Careful recording (including photographs) of injuries is essential, and standard diagrams should be available for this purpose (Figure 19.13).

> Box 19.19 **Diagnostic criteria for non-accidental injury**
>
> - Delay in seeking medical advice.
> - Account of the accident is vague and inconsistent among parties.
> - Discrepancy between the history and the degree of injury.
> - Abnormal parental behaviour, with lack of concern for the child.
> - Abnormal interaction between child and parents.
> - Bruising caused by finger tips, especially over upper arms, trunk, sides of face, ears or neck.
> - Bizarre injuries, e.g. bites, cigarette burns, rope marks.
> - Sharply demarcated burns in unusual areas.
> - Perioral injuries, e.g. torn frenulum.
> - Retinal haemorrhage.
> - Multiple subdural haemorrhage.
> - Ruptured internal organs with no history of major trauma.
> - Perianal or genital injury.
> - Long bone fractures in non-ambulant children.
> - Previous injuries, e.g. old scars, healing fractures.

Should relatives be present in the resuscitation room?

Families must have open access to their children and must be given complete information about the child's condition and prognosis as soon as it is known. This information must be passed on in a sensitive but frank way.

Presence of relatives in the resuscitation room during attempted resuscitation is a controversial issue. A survey in 1994 (British Association of Emergency Medicine/Royal College of Nursing)

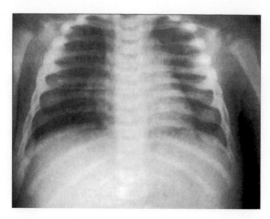

Figure 19.12 Chest radiograph showing multiple healing rib fractures after non-accidental injury.

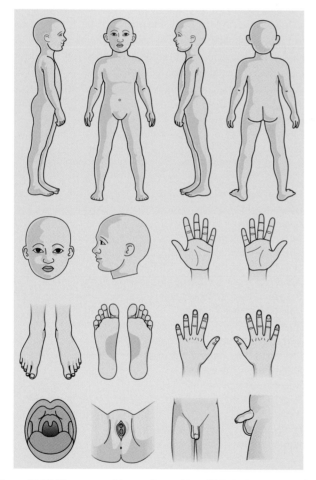

Figure 19.13 Diagram used for precise marking of injuries in a suspected case of non-accidental injury.

revealed that less than one-quarter of emergency departments allowed the relatives of children into the resuscitation room. It is now standard practice to at least offer parents the option of witnessing the resuscitation of their child (Box 19.20).

The view of many healthcare professionals, in contrast to the view of many relatives, is that the presence of relatives in the resuscitation room does more harm than good. However, there is little data to demonstrate any detrimental effect on the patient, relatives or staff of relatives' presence. Views among clinicians vary, with most emergency physicians and paediatricians in favour, and many physicians and anaesthetists against, often strongly so.

Relatives perceive several advantages in being present in the resuscitation room but there are potential disadvantages. The reality of the resuscitation may prove distressing, particularly if the relatives are uninformed, and they may physically or emotionally hinder the staff's efforts at resuscitation; subsequently, relatives may be disturbed by the memory of the attempt, although there is evidence that fantasy is worse than fact. Current evidence suggests that for many it is more distressing to be separated from a family member during these critical moments than to witness attempts at resuscitation.

In summary:

- offer relatives the chance to be present during resuscitation
- allocate a staff member to be with them at all times
- make it clear that if they interfere they will have to leave
- explain what is happening in terms that they can understand
- allow them to touch the child when it is safe to do so.

Summary

The injured child must be systematically assessed and every life-threatening emergency treated as soon as it is identified, following the '(C)-ABCDE' guidelines.

Those responsible for providing initial care for injured children must be familiar with the common patterns of injury and with their initial assessment, management and treatment. It is essential that good communication systems are in place so that the child can be assessed promptly by an experienced surgeon and, if necessary, transferred to a definitive paediatric care facility as soon as his or her condition is stabilised. The future development of major regional trauma centres and integrated prehospital critical care networks in the UK may further significantly improve the outcomes of children with complex patterns of injury.

Acknowledgements

The paediatric resuscitation chart is by P.A. Oakley and was derived from the guidelines of the Resuscitation Council UK. The radiographs were kindly provided by Drs B. Kendall, D. Shaw, C. Hall and D. Hatch, Hospital for Sick Children, Great Ormond Street, London.

Further reading

Advanced Life Support Group. (2004) *Advanced Paediatric Life Support: The Practical Approach*, 4th edn. Oxford: Blackwell Publishing.

Black JJM, Davies GD. (2005) International EMS systems: the United Kingdom. Resuscitation 64(1): 21–9.

Driscoll P, Skinner DV (eds). 1998) *Trauma Care Beyond the Resuscitation Room*. London: BMJ Books.

Lund CC, Bowder NC. (1944) The estimation of area of burns. Surg Gynecol Obstet 79: 353–60.

National Institute for Health and Clinical Excellence. (2007) Head Injury Guidelines. http://publications.nice.org.uk/head-injury-cg56

Resuscitation Council. (1996) *Should Relatives Witness Resuscitation?* London: Resuscitation Council.

Salter RB, Harris WR. (1963) Injuries involving the epiphyseal plate. Am J Bone Joint Surg 45: 587–622.

Skinner DV, Whimster F. (1999) *Trauma. A Companion to Bailey and Love's Short Practice of Surgery*. London: Arnold.

Stewart B, Lancaster G, Lawson J *et al.* (2004) Validation of the Alder Hey triage pain score. Arch Dis Child 89: 625–30.

Walls RN. (1999) *Manual of Emergency Airway Management. The Airway Course*, 3rd edn. Wellesley, MA: Airway Management Education Center.

CHAPTER 20

Trauma in the Elderly

Carl L. Gwinnutt and Michael A. Horan

Hope Hospital, Salford, UK

OVERVIEW

- The elderly are an increasing proportion of both the population and trauma patients.
- There are important differences in the physiological response to trauma in the elderly.
- The primary and secondary surveys must be conducted with an understanding of injuries that are common in the elderly.
- There is good evidence that with timely and aggressive intervention, outcome in the elderly can be improved.
- Patients with hip fractures must be cared for using currently established 'best practice' guidelines.

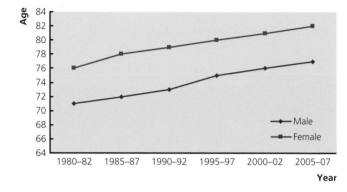

Figure 20.1 Increasing life expectancy from 1980 to 2007.

The morbidity and mortality of older people following trauma are greater than that of any other age group, regardless of the severity of their injuries. Although the elderly are seriously injured less often than any other sector of the population, the proportion is increasing as more active lifestyles are adopted (Figure 20.1). Fewer injuries are associated with motor vehicle accidents, falls being the main cause. This is because of changes in vision, vestibular function and proprioception, prolonged motor reaction time, and neurological and musculoskeletal diseases.

Until recently, the outcome of trauma care for elderly people was poor but it has become increasingly clear that early and aggressive therapeutic intervention, accompanied by invasive monitoring, can considerably improve it. Age alone accounts for little of the variance in outcome in intensive care units; the underlying pathophysiology is the major determinant. Consequently, to maximise survival in the elderly, clinicians need to focus on detecting and correcting physiological and metabolic derangements that accompany major trauma.

Primary survey and resuscitation

In most trauma systems, standardised anatomical and physiological criteria are used as a trigger to activate the trauma team. However, because of their lack of physiological reserve, the elderly may not meet the standard physiological criteria, thereby leading to an underestimation of the severity of their injuries. Consideration should be given to activating the trauma team for all patients over the age of 70 years with an Injury Severity Score (ISS) >15, irrespective of their haemodynamic status.

Airway management with protection of the cervical spine

Many older patients are edentulous but some are not and may have loose, inconveniently situated or very carious teeth. Resorption of the mandible and lax cheeks may make maintenance of the airway more difficult. Well-fitting dentures may be left in place initially, but the doctor dealing with the airway should record this and inform the team leader. If dentures are removed, they must be inspected to ensure they are complete, particularly if they have been fractured. Airway adjuncts must be used with care because the soft tissues of the oropharynx and nasopharynx are more prone to damage, particularly the turbinates, which may bleed profusely.

Intubation is generally straightforward, but care must be taken with the cervical spine because arthritis (osteoarthritis and rheumatoid disease) is the rule rather than the exception (Figure 20.2). Consequently, these trauma patients are particularly prone to cervical cord or nerve injury if subjected to excessive flexion of the neck or extension of the head. Occasionally, temporomandibular arthritis may limit mouth opening, making laryngoscopy difficult. As a result of a fall, injury to the cervical spine occurs more commonly between the craniocervical junction and C2, tends to involve

ABC of Major Trauma, Fourth Edition. Edited by David V. Skinner and Peter A. Driscoll.
© 2013 Blackwell Publishing Ltd. Published 2013 by Blackwell Publishing Ltd.

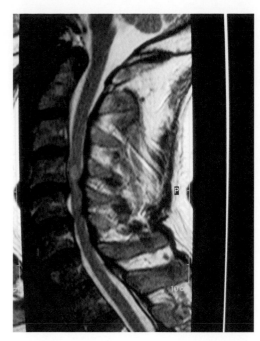

Figure 20.2 Magnetic resonance scan of the cervical spine showing severe degenerative changes.

more than one level and is unstable. Also, the cervical spine seems to be peculiarly vulnerable in falls associated with seizures. Full immobilisation of the cervical spine is therefore mandatory in these patients and if tracheal intubation is required, this must be achieved using manual inline immobilisation.

Breathing and ventilation

Lung function in older patients is affected by changes in the upper airway, chest wall, ventilatory muscles and lung parenchyma. Age-related changes in the upper airway render it more vulnerable to collapse and obstruction. The thorax becomes stiffer as a result of calcification of the costal cartilages, reduction in the intervertebral disc spaces and co-existing crush fractures of the vertebral bodies. Together, these produce an increase in the anteroposterior diameter of the chest and reduced rib excursion. The elastic recoil properties of the lung also decrease with age, which reduces the ease of ventilation and decreases compliance. In addition, there is an increase in the collapse of small airways during expiration, leading to non-uniform ventilation and air trapping. Collectively, these cause a small reduction in PaO_2. Such changes, together with an impaired mucociliary escalator, predispose elderly patients to atelectasis, pneumonia and hypoventilation.

For the reasons given above, it is often difficult to support ventilation with oxygen given by a facemask and hypoxia can develop rapidly. If there is any doubt about the adequacy of oxygenation, mechanical ventilation with 100% oxygen should be started early.

Pulse oximetry should be used routinely in all patients. Finger probes may give a poor reading in the elderly as a result of cold-induced vasoconstriction and shivering. Probes designed for the nose and earlobe are often more reliable. All intubated, ventilated patients must have their end-tidal carbon dioxide concentration ($ETCO_2$) monitored. This serves three key purposes: the presence of CO_2 in expired breath confirms that the tracheal tube is within the lower airway, it acts as a disconnect alarm and under normal circumstances, $ETCO_2$ closely matches $PaCO_2$, with a gradient of 0.7 kPa (5 mmHg) and it can be used as an indicator of the adequacy of alveolar ventilation. In the elderly patient, particularly those with chronic obstructive pulmonary disease, the gradient is increased (because of a reduced $ETCO_2$), and a gradual rising slope is seen on the capnograph trace during expiration, rather than a plateau. Therefore the $ETCO_2$ should be checked against analysis of an arterial blood sample as soon as possible (Box 20.1).

Pneumothoraces are produced more commonly in this age group, particularly in those patients with chronic lung diseases. The team leader should be constantly aware of this. In addition to frequent inspection of the chest for symmetry of movement, the development of surgical emphysema, equality of breath sounds and, in ventilated patients, airway pressures should all be monitored. Ventilation is adjusted to keep peak inspiratory pressures as low as possible to reduce the risk of barotrauma, particularly in emphysematous patients. In view of the serious potential problems that may arise in these patients, the help of an anaesthetist should be sought early.

Box 20.1 **Adequacy of alveolar ventilation**

In the ventilated patient, the $ETCO_2$ should be checked against analysis of an arterial blood sample as soon as possible to ensure adequacy of ventilation.

Circulation and control of haemorrhage

The incidence of ischaemic heart disease increases with age but its prevalence in old age is unknown (Table 20.1). Necropsy studies suggest a prevalence in those over 65 of about 60%, but in the living of similar age, estimates vary between 10% and 30%. Even in healthy people, advancing age is associated with cardiovascular changes. Increased stiffness of the arterial walls leads to an increase in systolic blood pressure and left ventricular hypertrophy. Resting cardiac output is maintained, but the ability to mount a compensatory tachycardia is reduced. Healthy old people compensate by increased venous return and raise cardiac output predominantly through the Starling mechanism. Consequently, reduction in intravascular volume may lead to a rapid reduction in cardiac output.

Table 20.1 Ageing and incidence of ischaemic heart disease (annual rate per 1000 population).

Age group	Men	Women
35–44	5	1
45–54	11	4
55–64	19	10
65–74	23	14
75–84	30	22
85–94	39	41

The initial fluid for resuscitation is warmed Ringer's lactate, but there must be continuous, accurate monitoring of the response in the elderly patient, because of the reduced tolerance of hypo-volaemia or fluid overload. It is important to remember that measures of pulse rate and indirect measurement of blood pressure give only limited information about intravascular volume. Furthermore, the jugular venous pulse and fullness of peripheral veins can be difficult to assess in the elderly and should not be relied on. This is particularly true in patients with heart disease, indwelling pacemakers, and those taking cardiovascular drugs. Consequently, early consideration should be given to invasive monitoring. Initially, central venous pressure can be monitored, with trends being more informative than absolute values. However, even this may be misleading in those with significant pulmonary and heart disease. Ideally, a pulmonary artery catheter is required but this may not be easily achieved within the emergency department. Early consideration must therefore be given to moving such patients to a suitable environment, for example the intensive care unit.

Direct measurement of arterial blood pressure is informative and more accurate, particularly at extremes, than using non-invasive devices. It is also relatively easy to perform. The waveform that can be displayed gives an indication of the systemic vascular resistance and myocardial contractility. A large artery, for example the femoral, is preferable for this purpose to the radial or dorsalis pedis, but the groin must always be examined for signs of previous vascular surgery. The presence of an arterial cannula will also allow frequent sampling of arterial blood without the need for repeated arterial puncture.

The urinary bladder should be catheterised to measure urine output, and a strict aseptic technique must be used. Ageing is usually associated with loss of renal cortical structures, a fall in the glomerular filtration rate, and decline in renal function by about 1 mL/min for each year after the age of 40 years. This may be compounded by the use of drugs, particularly angiotensin-converting enzyme inhibitors (ACEIs), non-steroidal anti-inflammatory drugs and diuretics that may further impair renal function. These changes make old people particularly vulnerable to incompetent fluid and metabolic management. Cardiac dysrhythmias and conduction abnormalities are common, even in apparently healthy old people. Adequate oxygenation should be ensured and cardiac contusions excluded before they are discounted.

Dysfunction of the central nervous system

Most confused, ill, old people are not demented. Confusion can be a feature of almost any illness in the aged, particularly infection, fluid and metabolic derangements, head injury, and as a result of medications or their withdrawal. In addition, multiple sensory impairments may lead to disorientation and inappropriate responses and make assessment difficult. Initial treatment is to ensure adequate cerebral perfusion with oxygenated blood, rather than to assume that confusion is the patient's normal mental state. In unconscious elderly patients, consider intracerebral haemorrhage as both the cause and effect of co-existing trauma, particularly if the patient is known to be taking anticoagulants.

Exposure

Patients must be completely undressed to ensure that all injuries are identified. It is, however, important to prevent the development or worsening of hypothermia. As soon as the examination is completed, the patient should be wrapped in blankets. Core temperature must be monitored rather than simply feeling the patient's peripheries to estimate body temperature. Infrared tympanic membrane thermometers are now widely available, but in the elderly patient it is important to ensure that the external auditory meatus is not occluded with wax.

Analgesia

Elderly people must not be denied adequate pain relief after trauma. Morphine is safe and effective provided that it is titrated in small doses (0.5–1.0 mg) intravenously. Intramuscular injections must be avoided as they are painful and absorption is unpredictable. Pethidine, buprenorphine (Temgesic) and non-steroidal anti-inflammatory drugs are less well tolerated and are best avoided. If antiemetics are administered, the dose should be reduced accordingly to avoid unwanted extrapyramidal side-effects.

Local anaesthetic techniques are often ignored but are effective when used to supplement systemic analgesics. A femoral nerve block is easily performed and useful in patients with fractures of the neck or shaft of the femur. Intercostal nerve blocks may provide relief from the pain of fractured ribs, particularly for patients who have to be transported around the hospital. An axillary nerve block can be used for forearm fractures, but is usually best delayed until after a comprehensive assessment of neurological function.

Secondary survey: AMPLE

A detailed history is particularly important and no source of information should be overlooked. The ambulance personnel will be able to give details of the immediate event and, when it occurred in the patient's home, may have brought medications with them. One member of the team should try to obtain hospital records and contact the general practitioner to find out about illnesses and medicines that may influence future management (see Chapter 13). Sometimes the patient may be able to give information directly while those with diabetes, on anticoagulants or on steroid hormones may be carrying a medication card.

Communicating with deaf patients may be particularly difficult. Check that any hearing aid is working and switched on. Shouting tends to use high-frequency sounds and may be counterproductive in patients with presbyacusis. The voice should be lowered and the patient, wearing spectacles if needed, should be in a position to watch the speaker's lips. Significant confusion can usually be assessed by checking that the patient knows where they are, what day it is and why they were brought to hospital. However, remember that even people who are not confused may not be able to co-operate because of pain and anxiety.

Injuries arise from the transfer of energy at rates and in amounts that exceed the tolerance of tissues. In old people, particularly women, bone strength may be appreciably reduced and fractures may occur after only modest transfers of energy. Age-related changes in other organs and tissues make them particularly vulnerable to injury, so a head-to-toe examination must be undertaken after even apparently minor injuries. This will also ensure the detection of coincident medical problems and the institution of appropriate treatment.

During physical examination, care should be taken to maintain the usual anatomical position for the particular patient. It is particularly important to avoid producing traction and compression neuropathies (especially in the operating room) that may compromise rehabilitation. Extreme vigilance must be exercised during 'log rolling', particularly if the patient is unconscious. The age-related changes described above make such patients vulnerable to iatrogenic damage to the cervical cord or nerve roots.

Consideration must also be given to the prevention of decubitus ulcers. Appropriate pressure-dispersing surfaces should be readily available and all patients with multiple injuries must be considered to be at high risk. Consequently, prevention must begin in the emergency department.

Initial X-ray examinations should include the standard three films of the cervical spine, chest and pelvis. Results from the National Emergency X-Radiography Utilisation Study (NEXUS) found that the cervical spine was twice as likely to be injured in the elderly as younger patients (Box 20.2). However, the NEXUS criteria were equally sensitive for clearing the cervical spine in both age groups. Unfortunately, co-existing medical illness and disease of bone and joints may make interpretation of X-rays difficult, and the advice of more experienced colleagues should be sought early.

Box 20.2 **Beware of pitfalls in interpretation of C spine views in the elderly**

- The cervical spine is twice as likely to be injured in the elderly as younger patients.
- Co-existing degenerative disease of bone and joints may make interpretation of X-rays difficult; advice of more experienced colleagues should be sought early.

Head injuries

As the brain ages, its dura becomes tightly adherent to the skull, which makes epidural (extradural) haematomas uncommon. A progressive loss of brain volume leads to an increase in the space around the brain that is thought to protect it from contusions, but makes subdural haematomas more likely. Patients over the age of 55 years who are anticoagulated have a higher frequency of isolated head trauma, more severe head injury and a higher mortality.

Even mild head injuries, particularly in patients with pre-existing cognitive impairment, may lead to permanent neurological damage. If there is a skull fracture and an associated hemiparesis, a traumatic intracranial haematoma should be assumed and not a stroke. Similarly, confusion lasting more than 12 hours after head injury,

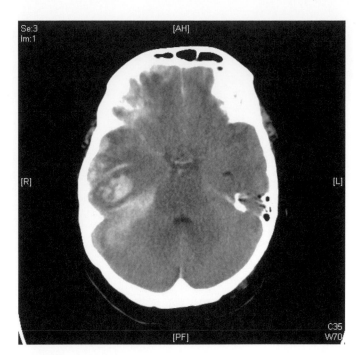

Figure 20.3 Despite the presence of a significant abnormality on CT scan, this patient had a GCS of 15.

even in a patient with no skull fracture, is an indication for a CT scan. Any deterioration demands immediate action and a CT scan should be obtained in all patients who are unconsciousness for more than 5 minutes after head injury (Figure 20.3). The outcome is extremely poor in elderly patients who have sustained head injuries sufficient to cause immediate coma that persists after correction of hypoxia and hypovolaemia. Neurosurgical intervention is not warranted for most of these patients.

Chest trauma

Rib fractures often complicate even mild blunt trauma to the chest in old people. The presence of fractured ribs on the chest X-ray is an important indicator of severity of injury and outcome, as mortality increases with increasing number of rib fractures (Figure 20.4). Because they are poorly tolerated, these patients must be watched carefully and the need for mechanical ventilation frequently reassessed. Those with more severe blunt chest trauma, such as those with penetrating injuries, are managed in the same way as younger patients.

Abdominal trauma

The principles of care for elderly patients with abdominal trauma follow those already outlined in Chapter 9 but it must be remembered that old people are intolerant of shock and unnecessary laparotomy. Their assessment therefore demands a sense of urgency and a high degree of clinical acumen.

Those who have a history or clinical evidence of previous major abdominal surgery should have a CT or ultrasound scan of the abdomen rather than diagnostic peritoneal lavage.

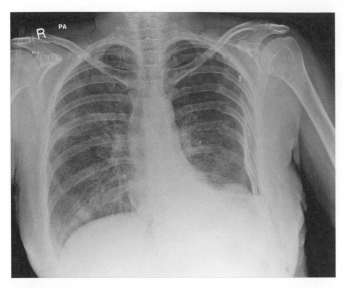

Figure 20.4 Chest X-ray showing multiple rib fractures on the left after relatively minor trauma.

Fractures

In old people with multiple injuries, fractures must be stabilised to permit optimal positioning and movement, both for immediate management and later rehabilitation. While isolated fractures of the humeral shaft are managed conservatively, there is no logic to such management in a patient with leg injuries who will need to use a walking frame or crutches for mobilisation. The aim of treatment should be to undertake the least invasive, most definitive procedure with a view to early mobilisation as soon as other problems permit. Prolonged inactivity and disuse may seriously limit the eventual functional outcome.

Hip fractures

This is an increasingly common problem in Europe. In the UK around 70,000 patients suffer a hip fracture each year (Figure 20.5),

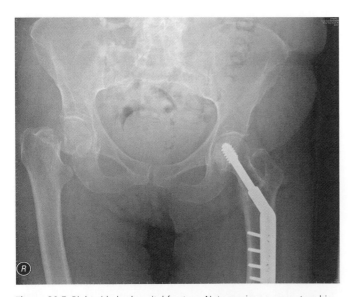

Figure 20.5 Right-sided subcapital fracture. Note previous surgery to a hip fracture on the other side.

increasing at approximately 5% per annum and projected to reach 120,000 cases per year by 2015. Seventy-five percent of patients are over 75 years of age and 80% are female. The average length of stay in hospital is 30 days, with a 30-day mortality of about 10%. Hip fractures account for 20% of all orthopaedic bed occupancy. There are now a number of recommendations for 'best practice' for the management of this increasing burden on healthcare. The following are based on the Scottish Intercollegiate Guidelines Network (SIGN) (Box 20.3).

1 Early assessment, within 1 h of arrival, by medical staff in the emergency department (ED). Whilst in the ED:
   • keep patients warm
   • give adequate analgesia
   • organise early radiology
   • assess and correct any fluid and electrolyte abnormalities
   • institute pressure sore prevention.
2 Diagnosis
   • Plain X-rays identify most fractures.
   • Magnetic resonance (MR) imaging is the investigation of choice if diagnosis is in doubt.
   • If MR is not available or feasible, repeat X-rays after 24–48 h.
3 Analgesia
   • Give appropriate and adequate analgesia before transfer of the patient from the ED.
   • Intravenous opioids, titrated to effect.
   • Local anaesthetic nerve blocks when appropriate.
4 Rapid transfer to the ward: 'fast tracking'
   • Within 1 h of arrival has been suggested but currently there is little evidence that this improves outcome.
   • Aim for within 2 h of arrival in the ED. Further delay increases length of hospital stay and inpatient mortality.
5 Minimise the delay to definitive surgery
   Operate as soon as possible, within 24 h of admission during daytime working hours, including weekends. Use a multidisciplinary team approach. Medical conditions delaying surgery increase 30-day mortality by a factor of 2.5. Non-medical delays cause:
   • distress to the patient
   • increased morbidity and mortality
   • reduced chance of successful fixation and rehabilitation
   • reduced functional recovery
   • increased risk of deep vein thrombosis and pulmonary embolism
   • prolonged hospital stay.
6 Postoperatively:
   • ensure appropriate thromboprophylaxis:
     – mechanical foot pumps
     – aspirin
     – heparin in high risk patients
   • review the adequacy of pain relief often
   • ensure prompt and appropriate correction of fluid and electrolyte imbalance
   • check oxygen saturation, give oxygen to all patients with hypoxaemia
   • check the state of nutrition using a screening tool (e.g. MUST)

- ensure secondary prevention of low trauma fractures (calcium, vitamin D, bisphosphonates) according to local policies.

Box 20.3 **Key recommendations of SIGN for patients with hip fracture**

- Early assessment, within 1 h of arrival, by medical staff in the ED.
- Rapid diagnosis by X-ray, MRI if any doubt.
- Analgesia before transfer of the patient from the ED.
- Rapid transfer to the ward.
- Minimise the delay to definitive surgery.
- Ensure appropriate thromboprophylaxis.

Rehabilitation

Some patients are not suitable for a rehabilitation programme, usually those who were previously immobile or were severely impaired, though improving independence with transfers is sometimes a worthwhile goal. Those who were previously fit and active often make rapid improvements after surgery and can be discharged directly from the trauma ward. Most other patients will benefit from a structured programme of rehabilitation delivered in hospital, in a community setting or at home, depending on resources and expertise. If screening for the state of nutrition was omitted, it needs to be done now. The adequacy of pain relief must be assessed frequently, as the need for analgesics will change over time. Also, depression is extremely common after hip fractures: it must be sought and treated.

Summary

Elderly patients have a particularly high mortality rate and are extremely vulnerable to less than optimal management. A system of trauma care must be prepared to cope with this group of patients and their special needs. The trauma team must be aware of the anatomical and physiological changes that accompany ageing and how these factors, together with the effects of co-existing illnesses and medications, make special demands on their skills. Oversights and thoughtlessness in initial management of patients may have serious adverse consequences on recovery and eventual hospital discharge.

Elderly patients should be informed of what is happening and, where possible, be encouraged to participate in treatment decisions. Not all old people are demented. This does not mean they should necessarily receive identical treatment to younger people; instead, they must be managed in a way that is appropriate to their needs in the light of the likely outcome.

Further reading

Jacobs DG. (2003) Special considerations in geriatric trauma. *Curr Opin Crit Care* 9: 535–9.

NHS Scotland. (2002) Scottish hip fracture audit. www.show.scot.nhs.uk/shfa.

Scottish Intercollegiate Guidelines Network. (2002) Prevention and management of hip fracture in older people. www.sign.ac.uk.

CHAPTER 21

Prehospital Trauma Care

John J. M. Black

John Radcliffe Hospital, Oxford, UK

OVERVIEW

- This chapter will review the principles of the prehospital management of severely injured patients.

- It will highlight the challenges of the delivery of such care in the operational environment.

- In 2011 the GMC approved the creation of the medical subspecialty of Prehospital Emergency Medicine, a new subspecialty of Emergency Medicine and Anaesthetics.

- Recruitment to national training programs is due to commence in 2012.

Major trauma remains the fourth leading cause of death in western countries and the leading cause of death in the first four decades of life. The incidence of trauma is particularly high in the younger population; an average of 36 life-years are lost per trauma death. Furthermore, trauma is also a major cause of debilitating long-term injuries. For each trauma fatality, there are two survivors with serious or permanent disability. Severe injury is not only a leading cause of death but also a large socioeconomic burden. In 1998, the estimated cost to the NHS of treating all injuries was £1.2 billion per annum. Reducing injuries is, therefore, a key government objective. With the phased introduction of trauma networks in England since 2010, the Department of Health aims to have reduced the mortality from major trauma by 20% by 2015.

Road traffic collisions (RTC) account for over a third of all deaths due to injury (Figure 21.1). In 2001–2003, there were (on average) 3460 traffic-related fatalities per annum in Great Britain. The incidence of severe trauma, as defined by an injury severity score (ISS) of 16 or greater, is estimated to be four per million per week. Given that the UK population in mid-2003 was in the region of 59.5 million, there are approximately 240 severely injured patients in the UK each week.

The principles for looking after a major trauma patient and the requirement to identify and effectively manage any immediately

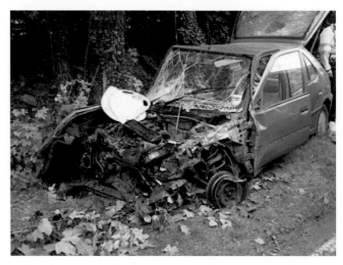

Figure 21.1 Car versus tree high-speed RTC. The driver was physically trapped by his lower legs due to engine compartment intrusion into the dash board and foot well.

life-threatening complications of injury are the same at the scene of injury as they are in the emergency department (ED). The constraints of the environment and the finite resources available at the scene of injury will make effective patient management challenging.

The latest National Confidential Enquiry into Patient Outcome and Death after Trauma (November 2007), highlights that clinical care at the scene can have a profound impact on patient prospects for survival and full functional recovery. It highlights for the first time the potential need for some severely injured patients to undergo critical care interventions prior to arrival in hospital if secondary injury is to be avoided. It also highlights the importance of the ambulance service personnel, supported if necessary by prehospital emergency physicians, correctly identifying life-threatening, time-critical injury patterns and appropriately directly transporting such patients to a hospital with the necessary surgical and critical care resources to manage complex injury. As trauma networks are established in England, the expectation is that all major trauma patients within a 45 minute drive time will be transported directly by the ambulance service to a major trauma centre.

ABC of Major Trauma, Fourth Edition. Edited by David V. Skinner and Peter A. Driscoll.
© 2013 Blackwell Publishing Ltd. Published 2013 by Blackwell Publishing Ltd.

Tasking and dispatch

Ambulance personnel will be tasked to attend a specific incident as soon as the geographical or general area of the incident has been identified from the 999 caller to the emergency services. This can now be established precisely within seconds when 999 calls are made from land lines. 999 calls may be passed from one emergency service to another (from police or fire and rescue to ambulance service) if a clinical response is deemed necessary from the initial information received.

Tasking of ambulance crews is increasingly done automatically through the use of dedicated software packages and mobile data terminals located within ambulances, radio-paging or by SMS texting using mobile phone networks. Clinical information may be updated by Tetra radio. The positioning of ambulances at predetermined standby locations known to receive a high density of calls, or at locations close to major roads, has also contributed to improved ambulance response times for medical and trauma emergencies.

The presence of a suitably trained clinician (usually a paramedic) working in an ambulance emergency operation control room is extremely important for early recognition of the potential for major trauma and for the dispatch of additional clinical resources when necessary.

By 2012, the ambulance service will endeavor to task a paramedic to initially assess and treat all potential major trauma emergencies.

A prehospital emergency physician may be dispatched if available, either by road or by helicopter to provide support for major trauma cases, either following receipt of key clinical information within ambulance control, or following an ambulance crew request, and for incidents occurring in geographically remote locations. Air ambulance, police and search and rescue helicopters are extremely valuable in rapidly confirming the incident location when accurate information is not immediately available to the emergency services.

Scene management

Scene safety (Box 21.1) is of paramount concern and it is essential that all clinicians who attend the incident are fully trained to risk assess the scene and understand command and control systems in use by the emergency services (Box 21.2)

The first priority for bystanders is to ensure their own safety, and to alert the emergency services as soon as the incident location has been established, even before the scene/casualties have been fully assessed. The widespread uptake of vehicle satellite navigation systems can facilitate this process.

Box 21.1 **The three tiers of safety**

- Yourself.
- The scene.
- The patient.

Box 21.2 **Roles and responsibilities of emergency services at the scene of major trauma**

Fire and rescue

- Save life.
- Rescue and extrication of casualties.
- Hazard management and containment.

Police

- Save life.
- Secure emergency service access and restrict bystander access to scene (cordon management).
- Preservation of evidence and investigation and prosecution of crime.

Ambulance service

- Save life.
- Triage and treatment of casualties.
- Appropriate transport of casualties to hospital

It is essential that all ambulance and medical personnel at the scene wear appropriate personal protective equipment (PPE) to reduce the risk of unnecessary injury. All personnel should wear high-visibility tabards that clearly state their role (doctor/paramedic/nurse) (Box 21.3).

Box 21.3 **Minimum PPE requirements**

- Identification badge.
- Suitable underclothing tailored for environmental temperature.
- High-visibility jacket with tabard (green letters/white background).
- Hard hat/head torch.
- Eye protection.
- Ear defenders.
- Water/oil-resistant steel-capped boots.
- Clinical gloves.
- Heavy-duty gloves (RTC in-vehicle care).
- Fireproof flight suit (as appropriate).

Moving traffic probably represents the greatest risk to all emergency service personnel present at the scene of an RTC, especially at night. Thresholds should be low for requesting road closure by the police. The fire service will park rescue appliances in fend-off position on fast-moving roads to provide a degree of protection to the RTC scene. Incidents occurring on the rail network are particularly hazardous, moving trains and high-tension electricity cables/live track being the main threats to rescuers and survivors.

When arriving at the scene, it is essential that clinical personnel receive a safety brief by the fire/ambulance/police incident commanders and safety officers and a situation report detailing the scale of the incident. The ambulance incident commander will

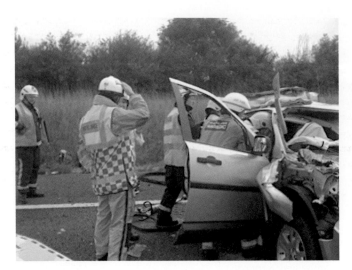

Figure 21.2 Command and control at an RTC. Ambulance and fire incident commanders can be identified from their tabards and helmet markings. The clinical teams are appropriately protected.

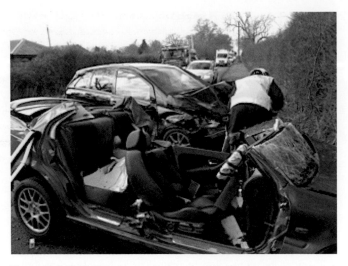

Figure 21.3 RTC. Note the massive intrusion into the driver's compartment from the front seat passenger compartment (left lateral pelvic compression and left torso injury, and foot well entrapment), and the presence of an un-deployed air bag, which was a potential hazard to the patient, fire and rescue personnel, and ambulance teams during extrication. The patient was released after removal of the roof and B post, and a dashboard roll.

indicate where clinical support is required and will summarise what other health resources are available (and *en route*) at the scene (Figure 21.2). He or she will identify the requirement for a medical incident commander in complex/major incidents and arrange for a suitably trained prehospital emergency physician to be mobilised to the scene.

It is particularly important when dealing with railway incidents that accurate information on the status of track and power supply is obtained from a competent authority. At a railway station, this will be the line controller; at other incidents this will be an immediate priority for the fire incident commander to establish.

Establishing the injury mechanism may provide useful information for predicting underlying injury patterns. The observations of witnesses and family members may provide invaluable clinical information regarding the preservation of consciousness, and any pre-existing co-morbid conditions and concurrent treatment. Initial estimates of vehicle speed at RTCs are notoriously unreliable; it takes specialist police investigation units up to 6 h to fully assess the scene of serious road traffic incidents. Establishing braking distances may much more usefully predict the presence of potentially serious occult injury, e.g. car versus tree injury mechanisms cause massive deceleration and correlate with the risk of shear injury to the viscera (aortic transection/hepatic lacerations).

Inspection of seatbelts, the deployment of airbags, impact protection systems and seatbelt pre-tensioners can provide valuable information about potential injury patterns. Airbags that have not deployed pose potential serious risk of injury to rescuers and may need to be actively managed by the use of restraints by fire and rescue personnel (Figure 21.3). Many regions of the UK will dispatch a fire service specialist technical rescue and extrication team to entrapment road traffic collisions.

Digital photographs of the scene (see Figure 21.3), taking care not to breach patient confidentiality, may provide invaluable handover information for the ED trauma team leader, especially when patients may appear deceptively well at first appearance.

Clinical management

Airway

Airway maintenance and treatment of ventilatory failure, thus preventing avoidable secondary hypoxic and hypercarbic neurological injury, are two of the fundamental clinical objectives of prehospital emergency medicine.

Nasal airways have an immensely important role in airway maintenance and their use is not contraindicated (in skilled hands) in the presence of a suspected base of skull fracture, although care will be required to ensure their safe insertion. Bilateral nasal airway placement, together with an oral airway, may be required to maintain airway patency in those with severe maxillo-facial/head injury. Vascularity of the nasal mucosa may limit their use in children. Once a definitive airway has been placed, the use of nasal tampons or epistats may help to control significant nasal haemorrhage from associated facial fractures.

Patient tolerance of an oral airway to maintain an airway usefully predicts the likely requirement for a definitive airway following significant injury, and therefore the potential requirement for rapid sequence induction (RSI) of anaesthesia.

Supraglottic devices also have a useful role as an airway adjunct in unconscious trauma patients, as well as being a useful device to provide assisted ventilation. They have now been widely introduced by England's ambulance services and are now used as the first line approach to assist the ventilation of patients in cardiac arrest. They may be much more effective than the use of a bag-valve-mask in adults, especially in the presence of distorted facial anatomy (e.g. maxillofacial and mandibular fractures).

Supraglottic devices, such as the LMA and I-gel, may also be useful for promptly assisting ventilation in unconscious patients, with partially preserved upper airway reflexes, who may be impossible to intubate without RSI. The I-Gel is a very simple device to insert, and does not require a cuff to be inflated to achieve a good seal with the glottis. These devices may be particularly valuable for assisted ventilation when access to the patient may be severely restricted (e.g. RTC entrapment). Endotracheal intubation via the mouth may be almost impossible in this scenario using conventional laryngoscopy (see below).

Supraglottic devices may also be helpful for supporting airway management in a confined space, working in collapsed structures (e.g. urban search and rescue [USAR] environments) as well as other hazardous environments, such as chemical incidents, where the constraints of personal protective equipment may also make endotracheal intubation particularly difficult.

The vast majority of severely injured patients with airway compromise and a potentially survivable injury pattern, will require rapid sequence induction of anaesthesia (RSI) to create optimal conditions for the establishment of a definitive airway.

Prehospital emergency anaesthesia

The indications for prehospital RSI in trauma are broadly similar to those in the ED resuscitation room (Box 21.4). Its main indications are impending or actual airway or breathing compromise, prolonged transport direct to a major trauma centre by road, or, the need for helicopter transport, where the transport of such patients is fraught with hazard without prior critical care intervention.

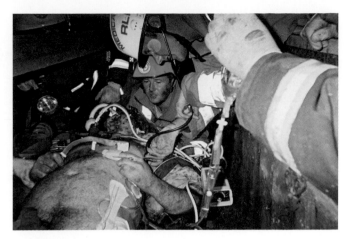

Figure 21.4 The risk-benefit of undertaking critical care interventions in a confined space requires careful assessment. This unconscious patient was intubated and ventilated prior to the overlying underground train being moved to enable patient rescue from the drainage pit.

Box 21.4 **Indications for prehospital RSI in trauma**

- Airway maintenance and protection.
- Ventilatory failure and controlled ventilation.
- Helicopter transport of the 'ABCD' physiologically compromised patient.
- Humanitarian reasons and anticipated clinical course.

However, the risks versus the benefits of RSI must be carefully balanced in each individual patient, when the resources and experience to support such interventions are usually finite, and therefore carry potentially greater risk in the prehospital environment (Figure 21.4).

Suboptimal patient positioning, adverse environmental conditions, abnormal upper airway anatomy and restricted patient access may make endotracheal intubation using conventional laryngoscopic techniques difficult because of inadequate glottic exposure and the need for blind intubation techniques. The use of a Macintosh laryngoscopic blade, augmented by a gum elastic bougie, is the current gold standard approach in the UK, but remains a challenging skill to acquire and maintain. A number of new indirect laryngoscopes potentially offer an attractive solution for particularly challenging trauma airways, and for those with limited exposure to emergency intubation. The training requirements for handling the device appear to be significantly less than those for the use of a Macintosh blade and gum elastic bougie. The author has had recent favourable emergency experience (50 cases) with one such device, the Airtraq laryngoscope, in the prehospital environment, as well as the ED, as both a primary laryngoscope and a rescue device.

Prior to undertaking prehospital RSI, it is important to give due consideration to the location in which to physically undertake

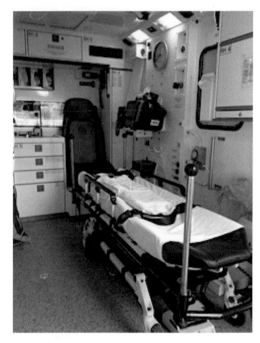

Figure 21.5 A modern modular-build ambulance, which has significantly improved patient access and a clinical environment for enhanced patient care. This vehicle is equipped with all necessary equipment to support critical care.

the procedure (see Fig 21.4). Unless absolutely essential, it may be safer not to undertake this where the patient was originally injured (e.g. under a train), but to undertake it adjacent to the ambulance/helicopter out of direct sunlight. Unless environmental conditions preclude this (e.g. heavy rain), it may be wise not to undertake RSI inside an ambulance because of the difficulty of securing adequate 360° access to the patient. Modern modular build ambulances, as opposed to van conversions, do, however, provide a much better clinical environment for improved patient access (Figure 21.5).

Surgical airway

Emergency cricothyroidotomy provides life-saving access to the airway in adults. In military medicine this is frequently used as the primary means of establishing a definitive airway in a tactical environment in unconscious spontaneously breathing patients with preserved upper airway reflexes, or in patients with life threatening major upper airway burns, but tends to be used as a rescue procedure for the failed airway in the civilian setting. It may also have a specific utility for RTC entrapment when adequate access to the upper airway may be impossible.

The author's preferred technique is to use a horizontal stab technique directly through the cricothyroid membrane unless the airway anatomy is distorted (by haematoma/surgical emphysema) in which case a 5 cm midline vertical incision is made through the skin and subcutaneous fat centred on a point four (patient) finger breadths above the sternal notch. The position of the cricothyroid membrane is confirmed by digital palpation through the wound and a horizontal incision is made through the cricothyroid membrane. The use of a tracheal hook in the latter scenario to lift and stabilise the cricoid cartilage, or the use of gum elastic bougie, may facilitate insertion of a cuffed ET tube (or tracheostomy tube) into the trachea The use of an uncut size 6 ET tube is important in major burns to the face/neck to accommodate later swelling, but care must be taken to avoid bronchial main stem intubation which can occur all too easily as the distance to the carina is usually no more than 5 to 7 cm distal to the cricothyroid membrane in most adults. The presence of a persistent air leak through the cricothyroidotomy wound, despite the inflated cuff in a spontaneously ventilating patient, may provide the first clue that this latter complication has occurred, and is easily managed by judicious withdrawal of the endotracheal tube from the right main bronchus.

The use of the Seldinger technique for cricothyroidotomy is usually not appropriate as this is likely to be a time-critical emergency intervention in most prehospital airway rescue scenarios.

Respiratory management

Pneumothorax

Simple pneumothorax that does not compromise oxygenation usually does not require prehospital drainage in spontaneously ventilating patients. Thresholds should be low for performing needle thoracocentesis (decompression) or ideally surgical thoracostomy in positively ventilated patients with signs of a significant chest injury (see below) because of the high risk of tension developing.

Tension pneumothorax is life threatening and is likely to recur following emergency decompression, especially in ventilated patients. Clinical diagnosis of tension is not straightforward in the prehospital environment and is usually a diagnosis of exclusion.

Thresholds for attempting decompression should be low in the presence of a high-risk injury with increasing *respiratory distress* (i.e. reported dyspnoea or tachypnoea). High-risk wounds include penetrating chest wounds (gunshot/blast/stab), the presence of multiple rib fractures, the presence of an external air leak through the wound on coughing (a confirmed pleural breach), progressive surgical emphysema or a sucking wound. The classic clinical signs of tension appear late and are pre-terminal. Access to prehospital thoracic ultrasound, if available, may reduce unnecessary thoracostomy rates by helping to rule-in pneumothorax.

Needle thoracocentesis (decompression)

Tension pneumothorax kills approximately 15% of combat casualties and usually takes at least 45–60 min to develop following penetrating chest trauma in spontaneously breathing casualties. These deaths are readily preventable. It can also occur following significant blunt chest trauma causing multiple rib fractures in spontaneously breathing patients, which also takes time to develop.

Lateral decompression of the chest in the axillary 'triangle of safety' is much safer than the classically taught anterior approach because of the latter's proximity to central mediastinal vascular structures. The triangle of safety is delineated by the axillary apex, nipple and fifth intercostal space in the mid-axillary line. The position of the mediastinum is unpredictable in severe bilateral chest injury. The author's preferred landmarks for decompression and thoracostomy this to be done one hand's breadth below the axilla (above the line of the nipple) in the anterior axillary line with the ipsilateral upper limb abducted to 90°. Body armour worn by police and military personnel in tactical environments may also make emergency access to the front of the chest difficult and impractical in this type of environment. This is the same landmark for chest drain insertion.

NEEDLE THORACOCENTESIS: TECHNIQUE   The use of a 12 G needle over at least a 2 inch cannula (e.g. Medicut) attached to a saline-filled syringe using a similar technique for an intrapleural pleural block is by far the safest method for undertaking emergency needle decompression of the chest in the prehospital environment. This method involves inserting the cannula through the skin, flushing the cannula with saline within the subcutaneous tissues to eject any skin plug, removing the syringe plunger from the syringe barrel, and then advancing the cannula until fluid within the attached syringe barrel siphons passively into the pleural space (which will occur as soon as the patent cannula enters the pleural space); the presence of bubbling confirms the presence of tension. This method is recommended as it provides visual confirmation of the presence of tension and prevents the needle being advanced unnecessarily deeply into the chest, which carries a significant risk of avoidable injury to the underlying lung/mediastinal structures. Needle decompression may fail as many standard IV cannulae are too short to reach the pleural space in muscular patients and they frequently become blocked by skin/subcutaneous fat and clot.

As these cannulae frequently block/kink post insertion, there is a strong argument for removing the cannula post insertion and repeat needling the chest (as above) should recurrent tension be suspected. All spontaneously breathing patients who have developed a confirmed tension pneumothorax will require chest drain insertion as soon as this can be safely achieved, usually in a hospital setting.

Finger thoracostomy

The main indication for finger thoracostomy in prehospital environment is to prevent tension pneumothorax from developing in chest-injured patients who require positive pressure (assisted) ventilation. It may also need to be undertaken should needle decompression fail in spontaneously breathing patients and there is a high clinical suspicion of tension. If this procedure is undertaken in a spontaneously breathing patient, it *must* be followed by chest drain insertion unless the patient is ventilated as this procedure will have effectively created an open (sucking) pneumothorax. Alternative options would be to apply a chest seal with a low profile outlet valve (e.g. Brolin/Russell) over the wound, or a simple occlusive dressing with close monitoring for recurrent tension (Figure 21.6).

The risks of undertaking blind finger thoracostomy in the presence of rib fractures is not without significant serological risk to the operator and the author has had recent favourable experience using 11.5 mm Thoracoport to facilitate pleural venting in positively pressure ventilated patients (see below and Figure 21.7).

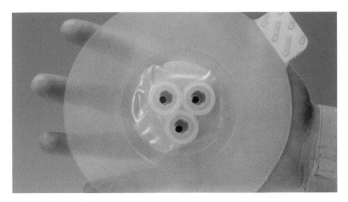

Figure 21.6 Chest seal (Brolin) with a low profile outlet valve designed to occlude large chest wall defects and sucking chest wounds. Its early application to large defects and sucking wounds may be life saving.

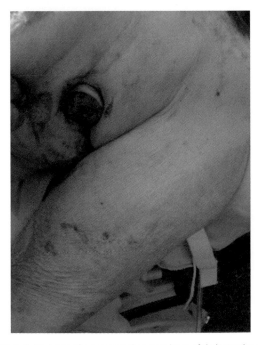

Figure 21.7 A 10.5 mm Thoracoport that may be useful alternative to open finger thoracostomy to achieve emergency pleural decompression in ventilated patients (see text).

Tube thoracostomy

Chest drain insertion is rarely undertaken prehospital care unless field care is prolonged (isolated/remote locations) or if there is a requirement for the casualty to be evacuated by helicopter at high altitude in mountainous regions. The principle reason for undertaking it is to prevent tension pneumothorax from recurring. There is no benefit in draining a haemothorax during prehospital management, and the real potential for harm (loss of clot and resulting persistent haemorrhage). Thoracostomy alone is usually sufficient in ventilated patients in urban settings with short transport times to hospital.

The standard technique for tube thoracostomy, either under procedural sedation (ketamine 0.5 -1.0 mgs/kg) or following emergency anaesthesia, is to incise the skin 3-5 cm down to rib using a combination of sharp and blunt dissection using 8 inch straight Spencer Wells forceps and a finger sweep to enter the pleural cavity (Figure 21.8).

An alternative method, which the author favours, is the use of a 10.5 mm Thoracoport, designed for minimally invasive thoracic surgical procedures (Figure 21.9) which can be used not only to facilitate the passage of the chest drain through the tissues of the chest wall, but also for emergency decompression of the chest in both spontaneously breathing and ventilated patients (as above).

The advantage of using a Thoracoport for both emergency decompression and chest drain insertion is that it can be rapidly and safely performed, it provides very effective pleural decompression (venting) through a short skin incision, and there is no need to expose the operator's gloved finger to fractured ribs and potentially serious blood-borne infection.

The use of percutaneous (Seldinger) chest drain kits in prehospital care has not been formally evaluated yet in the UK but may be an attractive alternative to open chest drain insertion techniques in adults, and also in small children where the size of the intercostal space may preclude traditional open thoracostomy techniques. A size 18 Ch chest tube will prevent tension occurring in

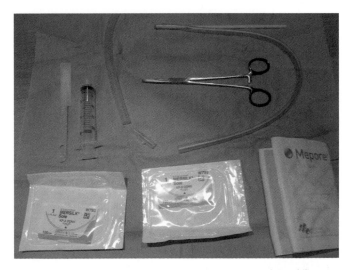

Figure 21.8 Chest drain insertion kit as supplied on National Capability Mass Casualty Equipment Vehicles. A vented chest drainage system is also supplied. A percutaneous set with size 12 and 18Ch drains is also supplied for use in children.

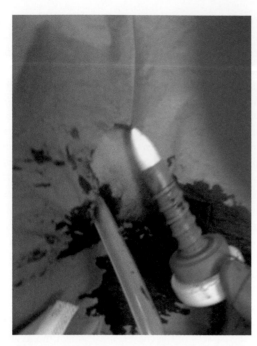

Figure 21.9 A10.5 mm Thoracoport used to facilitate chest drain insertion – in conscious patients the insertion of the drain through the chest through a surgically created track may be the most technically challenging part of the procedure – the use of a thoracoport transforms this part of the procedure.

most clinical scenarios with a small to moderate air leak from the underlying lung.

Open pneumothorax
Sucking wounds should be immediately sealed, ideally by an improvised three-sided dressing or specifically designed chest seals incorporating an outlet one way valve (see Figure 21.6). Hydrogel based dressings can also be used to rapidly occlude sucking wounds and to augment the stickiness of these types of chest seals in tactical environments if necessary (sweating can compromise the effectiveness of these dressings).

In the absence of available chest seals, all penetrating wounds should be packed/covered with an occlusive dressing and should respiratory distress occur, the chest should be decompressed/vented as above (to rule out tension pneumothorax) and subsequently formally drained as circumstances permit.

Large open defects in the chest wall should likewise be covered with an occlusive dressing or chest seal to prevent asphyxia. Formal pleural drainage will subsequently be required at the earliest opportunity in the presence of an air leak from the underlying lung. Should there be suspicion of tension developing prior to formal pleural drainage, these occlusive dressings should be temporarily removed and the wound track gently digitally explored if required to achieve chest decompression.

Circulation
Catastrophic haemorrhage control
Fifty percent of avoidable deaths following penetrating trauma and blast injuries occur from catastrophic but potentially compressible,

and therefore potentially immediately manageable, haemorrhage from the limbs. This is the overwhelming initial clincal priority when assessing patients who have sustained penetrating trauma (stab/gunshot) or blast injuries (Box 21.5).

> Box 21.5 **Clinical priorities for major trauma: <C>ABC**
>
> - <C>atastrophic compressible external haemorrhage control
> - Airway
> - Breathing
> - Circulation

The re-introduction of the immediate use of tourniquets, and the development elasticated compression field dressings, that can provide truly effective circumferential compression of arterial bleeding, has made a significant contribution to the management of these patients in recent military conflicts. Such patients are now reaching military field hospitals alive, even after sustaining multiple upper and lower limb traumatic amputations, when previously they would have bled to death shortly after injury. Recent combat experience has confirmed that 7% of casualties may require the application of more than one tourniquet per limb, especially when used for traumatic above knee amputation.

Catastrophic haemorrhage from penetrating wounds to junctional areas (groins/axilla and neck) can be particularly difficult to control by direct pressure alone. Foley balloon catheters can be particularly useful for emergency control of bleeding from discrete penetrating wounds to these areas (stab/shrapnel/gunshot). For more extensive open wounds with or without soft tissue loss, topical haemostatic agents when supplemented with direct pressure have been proven to be of particular value when rapidly applied in tactical environments. Topical haemostatic dressings are *not* a substitute for direct pressure but may help to control bleeding from transected major vessels when applied appropriately. Celox Gauze (a chitosan-covered gauze dressing that can be used to pack actively bleeding wounds) is currently being used by the UK MOD on operations in Afghanistan. These types of products are also of particular value when applied early to extensive blast injury wounds with significant soft tissue disruption; these patients become coagulopathic extremely quickly, even in the absence of crystalloid/colloid transfusion.

Volume expansion
Inappropriate administration of IV fluids during prehospital care can contribute to haemodynamic instability, an excessive systemic anti-inflammatory response to trauma, coagulopathy and hypothermia, and may contribute to late deaths from multiple organ failure.

Early definitive damage control surgery is the key to survival for severely injured patients. The author has found the assessment of central capillary refill using the mucous membranes of the gums helpful clinically when assessing the adequacy of tissue perfusion in all types of prehospital environments in adults and children.

Moderate hypotension (60–90 mmHg) is reasonably well tolerated for relatively short times (1–2 h) in conscious patients and may contribute to clot stabilisation and haemorrhage control, at least initially. Severe hypotension (blood pressure [BP] <60 mmHg) is poorly tolerated and there is little option in this scenario but to volume expand until definitive surgical intervention. This is particularly important in the presence of concomitant head injury. The ideal volume expander in hospital is (fresh) blood combined with platelets and fresh frozen plasma (FFP) in coagulopathic and acidotic patients but this is rarely achievable prehospital. Medical emergency teams responding to combat casualties in Afghanistan are now transfusing patients *en route* to field hospitals using packed cells and FFP in the hope of aggressively managing traumatic coagulopathy and blood loss, with the aim of supporting the patient in producing high-quality clot to address non-compressible haemorrhage, and limiting metabolic acidosis. In the UK 0.9% saline is the most frequently used crystalloid by the ambulance service for volume expansion.

The international multicenter randomized controlled CRASH 2 trial has recently confirmed the value of the early administration of tranexamic acid in improving major trauma survival and this has recently been approved for prehospital civilian paramedic use in 2012.

Current UK consensus guidelines adopted by the National Institute of Health and Clinical Excellence (NICE 2004) recommend volume expanding patients during prehospital care using 250 mL boluses of normal saline, titrating to the presence or absence of the radial pulse. There is now increasing evidence to support the use of small aliquots of hypertonic saline for volume expansion in hypotensive patients with significant head injury.

Should gaining vascular access be problematic in adults, as well as in children, the intraosseous (IO) route provides an attractive and simple means of securing this, and should be obtained in critically inured patients as rapidly as possible. There are a number of IO systems that have recently been developed for use in adults that now make this readily and rapidly achievable (Figure 21.10).

Intraosseous devices may also be of particular value when working in hazardous environments as the constraints of PPE can make IV cannulation technically challenging (Figure 21.11). IO access alone can be used for volume expansion and drug administration, and these systems provide adequate vascular access sufficient for emergency anaesthesia to be undertaken promptly in field conditions when necessary.

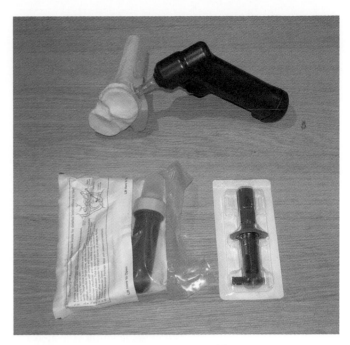

Figure 21.10 Adult intraosseus (IO) sytems used for securing emergency vascular access via bone medullary cavities: EZIO (top), FAST 1 (lower right – sternum only) and bone injection gun (lower left). EZIO now the most widely used system by ambulance services in England.

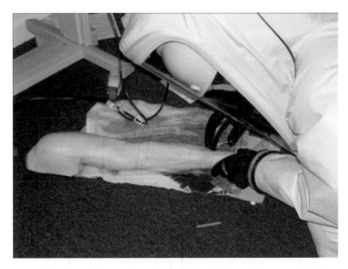

Figure 21.11 Establishing emergency peripheral intravenous access in the prehospital environment can be challenging: in this training exercise a Hazardous Area Response Team (HART) clinician is attempting to undertake IV cannulation while wearing breathing apparatus inside a chemical suit.

Head injury

All patients with potentially significant head injury, who may require neurosurgical care, should ideally be directly transported to a major trauma centre with on-site neurosurgical facilities. Evacuation of intracranial haematoma is time critical following head injury. Such patients may require RSI and controlled ventilation prior to transport from the scene of injury in order to prevent avoidable secondary hypoxic/hypercarbic injury. If this level of care is not available at the scene, then patients should be transported to the nearest ED (designated Trauma Unit) for stabilisation and critical care. Subsequent secondary inter-hospital transfer of such

patients to a regional neurosurgical centres should take place as soon as possible. It is essential that such inter-hospital transfers are prioritised by the ambulance service as 'time critical' as the therapeutic window for neurosurgery and neurosurgical intensive care to achieve optimal clinical outcomes for patients with intracranial haematoma is 4–6 hours following injury.

Spinal management

It is important to avoid unnecessary spinal movements in patients at high risk of spinal injury. Unconscious head-injured patients are particularly at high risk. Long boards are suitable devices for vehicular extrication but scoop type orthopaedic stretchers (OSS) are preferable for packaging as they avoid direct (midline) pressure over the spine and may thus provide more comfortable support for conscious spinal injury patients. OSS also obviate the requirement in the ED for formal log rolling which may reduce risk of clot dislodgement in patients with major pelvic disruption.

The risks of unstable spinal column injury are very low in isolated penetrating trauma, and the routine use of spinal packaging is unnecessary in these cases, which may lead to unnecessary extended on-scene times. This may be important in the context of time-critical, life-threatening penetrating wounds to head, neck, trunk and proximal extremities, as this may delay time to definitive surgical care.

Although the routine use of cervical collars is currently part of routine prehospital trauma clinical practice in patients who have sustained significant blunt head and neck injuries, their value and efficacy in preventing secondary spinal cord injury continues to be questioned. Alternative approaches in cooperative patients and unconscious patients, is the use of head blocks and tape only. Semi–rigid cervical collars are uncomfortable and are therefore frequently poorly tolerated (resulting in increased spinal movements), they elevate intracranial pressure when tightly fitting and can cause skin necrosis if not promptly removed after arrival in hospital. This area of ambulance clinical practice, which remains significantly influenced by medico-legal concerns, is currently under review.

Splintage and packaging

As part of haemorrhage control strategy, all femoral shaft fractures should be reduced and held in traction splints (Figure 21.12). All suspected pelvic fractures, which should be treated on the basis of injury mechanism, as well as physical findings, should be stabilised at the earliest opportunity with a pelvic binder (Figure 21.13). It is never appropriate to assess pelvic stability clinically by distraction because of the unacceptable risk of precipitating catastrophic haemorrhage by disrupting previously formed clot. This is best assessed in hospital using plain radiography initially augmented by computed tomography (CT).

Any fracture or dislocation of major joints compromising neurovascular status of a limb should be reduced at the earliest opportunity, using procedural sedation if necessary. In shocked patients ketamine (0.1–0.5 mg/kg) IV is an attractive option for achieving this.

Uncomplicated distal limb fractures should be supported using simple splints and triangular bandages.

All IV lines, ET tubes and ventilation tubing and monitoring cables must be secured to avoid clinical compromise during transport to hospital. Oxygen requirements must be anticipated and adequate provision made at all times. The multiple oxygen delivery systems that are now carried by England's ambulance services enable multiple casualties to receive oxygen simultaneously (see Chapter 28).

Maintenance of core temperature

Multiply injured patients with major trauma may rapidly develop coagulopathy as part of a systemic inflammatory response to

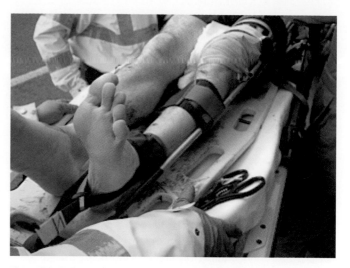

Figure 21.12 Femoral traction splint and an elasticated compression field dressing has been applied to a left femoral shaft fracture and open knee injury immediately post extrication following an RTC.

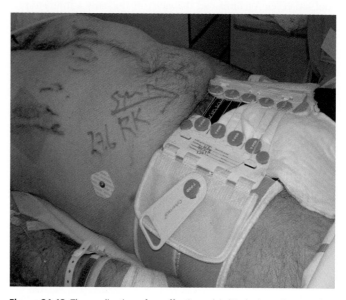

Figure 21.13 The application of an effective pelvic binder in patients with high energy pelvic injury during prehospital trauma care may be life saving and application thresholds should be low. The South Central Ambulance Service now carry pelvic binders on all front line emergency ambulances.

trauma. Severely injured, non-ambulant patients will rapidly become hypothermic, even in hot environments. This will exacerbate coagulopathy. Core temperatures below 35 °C on admission to hospital is associated with excess mortality in patients with Injury Severity Score > 15. This must be anticipated and actively managed. The use of survival blankets and skull caps can significantly reduce avoidable heat loss in these patients in all environments.

Monitoring

All physiologically compromised patients must have their vital signs recorded regularly – ideally every 3–5 min in severely compromised patients, preferably using automated systems. The minimum requirement is for non-invasive blood pressure, continuous surface electrocardiogram (ECG) and heart rate (HR), oxygen saturation (SaO_2) and respiratory rate, and in ventilated patients, end-tidal carbon dioxide. It is important that this data is captured for handover and for clinical governance purposes.

It is essential that physically entrapped and crushed patients have continuous ECG monitoring during release to monitor for signs for hyperkalaemia and arrhythmias as this may require prompt emergency treatment during reperfusion.

Road traffic crash entrapment

Entrapment at road traffic crashes will significantly extend the duration of prehospital care for these patients. For non-trapped patients in a urban environment, the average duration of the prehospital care phase is 45 min. For trapped patients, the 'golden hour' is a prehospital event.

The aim of the fire and rescue service will be to release the casualty as rapidly as possible, ideally within 20 min of arrival. One of the early key roles for ambulance and medical personnel will be to identify potentially life-threatening injury patterns and define an extrication time window for the fire and rescue extrication team. It is important that there is close communication and co-ordination between the health and the extrication teams. A second extrication plan (plan B) should be agreed in case the patient's condition deteriorates during the extrication process.

It is essential that the clinical team supporting the entrapped patient does not become a hindrance to extrication. It is important that all physiologically compromised and trapped patients are closely monitored; a member of the team will usually be placed inside the vehicle to assess, monitor and reassure, and to treat life-threatening complications of injury. All physically trapped patients should have the following vital signs recorded automatically every 3–5 min: non-invasive blood pressure, continuous surface three-lead ECG and pulse rate, SaO_2 and respiratory rate. ECG monitoring is especially important during release of crushed limbs/torso when the early signs of hyperkalaemia/cardiovascular collapse can be identified promptly and treated.

During extrication the fire and rescue service will endeavour to create space around the casualty to facilitate patient assessment and treatment. Only truly life-threatening injuries, for example airway obstruction, ventilatory failure or significant uncontrolled haemorrhage, should be treated *in situ* inside the vehicle by the simplest means. The use of supplementary oxygen via a non-rebreathing mask, airway adjuncts and supraglottic devices (see above) will frequently suffice in this setting. There may be an occasional role for the selective use of a limb arterial tourniquet if there is difficulty controlling external haemorrhage by direct pressure during extrication (e.g. lower limb open fractures in foot well entrapment) or during the release/reperfusion of a severely mangled/crushed extremity. Tourniquets applied below the elbow/knee are unlikely to be effective and should rarely be required.

Critical care can usually only be effectively and safely delivered with an acceptable degree of risk once $360°$ access to the patient has been established, i.e. after the patient has been released from the vehicle and placed on an ambulance trolley. Establishing a definitive airway will rarely be required inside a vehicle but if so, surgical cricothyroidotomy may be the simplest and fastest means of achieving this.

Unnecessary movements of the spine should be avoided in stable patients but compromise may be necessary in severely injured and unconscious patients; the key indication for potentially compromising spinal care is failure to effectively treat hypoxia inside the vehicle. In-line manual immobilisation and cervical collar use may also facilitate airway maintenance in unconscious patients. The use of an extrication long board may offer the simplest and most rapid means of extrication. It should be remembered that long boards are designed to facilitate extrication, and should not be used routinely for spinal immobilisation of ambulant patients, because of the very real risk of decubitus ulceration, and the needless pain and distress they cause conscious patients, unless appropriately padded. Kendrick type spinal immobilisation devices may have a role in stable patients but are potentially time consuming to apply and are cumbersome to remove in the ED (the use of an OSS may be helpful).

The extrication of conscious patients with long bone or multiple fractures may be facilitated by judicious use of procedural sedation – the use of an analgesic dose of ketamine (0.1–0.5 mg/kg) combined with a very small dose of midazolam (1–2 mg) can dramatically shorten the extrication times of distressed patients in considerable pain. It is essential that the clinical and extrication teams work in a co-ordinated way once in-vehicle sedation has been undertaken to ensure timely release from the vehicle.

During extrication, the requirement for general anaesthesia for safe onward transport to the most appropriate hospital may have been identified. The prehospital emergency physician must ensure that appropriate concomitant activity takes place to ensure that this can be promptly and safely undertaken at a suitable location following release from the vehicle.

Emergency department pre-arrival alert

An ED pre-arrival alert call should be made for every patient with a high-risk injury mechanism, and for physiologically compromised patients and those with a severe injury to more than one body region (Box 21.6). These calls should be made on a dedicated recorded telephone lines/radio channels for clinical governance and audit purposes.

The aim is to prevent the patient's management stalling following arrival in hospital by ensuring that a trauma team is assembled in good time. This should include a request for any other resource deemed necessary at the scene, including blood/clotting factors (activation of a massive transfusion protocol), and any other senior surgeon whose early presence in the ED is likely to facilitate patient care. The pre-arrival alert should clearly state the requirement for trauma team activation and should include estimated time and mode of arrival.

Mode of transport

The aim of any prehospital care system is to get the right patient to the right hospital in the best possible condition as rapidly as

Box 21.6 South Central Ambulance Service emergency department pre-arrival alert criteria for trauma

Physiological findings

- Airway obstruction.
- Respiratory distress/failure.
- Signs of shock.
- AVPU score P or less or cerebral irritation.

Mechanism and injury patterns irrespective of physiological status

- Patients requiring a tourniquet to control catastrophic extremity haemorrhage.
- Severe injury to more than one body region.
- Potential airway burn, major burns (>20 % BSA).
- Severe maxillo-facial injury.
- Progressive surgical emphysema.
- Presence of open fracture, extremity traumatic amputation, or multiple long bone fractures.
- Penetrating injury to head/neck or torso.
- Gunshot or blast injury to any body region.
- Spinal cord injury (paraplegia/quadriplegia).
- Fall from height from first floor or above.
- Prolonged physical RTC entrapment (>1 hour).
- RTC vehicle ejection or death of same vehicle occupant at scene.
- Near drowning.

Box 21.7 Patient handover system (ATMIST)

- **A**ge,
- **T**ime of incident.
- **M**echanism of Injury.
- **I**njuries identified top to toe
- **T**reatment

Clinical documentation (patient report forms) should be completed as soon as possible, and all physiological data from patient monitoring systems should be downloaded/printed out, and should form part of the inpatient clinical records.

In stable patients that have received all necessary resuscitation room interventions (for e.g. RSI) prehospital it may be appropriate in selected cases to bypass the ED and directly transfer the patient to CT scanner for handover and head to pelvis CT.

Future developments in prehospital trauma care

The UK ambulance service is one of the most developed in the world and continues to secure increasing resources, modern well-equipped ambulance vehicles and equipment. Clinical practice is being standardised with the implementation of evidence-based clinical guidelines through the Joint Royal Colleges Clinical Liaison Committee. New clinical performance indicators are being developed and introduced across ambulance services in England that will enable the quality of care to be objectively assessed for the first time.

Following the publication in 2007 of the NCEPOD report entitled *Trauma: Who Cares?*, which identified various shortcomings in NHS trauma care, a number of significant whole-systems issues for trauma care have now been identified and are being addressed. In order to drive through the required changes, the Department of Health has appointed a new national director for trauma who has been charged with reviewing trauma care in England with a view to improving the outcomes of patients with major trauma, as well as the care of the elderly who have sustained frailty related fractures.

This has lead to the role out of trauma networks throughout England with each region of England having dedicated regional major trauma centres, which will support a network of district general hospitals that have been approved and designated as trauma units. This phased implementation is due to be completed during 2012. This has led to the recognition that further significant investment in ambulance service clinical capability will be required for the successful implementation of these new clinical networks.

Most of the prehospital care delivered by physicians in the UK is currently undertaken on a voluntary and *ad hoc* basis. Following the merger of England's ambulance services into 11 new ambulance service trusts covering approximately 4–11 million people each, opportunities now exist to further integrate voluntary immediate medical care schemes (BASICS) into commissioned ambulance service operations to provide robust, consistent round-the-clock care for critically ill and injured patients. Such systems will provide much enhanced direct access to tertiary centre expertise for both critical injury and illness.

possible. Over the last 10 years there has been a significant growth in charity-funded air ambulance operations; all parts of the UK now have access to such a service during daylight. Decision making around which patients to transport by air is potentially complex and should be influenced by the environment and circumstance of injury, geographical remoteness, the physiological status of the patient, the presence or absence of an on-scene critical care capability, and the resources and proximity of adjacent hospitals

Although regional air ambulance operations are currently daylight only operations in the UK, a number of operations in England are considering developing night time capability in order to effectively address clinical need 24 h a day

Handover

Patient care must be handed over in an effective and systematic way and all members of the trauma team should be in a position to receive this information collectively when the patient is handed over by the ambulance service. The composition of the trauma team must be agreed and standardised and the team leader should be of the consultant grade.

Handover should be undertaken after the patient has been transferred from the ambulance to the ED resuscitation room trolley and the airway handed over and ventilation has been confirmed in ventilated patients. It should be succinct, readily audible to the whole team, and directed at the trauma team leader (Box 21.7).

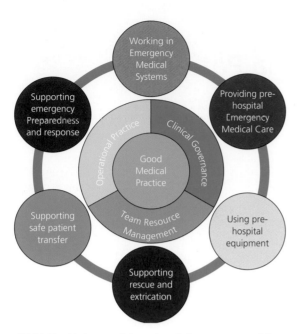

Figure 21.14 The 10 themes of the prehospital emergency medicine subspecialty curriculum.

In May 2009 a new Intercollegiate Training Board for Prehospital Emergency Medicine (IBTPHEM) came into being following the support of the Academy of Royal Medical Colleges. This board has broad representation from all the royal medical colleges, postgraduate deans and the UK Departments of Health. Its remit has been to oversee the application to General Medical Council for the new medical subspecialty of prehospital emergency medicine, the development of the core curriculum and assessment framework (Figure 21.14), and future national training programme accreditation. First recruitment to the national training programs is anticipated in commence in August 2013. Further information is available at the IBTPHEM website at www.IBTPHEM.org.uk.

Fully trained and accredited prehospital emergency physicians of the future would be well placed to provide regionally based high-level clinical care to ambulance services for patients with complex clinical needs 24 h a day. From this pool would also come a cadre of suitable trained physicians to provide management and clinical leadership as ambulance foundation trusts medical directors of the future.

Following the bombing incidents in London in July 2005, it is now accepted that ambulance clinical teams will occasionally need to deploy into potentially hazardous environments in order to save lives. Specific training, additional personal protective equipment and equipment are needed to enable clinicians to operate safely and effectively in these types of environments (Box 21.8).

Box 21.8 Hazardous environments

- Non-terrorist Hazardous Materials Incidents (HAZMAT)
- Chemical, biological radiological and nuclear and explosive incidents.
- Urban search and rescue (casualty care in collapsed structures).
- Firearm incidents.
- On- and off-shore terrorism.

Ambulance service Hazardous Area Response Teams (HART), which have been developed to respond to potentially hazardous incidents, were piloted in London in 2008 and have been rolled out to all other regions within England and Wales following further critical evaluation during 2009–2012. The initial focus for these HART teams has been on chemical incident scenarios and casualty care in USAR type incidents. The scope of practice of these teams is likely to be extended in the near future to address other current emergency care capability gaps for the other types of hazardous incidents listed. Appropriate prehospital emergency physician clinical support for HART teams is likely to be important in the future.

Further reading

Black JJM, Gareth GD. (2005) International EMS Systems: UK. Resuscitation 64: 21–9.

Black JJM, Ward ME, Lockey DJ. (2004) Appropriate use of helicopters to transport trauma patients from incident scene to hospital in the United Kingdom: an algorithm. Emerg Med J 21: 355–61.

Bulger EM, Maier RV. (2007) Prehospital care of the injured: what's new? Surg Clin North Am 87: 37–53.

Findlay G, Martin I, Carter S, et al. (2007) *Trauma: Who Cares?* London: National Confidential Enquiry into Patient Outcome and Death.

Gabriel EJ, Ghajar J, Jagoda A, et al. (2002) Guidelines for prehospital management of traumatic brain injury. J Neurotrauma 19: 111–74.

National Institute for Health and Clinical Excellence. (2004) Prehospital initiation of fluid replacement therapy in trauma. A technology appraisal. www.nice.org.uk/TA074guidance.

Royal College of Surgeons of England and the British Orthopaedic Society. (2000) *Better Care for the Severely Injured.* London: Royal College of Surgeons of England and the British Orthopaedic Society.

CHAPTER 22

Transfer of the Trauma Patient

Carl L. Gwinnutt[1] and Alastair W. Wilson[2]

[1]Hope Hospital, Salford, UK
[2]Royal London Hospital, London, UK

OVERVIEW

- Correct packaging of trauma patients reduces the risk of further harm during transfer.

- During secondary transfer, patients need the same standard of care that they would receive in a critical care environment.

- Transfers are best conducted by dedicated, trained, transfer teams.

- Ensure that provision is made for all requirements, of both patient and accompanying staff, during the transfer and checked before departure.

- Documentation of vital signs, interventions and events during the journey is essential.

- On arrival, a structured, verbal and written handover must be delivered to the receiving team.

Box 22.1 **Pretransportation check**

Before transportation check that:

- the airway is clear and secure and the spine is stabilised
- breathing is normal and ventilation symmetrical
- any intravenous lines are running adequately
- all monitors are functioning
- drugs and equipment are accessible.

The term 'primary transfer' is used to indicate the movement of a patient from the scene of an incident to hospital. Secondary transfer refers to the movement of a patient between hospitals, usually for more specialised care such as neurosurgery or intensive care. Although the two types of transfer are very different, the fundamental principle of 'do no further harm' should govern both.

Primary transfer

Primary transfer deals predominantly with prehospital emergencies. Timing, type of transport and destination are determined by the patient's injuries and their response to resuscitation. At the scene, time taken to clear and secure the airway, institute effective ventilation, control external bleeding and splint the spine and limbs is time well spent (Box 22.1). Such actions help to minimise complications and reduce the need for intervention during the journey to hospital. A 'scene time' of 15 min is optimal to achieve hospital arrival times for definitive care well within the 'golden hour'. The 'platinum 10 minutes', as used by the British Association of Immediate Care, is an even better target.

Failure to achieve haemodynamic stability at the scene, often because of uncontrollable bleeding, is an indication for transport to hospital by the fastest possible means. A doctor present at the accident scene can potentially undertake more interventions than a paramedic alone, but it is unnecessary to utilise every skill in an attempt to restore normal physiology and thereby delay transfer to definitive care. Unless the victim is trapped, cannulation should be attempted *en route* and fluid administration should be titrated against return of a radial pulse. The greater interventional and diagnostic skills of a doctor should be employed to direct the patient to a hospital capable of dealing with the patient's injuries. This may not be the nearest hospital. There is considerable evidence to show that the selection of the right hospital at the beginning is extremely important for patient outcome.

Packaging and stabilisation

During any treatment, but particularly during primary transfer of the injured patient, all movement is potentially harmful. It encourages haemorrhage and worsens any cardiorespiratory instability. Movement of a fractured limb is painful and may result in neurovascular damage. Movement of the head, neck or thorax in the presence of injury to the vertebral column may cause or exacerbate injury to the spinal cord. Even in a fully immobilised patient, internal organs are at risk of further damage from forces of inertia when an ambulance brakes, accelerates or corners. There is also the potential for secondary injury when stretchers are manhandled into and out of vehicles. From start to finish the journey should be as smooth as possible.

During the transfer, the whole spine must be protected if a spinal injury has not been excluded. This precludes the use of the lateral

ABC of Major Trauma, Fourth Edition. Edited by David V. Skinner and Peter A. Driscoll.
© 2013 Blackwell Publishing Ltd. Published 2013 by Blackwell Publishing Ltd.

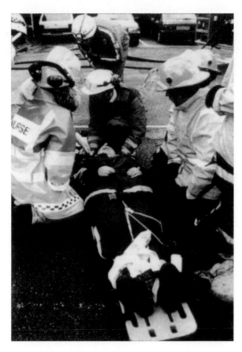

Figure 22.1 Patient immobilised on long spine board.

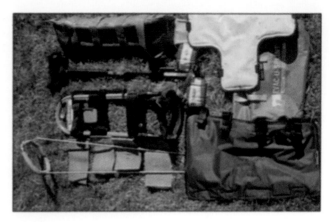

Figure 22.2 Variety of limb splints.

position so most patients are placed supine. Immobilisation of the spine is best achieved using a vacuum mattress. If this type of device is not available, a long spine board (Figure 22.1) can be used, bearing in mind that pressure sores develop rapidly. Whatever device is used, it must be capable of allowing the patient to be tipped or turned if he or she starts to vomit.

Patients with a known head injury and who are not hypotensive should be positioned slightly head up to help reduce intracranial pressure. Although this orientation can be difficult to maintain when entering or leaving an ambulance, it is essential to ensure that they are not tipped head down. The greatest forces on a patient during transfer are those from deceleration under braking. Ideally the patient should travel in the ambulance feet first, because these forces will then be least damaging to the brain. This has practical implications, as equipment and the accompanying personnel are then concentrated at the rear of the vehicle. Pregnant patients should be positioned in such a way as to displace the uterus to the left during transfer, to prevent supine hypotension syndrome (see Chapter 18).

Confused, combative patients should be transported only when the cause has been identified and treated. Great care must be taken to eliminate cerebral hypoxia or hypoglycaemia as the cause. Head-injured patients with a Glasgow Coma Score less than 9 should be intubated and ventilated prior to transfer. However, this is usually possible only when a doctor familiar with anaesthetic techniques and trained to cope with the particular difficulties of applying these skills in the prehospital setting is present at the scene. Similarly, any patient who is unconscious and tolerating an oropharyngeal airway, has airway burns or has impending respiratory failure should be intubated and ventilated before transportation.

If intubation has to be attempted during an ambulance journey, the vehicle will need to stop for the safety of all concerned, thereby prolonging the transfer. Therefore the airway should be secured before transfer. Actual or suspected injury to the cervical spine is not a contraindication to intubation, but makes the procedure more difficult. In cases where difficulties are anticipated and there is a risk that intubation and ventilation may fail, the doctor must be capable of creating a surgical airway. Where an individual possessing all of these skills is not immediately available, the airway must be maintained using basic techniques, high-flow oxygen given and the patient transferred rapidly to hospital.

All intravenous cannulae must be secured. In the prehospital environment, they are often inserted in the antecubital fossa and an Armback splint will keep the arm straight and ensure the intravenous line continues to function. Although central venous access is seldom indicated at the scene of an accident, the external jugular vein is becoming increasingly used. All connections must be checked to prevent disconnection and the risk of air embolism.

Limb splintage

The aim of splinting is to reduce blood loss, prevent soft tissue damage and provide pain relief. A variety of non-compromising traction splints are available that allow inspection of the limb and palpation of pulses (Figure 22.2). Conforming vacuum splints that can be moulded around limbs are helpful. Whole-body splinting can to some extent be achieved with the semi-rigid Vacumat. The use of the pneumatic anti-shock garment (PASG) remains controversial in trauma patients and it is now used infrequently in civilian practice. It is of limited use for controlling haemorrhage, but may help to stabilise an unstable pelvic fracture.

Transportation

The transport phase must not be regarded as a therapeutic vacuum. One of the most important tasks of the medical attendant during transportation is the continued assessment and monitoring of the patient to allow the detection and treatment of problems that develop with the patient or equipment.

On the way into hospital from the scene of an accident, monitoring is most commonly achieved using non-invasive devices to supplement clinical observation. Monitoring of respiratory rate, pulse oximetry, heart rate, blood pressure and electrocardiogram

(ECG) should be regarded as standard. If the patient is intubated and ventilated, end-tidal carbon dioxide and airway pressures must also be monitored. The level of consciousness in the unsedated patient must be assessed regularly.

Box 22.2 Essential information given *en route* to the receiving hospital

- The number of patients.
- Age and sex of the patients.
- Mechanism of injury.
- Vital signs at the scene.
- Initial findings on assessment.
- Procedures at scene.
- Response to treatment given.
- Estimated time of arrival.

Remember, it is crucially important to relay all vital information to the receiving hospital (Box 22.2).

Ideally, the patient should be positioned with their head next to the attendant's seat with enough room to gain access to the airway, to allow suction of the tracheal tube or, in an emergency, to identify and relieve a tension pneumothorax in a ventilated patient. Intravenous lines should be checked regularly and replaced when necessary. If there is cardiac arrest, cardiopulmonary resuscitation is almost impossible for a single operator. Two attendants allow effective therapeutic intervention.

Secondary transfer

Ideally, no patient should undergo secondary transfer. However, transfers do occur for specialised surgical care, investigations or for intensive care facilities (Box 22.3). As all patients undergoing secondary transfer have had the benefit of medical intervention within hospital, there is no place for the transfer of an unstable patient; patients deteriorate during transfer and treatment in the back of a moving ambulance is exceedingly difficult. Therefore it is essential that the patient has been fully assessed, treated and is haemodynamically stable, but not necessarily normal (for example,

---

Box 22.3 Reasons for secondary transfers

Specialised surgical care

- Neurosurgery.
- Plastic or burns surgery.
- Cardiac surgery.
- Spinal surgery.
- Paediatric surgery.

Specialised investigations

- CT scanning.
- Magnetic resonance imaging.
- Intensive care facilities.
- Specialised organ support.

---

the patient with penetrating trauma) before movement. Any intervention that may be required *en route* must be performed before departure. The decision to transfer a patient to another hospital must be made by senior medical personnel on the basis that the benefits to the patient outweigh any potential risks of the transfer.

The aim during secondary transfer is to provide the patient with the same standard of care that they would receive in an intensive care environment. To encourage this standard of care, the Intensive Care Society has produced a document entitled *Guidelines for Transport of the Critically Ill Adult* upon which many of the following recommendations are based.

Wherever possible, a dedicated team should undertake the transfer; a senior clinician and nurse should be identified as responsible in each hospital for the organisation of such a team. Those engaged with transfers on a regular basis should be encouraged to attend a recognised course, for example Safe Transfer and Retrieval (STaR) (www.alsg.org).

Before undertaking secondary transfer, it may be possible to rule out injury to the spine. If not, the patient should be fully immobilised using a vacuum mattress in preference to a long spinal board. The latter should only be used for short journeys and then padded adequately to prevent the development of pressure sores. Ventilation and gas exchange must be optimised and stabilised as demonstrated by arterial blood gas analysis. Heart rate, blood pressure, urine output, central venous pressure and occasionally pulmonary artery pressure are monitored to help maintain cardiovascular stability. If inotropic drugs are being given before departure, they will almost certainly have to be continued throughout the transfer. Despite the best preparations, the critically ill patient will be susceptible to the accelerative forces exerted during transportation, particularly at high speed, which can cause hypertension, arrhythmias and hypoxia. Aim to move these patients at normal road speed to minimise complications.

All patients will require an increased inspired oxygen concentration during transfer. A patient breathing spontaneously via a reservoir mask or being ventilated manually will require an oxygen flow of 12–15 L/min and a full, size D oxygen cylinder will only last about 20 min at these flow rates. Portable mechanical ventilators are more efficient despite using cylinder oxygen to both supply the patient and power the ventilator. They can usually be set to provide either 100% oxygen or an air mix that has a fraction of inspired oxygen (FiO_2) of about 45%. For an average adult, a size D oxygen cylinder will last approximately 40 min delivering 100% oxygen and double this in air mix mode. Adequate reserves must be available and will clearly depend on the anticipated duration of the transfer. As a rule of thumb, calculate the volume of oxygen required and take the same volume again as a reserve. Any ventilator must have disconnection and high-pressure alarms. Variable inspiratory/expiratory (I/E) ratios, pressure controlled ventilation and positive end-expiratory pressure (PEEP) will be required in patients with severe lung injury or acute respiratory distress syndrome (ARDS). Humidification, using a heat and moisture exchange (HME) device, should be provided on long journeys to reduce the risk of secretions becoming inspissated and difficult to remove with suction. Patients with a simple pneumothorax or haemothorax should have a large-bore chest drain inserted and connected to a (non-fluid) drainage system before transport. Chest drains must never be clamped.

Pain control

Pain should be controlled with intravenous analgesics, given as a continuous infusion to help maintain haemodynamic stability. Fractures should be immobilised in hospital before transfer by applying external fixators or appropriate splintage. Where there is a fracture of the pelvis the application of an external fixation device or C clamp will significantly reduce the risk of further blood loss and make transfer of the patient much safer.

Personnel and monitoring

Once secondary transfer of a patient has been deemed necessary and the destination determined, arrangements should be made between the senior medical staff responsible for initiating and receiving the transfer. The referring doctor is responsible for ensuring that the patient is stable and any treatment or investigations requested by the receiving specialist prior to transfer have been performed.

Accompanying personnel must be adequate in number as well as skill and experience. Ideally there should be two experienced attendants: one a doctor trained in intensive care medicine, anaesthesia or other acute specialty with the skills to carry out resuscitation, ventilation and organ support, and the other a healthcare professional trained in intensive care procedures and familiar with the transfer equipment.

The referring doctor must fully brief the attendants and confirm that they have the patient's records (or a copy), with the results of all investigations, X-rays and CT or MRI scans, and any cross-matched blood that is available. Where possible, communication should be maintained between the transfer team and the receiving hospital: a mobile phone is recommended. Be clear about the destination in the receiving hospital. If the hospital is unfamiliar territory, arrange to have someone meet the ambulance at the hospital entrance or for the local ambulance service to act as guides. The final duty of the referring doctor is to ensure that the receiving hospital is aware of the estimated time of arrival, so that arrangements can be made to receive the patient.

The minimum standards for monitoring during transfer include the continuous presence of appropriately trained staff, ECG, non-invasive blood pressure, oxygen saturation, end-tidal carbon dioxide and temperature. Ideally, a suitably equipped transport trolley containing all equipment and compatible with the local ambulance service systems should be used. Invasive monitoring of blood pressure should be used in the majority of patients and central venous pressure and urinary output are also often monitored during secondary transfer. In mechanically ventilated patients, the oxygen supply, inspired oxygen concentration, ventilator settings and airway pressures should also be monitored. When indicated, intracranial pressure monitoring may be required. Hypothermia is a common complication of transfers and is easier to prevent than treat. All patients should have their temperature monitored, and active warming should be used in all but

the shortest journeys. In the intubated, ventilated patient, the adequacy of sedation, analgesia and muscle relaxation must be assessed regularly. Whenever possible, if not already present, a nasogastric or orogastric tube should be inserted and suctioned regularly to reduce the risk of regurgitation and motion-induced vomiting.

Supplies

Provision should be made for all requirements during transfer, including adequate amounts of intravenous fluid, blood, supplementary drugs, oxygen and equipment for reintubation and replacement of intravenous cannulae. Drugs should be taken in labelled, prefilled syringes. In a moving ambulance, attempts to draw up drugs from ampoules are inaccurate, potentially dangerous and usually rendered unsterile. Where drugs are administered by infusion pump, the rate, syringe volume and battery status should be checked regularly. Always take spares.

The transfer team must also be adequately equipped to cope, particularly in bad weather and with protective clothing if appropriate. A mobile phone allows communication with base and the receiving unit. On long journeys, take adequate refreshments, ensure a lift home is organised and take sufficient money and credit cards in case of delays (Box 22.4).

Box 22.4 **PERSONAL equipment**

- **P**hone.
- **E**nquiry number and name.
- **R**evenue (and credit card).
- **S**afe clothing.
- **O**rganised route.
- **N**utrition.
- **A**–Z.
- **L**ift home

Documentation during transfer

Adequate documentation is essential to provide the receiving hospital with a record of events during the journey. Ensure that all physiological parameters and significant events are recorded along with any drugs and fluids administered. This can be difficult to achieve in a moving ambulance but many modern monitors store the relevant data and allow subsequent retrieval. Standard documentation or prepared sheets are also useful, because they act as an *aide mémoire* and allow subsequent audit.

Land ambulances

A compromise between speed and safety is required. The speed of an ambulance flashing a blue light is only marginally faster than its routine speed. Two-tone sirens terrify patients, as well as passing motorists. Attempting to maintain a high speed in traffic may simply result in great acceleration and deceleration forces. These cause significant cardiovascular and respiratory disturbances in the patient and motion sickness in the attending personnel. Vertical forces from unevenness in road surfaces can be minimised by the use of a 'floating' stretcher, but some conscious patients find this very nauseating. Space is at a premium in an ambulance, with few facilities for extra equipment. Care must be taken to secure all equipment, particularly oxygen cylinders. Staff should remain seated at all times during the journey and everything must be within their reach, so that they do not have to remove their seatbelts and move around during the journey (Figure 22.3).

Most ambulances are inherently cold but carry heating devices: one may simply need to ask for the heating to be switched on! Emphasis is placed on preventing heat loss by warming all intravenous fluids, using an HME on breathing circuits and minimising exposure of the patient.

Air ambulances

The designated medical helicopter is the most expensive part of the transfer armamentarium and should be used with care. The crew should be trained to the highest possible level and must act as the extended arm of the hospital. A helicopter can be used for both primary and secondary transfers, over long and short distances and therefore must be capable of allowing all monitoring facilities to be available during flight (Figure 22.4).

Helicopters that are not specifically designed for medical transportation (police or military aircraft) may have only minimal 'carry-on' medical equipment (Box 22.5). The use of monitoring and defibrillation equipment can interfere with aircraft avionics and only that which has been tested and found compatible should be used. Some helicopters are cramped, making management of the patient difficult. Anticipating potential problems is even more important than during land transport and potential problems are best solved before lift-off (Box 22.6). Ensure that all the necessary equipment, and space to cope with emergencies, are available during flight.

Helicopters are noisy, making communication difficult and use of a stethoscope impossible. Headphones should be put on the patient's head to allow reassuring conversation. The patient must be kept warm and comfortable during the flight. If a long journey is expected an antiemetic may be given to prevent air sickness and the stomach kept empty by gastric aspiration.

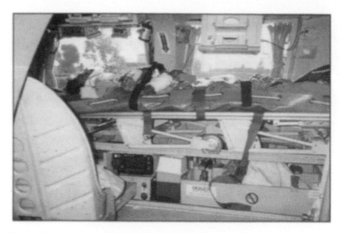

Figure 22.4 Interior of medical helicopter.

Box 22.5 **Equipment carried on medical helicopters**

- Non-invasive blood pressure monitor.
- Electrocardiograph and heart rate monitor.
- Invasive blood pressure monitors.
- Temperature monitors.
- Pulse oximeter and pulse rate monitor.
- Capnograph.
- Defibrillator.
- Syringe drivers and infusion pumps.
- Ventilators.
- Suction.

Box 22.6 **Indications and contraindications for helicopter transport**

Indications

Primary transfer

- Need for specialist trauma centre care.
- Long distances.
- Obstruction to land transport by traffic.
- Obscure or inaccessible accident sites.
- Transportation of medical staff or equipment to accident scene.

Secondary transfer

- Transfer for specialised surgery.
- Long distances.
- For intensive care.

Contraindications

- Poor weather.
- Difficulty in landing because of obstruction or poor lighting.
- Patient's injuries do not warrant care in specialised unit.
- Patient is violent or has psychiatric problems.
- The incident is close to the hospital most appropriate for the patient's needs.

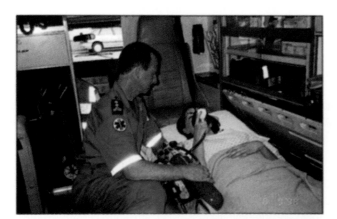

Figure 22.3 Interior of land ambulance.

Communication and handover

Once the patient's transfer to hospital is under way, staff in the receiving hospital must be informed of the patient's impending arrival and condition by the ambulance staff or the accompanying medical attendant. In the light of this information, staff in the emergency department can prepare the resuscitation room and call the trauma team (see Chapter 1).

On arrival at the receiving unit, there should be a structured verbal and written handover to the receiving medical and nursing teams. Start by introducing yourself and the patient and indicate any problems that need immediate attention. Subsequently, give details of the mechanism and time of injury, the patient's initial condition, injuries and other problems identified, treatment given and their response, investigations, results and any further treatment given. All documentation should be handed over and equipment retrieved before leaving.

On returning home, consider the need for debriefing, especially after complicated transfers, audit and reporting any critical incidents.

Summary

The underlying principle of any transfer is to do no further harm. Patient transfer from the scene of an accident to hospital must be accomplished with the minimum of delay and with resuscitation ongoing during transportation if necessary. Patients being transferred from a primary receiving centre to another hospital must be thoroughly resuscitated and stabilised before departure. The decision to transfer must be made by senior medical staff at both ends of the journey. Staff trained and experienced in transferring critically ill patients should accompany the patient. The aim should be to provide a level of care they would otherwise receive in the intensive care unit.

Further reading

Advanced Life Support Group. (2002) *Safe Transfer and Retrieval: The Practical Approach*. London: BMJ Books.

Intensive Care Society. (2002) *Guidelines for Transport of the Critically Ill Adult*. London: Intensive Care Society.

Lennon K, Davies S, Oakley P. (2003) Inter- and intra-hospital transfer of the trauma patient. In: Gwinnutt C, Driscoll P (eds) *Trauma Resuscitation: The Team Approach*, 2nd Oxford: Bios Scientific Publishers.

Morton NS, Pollack MM, Wallace PGM (eds). (1997) *Stabilisation and Transport of the Critically Ill*. London: Churchill Livingstone.

Neuroanaesthesia Society of Great Britain and Ireland and Association of Anaesthetists of Great Britain and Ireland. (1996) *Recommendations for the Transfer of Patients with Acute Head Injuries to Neurosurgical Units*. London: Association of Anaesthetists of Great Britain and Ireland.

Nicholl J, Hughes S, Dixon S, Yates D. (1998) The costs and benefits of paramedic skills in pre-hospital trauma care. *Health Technol Assess* 2: 17.

CHAPTER 23

Management of Severe Burns

Oliver Fenton,[1] Colin Robertson[2] and Orla Austin[1]

[1]Pinderfields Hospital, Wakefield, UK
[2]Royal Infirmary of Edinburgh, Edinburgh, UK

> ## OVERVIEW
>
> - The management of severe burn injuries begins at the scene.
> - The ABC approach applies in burns, as with other injuries.
> - Use cold soaks briefly – avoid hyperthermia.
> - Remove hot but not adherent clothing.
> - Consider the special needs for new thermal burns.

At the scene of a fire, first aid procedures are often life saving. We begin this chapter with instructions for medical staff on preparing a victim for evacuation to a burns unit. Always remember that however dramatic a major burn may look, there may be other more important injuries and ATLS principles always apply.

Evacuation from the scene

Under the direction of the fire service, and ensuring the safety of the rescuers, the patient should be removed from the scene of injury to a place of safety and fresh air.

Flames and heat track upwards, potentially burning the most important parts of the body, the face and hands, so keep the patient supine and rolled or covered with a heavy blanket, coat or rug to extinguish any residual flames. Take care not to get burnt yourself, especially if dealing with petrol burns or self-immolation, but you do want to bring down the contact temperature with the skin as quickly as possible – thermal injury is the product of the contact temperature and the length of time for which it is applied.

If the clothing is still smouldering or hot, apply large amounts of cold water. Clothing saturated with boiling liquids or steam should be removed rapidly, but do not remove burnt clothing that is adherent to the skin. Cover burnt areas with clean (sterile if available) towels or sheets and ensure that the patient is kept warm. **Do not apply cold wet soaks for longer than a few minutes or use them during transit**, because this will not provide any pain relief for patients with full-thickness burns and can cause profound

hypothermia, especially in children. Bringing the initial contact temperature down as quickly as possible is important, but not at the expense of producing hypothermia.

Evacuate the patient to the receiving hospital as quickly as possible. In patients with severe burns or those who have been exposed to smoke or fumes, high-flow oxygen through a facemask should be given during transit. Alert the receiving emergency department by radio or telephone. Advise them of the number and ages of the patients, the severity of their burns and the estimated time of arrival.

Reception and resuscitation

The primary assessment, investigation and treatment of a patient with severe burns should be a continuous and integrated process rather than a stepwise progression. While assessment is being performed, a member of staff must obtain the necessary information about the incident from the ambulance crew and other emergency services (Box 23.1). This should then be conveyed to the senior doctor in charge of the patient.

> Box 23.1 **Necessary information about the incident**
>
> - Its nature (house fire, blast, release of steam or hot gas, etc.)
> - If possible, the nature of burning materials (furniture, polyurethane foam, polyvinyl chloride, etc.)
> - Was there any explosion?
> - Was the patient in an enclosed space?
> - For how long was the patient exposed to smoke or fire?
> - Did the patient have to jump from a height to escape the fire?
> - The time elapsed from burn/injury/smoke inhalation to arrival in hospital

Management of the airway

Rapidly examine the patient for clinical evidence of smoke inhalation and thermal injury to the respiratory tract (Box 23.2). In patients with one or more of the features described, respiratory obstruction from pharyngeal or laryngeal oedema may develop rapidly. Patients exposed to steam or hot vapours are at particular risk of damage to the upper airways. Stridor, difficulty in swallowing

---

ABC of Major Trauma, Fourth Edition. Edited by David V. Skinner and Peter A. Driscoll.
© 2013 Blackwell Publishing Ltd. Published 2013 by Blackwell Publishing Ltd.

and drooling of saliva are signs of epiglottis swelling. In such patients, examination and early endotracheal intubation, performed by an experienced doctor with anaesthetic training, are essential (Box 23.3). Mucosal swelling of the oropharynx and epiglottis can be extremely rapid and delay can render tracheostomy necessary.

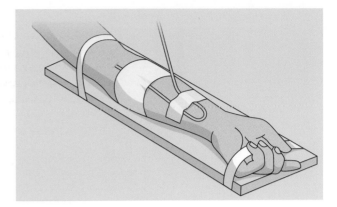

Figure 23.1 Intravenous cannulation.

Box 23.2 Clinical features indicating smoke or thermal injury to respiratory tract

- Altered consciousness
- Direct burns to face or oropharynx
- Hoarseness, stridor
- Soot in nostrils or sputum
- Expiratory rhonchi
- Dysphagia
- Dribbling, drooling of saliva

Box 23.3 Immediate investigations in the patient with severe burns

- Peak expiratory flow (if possible)
- Arterial blood gas tensions
- Carboxyhaemoglobin concentration
- Blood grouping and cross-matching
- Packed cell volume
- Urea and electrolyte concentrations
- 12-lead electrocardiography
- Chest radiography

If complete respiratory obstruction has already occurred or intubation is unsuccessful, or both, immediate cricothyrotomy or 'mini' tracheostomy is required, then formal tracheostomy. It should be emphasised, however, that in patients with severe burns the tracheostomy site is an important site of infection.

All patients suspected of having thermal or smoke injury to the respiratory tract should be given humidified high-flow oxygen, with an inspired oxygen concentration (FiO_2) of at least 40–60%, through a facemask. If bronchospasm is present give the patient a β_2 agonist (such as salbutamol or terbutaline) with an oxygen-powered nebuliser.

Frequent repeated clinical assessment of the airway and ventilation is mandatory in patients with all types of injuries caused by fire, with further measurements of arterial blood gas tensions, carboxyhaemoglobin and, if the patient can comply, peak expiratory flow. Note that values for oxygen saturation measured by pulse oximetry may be erroneous in the presence of carboxyhaemoglobin.

Intravenous access

Establishing adequate intravenous access must not be delayed. The fluid losses in major burns can be very large, and inadequate early fluid resuscitation can have serious consequences. Insert and secure one or more large-bore (needle gauge 14–16) intravenous cannulae

(Figure 23.1). If possible, use 10–15 cm cannulae to reduce the risk of dislodgement. The normal and easiest sites for percutaneous insertion of intravenous cannulae are the forearms and antecubital fossae. Narrow-bore cannulae inserted into small veins on the back of the hands are of little practical value. Occasionally, alternative sites such as the external jugular and femoral veins or the long saphenous vein at the ankle must be used, although the saphenous vein is prone to early occlusion.

Intravenous cutdown in the cubital fossae or on the long saphenous vein in the groin may be required if percutaneous intravenous access cannot be performed. This approach can be made through burnt skin, but do not attempt to suture the resulting gaping wound. If possible, before attaching the tubing of the intravenous drip, take enough blood through the cannula for cross-matching and determining blood group, packed cell volume, and urea and electrolyte concentrations.

Intravenous fluid requirements

For rapid assessment, the 'rule of nine' is useful (Figure 23.2). Do not include areas of simple erythema in the estimate. The size of small burns can be judged roughly by considering the palmar surface of the patient's closed hand as about 1% of the total body surface area. Use your own hand to map out the burnt area, and then make allowances for the size of your hand compared with the patient's; for example, it would be three times the size of a 1-year-old child's and twice the size of a 5-year old-child's. The result can be cross-checked by mapping the size of the unburnt area. In patients with very large burns it is simpler to measure the unburnt area and then subtract from 100.

Start treatment with intravenous fluids; fluid resuscitation is carried out according to the Parkland formula. This uses crystalloids, usually Hartmann's solution, as the main initial intravenous fluid, and is given at the rate of 0.25 mL/h/%burn/kg in the first 8 h (Box 23.4).

Box 23.4 Fluid replacement: Parkland formula

4 mL Hartmann's solution per 1% burn per kg bodyweight: half in first 8 h post burn, half in the next 16 h = 0.25 mL/h/% burn/kg in first 8 h from time of burn

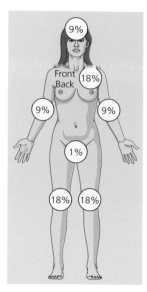

Figure 23.2 The 'rule of nine' is useful for rapid assessment of the body surface area affected by burns.

Patients with full-thickness burns that cover more than 10% of the body surface area may need a transfusion of red blood cells in addition to fluid replacement. As a rule of thumb, each 10% of full-thickness burn will drop the haemoglobin by at least a gram, from a combination of direct thermal injury, damage to red blood cells passing through injured blood vessels, and possible systemic haemolytic effects. A blood transfusion can be given in place of the fluid requirement for that period. However, since most full-thickness burns are taken to theatre for early excision and grafting, transfusion is usually given in theatre or in response to a haemoglobin level.

Insert a urinary catheter and start hourly measurements of urine volume. Note the colour and consistency of the initial urine in patients with severe flame or high-voltage electrical burns. The urine may be a treacly black, indicating haemoglobinuria (Figure 23.3) or myoglobinuria, or both. This is of prognostic importance for subsequent renal function.

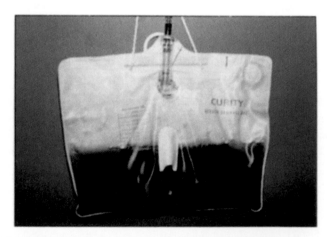

Figure 23.3 Urine from patient with electrical burns that indicates haemoglobinuria.

In elderly patients, patients with cardiorespiratory disease and patients who have delayed presentation, consider inserting a central venous pressure line if you are experienced in the technique. This can play an important part in subsequent restoration of volume in a patient with a severe burn. The risks of infection related to a central line are small in the early stages. With current methods of line management, these risks are outweighed by the importance of the line for monitoring and access.

The rate of intravenous fluid replacement should be tailored by the above guideline and the clinical response of the patient in terms of haemodynamic variables and urine output. The aim in adults is to achieve a urine output of 0.5–1.0 mL/kg/h.

Analgesia and reassurance

Severe burns cause both pain and distress. Analgesia and reassurance should be given as soon as possible. Treatment for pain in patients with severe burns must be tailored to the patient's individual requirements. Full-thickness burns, if present, are pain free, but all patients will be frightened and distressed, and constant reassurance and communication are vital (Box 23.5).

> Box 23.5 **Pain relief in patients with severe burns**
>
> - Entonox – for conscious, co-operative patients, especially in the prehospital phase
> - Opioids – give intravenously in small aliquots titrated to the patient's clinical response

A mixture of 50% nitrous oxide and 50% oxygen (Entonox) given by an on-demand system with a tight-fitting facemask can provide simple and effective analgesia, particularly before arrival in hospital. Subsequently, if required, an opioid such as Cyclimorph (cyclizine and morphine) should be given intravenously in aliquots of 1 mg at a dose carefully titrated to the clinical response.

Reassessment

The airway

Confirm that the patient's airway is secure and that ventilation is adequate. Repeat the measurements of arterial blood gas tensions and the analysis of carboxyhaemoglobin concentrations, which give an approximate guide to the amount of smoke inhaled; concentrations at the time of exposure can be predicted by using the nomogram shown in Figure 23.4. For example, if the carboxyhaemoglobin concentration is 30% at 1 h after exposure, the concentration at exposure would have been about 37%.

Clinical features of carbon monoxide poisoning correlate only moderately well with carboxyhaemoglobin concentrations but alteration of the conscious state should be regarded with suspicion. The so-called 'classic' feature of cherry red mucous membranes is a rarely seen, totally unreliable clinical sign.

Treatment with hyperbaric oxygen may be indicated in patients with carboxyhaemoglobinaemia, particularly if they are or have been unconscious, have cardiac or neurological symptoms, or are central venous pressure (if indicated), urine output, packed cell volume and peripheral perfusion and the trends in these values provide additional guidance for adjusting the rate of infusion. Fluid replacement should not be limited in patients with burns and inhalation injury. Indeed, increased fluids are often needed to maintain the systemic circulation and optimise cardiac and renal function.

The burns

Pending the patient's transfer from the emergency department to the ward or specialist burns unit, the burnt area should be covered with a sterile, warm, non-adherent dressing. A layer of Clingfilm covered by a dry sheet and blanket is effective. Never transfer a patient in wet sheets or towels, because this can lead to hypothermia, with occasional fatal consequences.

Deep circumferential burns over the limbs, neck and chest can produce a tourniquet-like effect because the damaged skin is unable to expand as tissue oedema develops. If this occurs, escharotomies (longitudinal incisions of the skin) are required to permit adequate circulation and ventilation. Escharotomy is also required if circumferential neck burns make intubation difficult. It is often necessary to do escharotomies before transfer. The affected part should be incised under sterile conditions on both sides, just as a plaster of Paris cast is bivalved. Ensure that the entire length of the constriction is released. In the hand, take the incisions right to the tips of affected digits.

If escharotomy of the chest is required, make vertical incisions along anterior and posterior axillary lines (Figure 23.6). If sufficient chest expansion does not occur, further incisions in the midline and midclavicular lines and transverse incisions may be needed.

Escharotomy does not require anaesthesia as the burns are full thickness. If it does cause pain then escharotomy is probably not indicated. Failure to do an early escharotomy can lead to the loss of a limb; therefore, if doubtful, always err on the side of escharotomy. The incisions do not cause any additional scarring as the burns are full thickness. Substantial bleeding occurs from the wounds, and sterile absorbent dressings should be applied and, if necessary, blood replacement given. Ensure that the patient is adequately protected against tetanus.

Lethal burns

Improvement in the management of burns in intensive care is resulting in some patients surviving burns of more than 90% of the total body surface area. However, few patients survive full-thickness burns of more than 70% of the total body surface area. As a rough guide, if the patient's age added to the percentage of the body surface area of the burn exceeds 100, the chances of survival are less than 50%. Any decision not to treat a patient with a lethal burn aggressively must be taken by a consultant with experience in burns. If aggressive resuscitation is not to be instituted in a patient, the other aspects of reassurance and analgesia are of even greater importance. Remember that even patients with 100% full-thickness burns are usually conscious and sentient.

General aspects

Ask the patient and the relatives about pre-existing medical conditions, especially if these may be relevant to the therapeutic

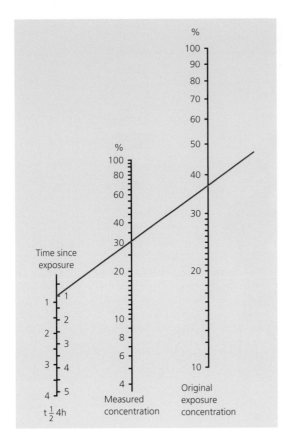

Figure 23.4 Nomogram for calculating carboxyhaemoglobin concentration at time of exposure. Time since exposure is given in two scales for the effects of previous oxygen administration on the half-life of carboxyhaemoglobin (left scale assumes a half-life of 3 h). (Reproduced from Clark CJ, *et al.* (1991) Lancet: 1332–5.)

pregnant. Early consultation with local hyperbaric specialists is recommended.

Other toxic gases, such as hydrogen cyanide, hydrogen sulphide and hydrogen chloride, are often produced in fires. They may cause local irritation to both upper and lower airways as well as acting systemically as direct cellular poisons. Few laboratories can provide cyanide concentrations in an emergency but a severe metabolic acidosis, high lactate concentration and an increased anion gap suggest cyanide poisoning if there is an appropriate history of exposure. In these patients, emergency resuscitation with assisted ventilation is required and the use of cyanide antidotes, such as sodium thiosulphate with amyl nitrite (for enhanced distribution) and dicobalt edentate, should be considered. Ensure that deep circumferential burns of the thorax are not causing restriction in chest expansion and hence ventilation (see below).

Treatment with fluids

The rule of nine, used in the rapid assessment of burn injury, can result in overestimation of the extent of the burn. More accurate assessment can be made with Lund and Browder charts (Figure 23.5) and the rate of fluid replacement adjusted accordingly.

Formulae for intravenous fluid requirements are only rough guides and need modification according to the patient's clinical state. Regular checks and recording of heart rate, blood pressure,

CHART FOR ESTIMATING SEVERITY OF BURN WOUND

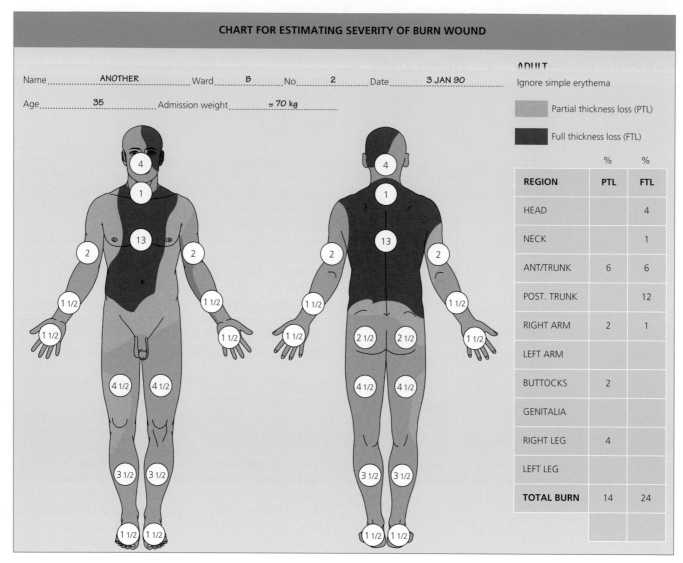

Figure 23.5 Lund and Browder chart.

intervention being performed – for example, obstructive airways disease and ischaemic heart disease. Consider the possibility of underlying medical conditions that may have led to the burn injury such as epilepsy, a cerebrovascular episode, hypoglycaemia, drug or alcohol overdose.

In elderly patients, patients with known ischaemic heart disease and all patients with a carboxyhaemoglobin concentration greater that 15%, obtain a 12-lead electrocardiogram and attach a cardiac monitor. Myocardial ischaemia or infarction and arrhythmias occur commonly and often do not have their usual clinical features. Consider the possibility of non-accidental injury in children. Do not give prophylaxis with antibiotics or steroids. Depending on local policies, discuss the patient's management with the burns or plastic surgical receiving team.

If the patient is being moved within the hospital or to another referral hospital, adequate intravenous fluids and analgesics should be transported along with him or her. All patients suspected of having inhaled smoke or requiring additional care of the airway

must be escorted by an experienced anaesthetist with appropriate equipment. Make clear, concise notes, which must accompany the patient and should include the size of the burn, the weight of the patient, the time when intravenous fluids were started, which drugs were given for pain relief and at what dose and time they were given, the urine and fluids chart, and details of special problems (Box 23.6).

Box 23.6 **Information required by burns unit**

- Name, age and sex of patient
- Percentage of body surface area covered by burns
- Depth of burns
- Any 'special' areas affected, such as the face, head and perineum
- Time of injury
- Presence of respiratory problems
- Associated injuries
- Medical history
- Treatment instituted and response

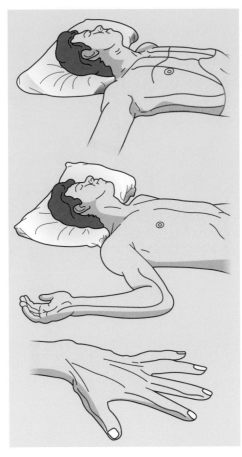

Figure 23.6 Escharotomy of the chest, arm and fingers.

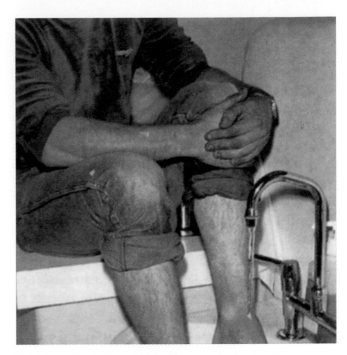

Figure 23.7 Chemical burn being copiously washed under a tap.

Chemical burns

In an emergency, all chemical burns can be treated with copious quantities of water and a bar of soap applied as soon as possible after the injury (Figure 23.7).

Although there are specific treatments for certain chemicals (see below), these may be difficult to recall with accuracy in a confused environment and water and soap applied urgently in sufficient quantity for sufficient time will cover all eventualities. Running water should be applied for at least 20 min and should be lukewarm rather than cold if possible. The soap is not always necessary, but will overcome difficulties with organic chemicals (such as phenol) that may not be soluble in water.

In most factories that deal with dangerous chemicals, buffer solutions are available and procedures exist for neutralising specific agents. In some cases, however, these injuries may be first seen in an emergency department and some of those from more common substances will benefit from specific treatment.

Hydrofluoric acid

Hydrofluoric acid is used in the glass industry and for cleaning pipes and is both toxic and painful. It can be neutralised by calcium gluconate gel or, in more severe cases, the calcium gluconate may be injected as a 10% solution under the skin to prevent further tissue damage and relieve the pain. Since even a very small percentage area burn may be fatal, early excision and grafting are usually undertaken.

Phenol (carbolic acid)

Phenol is an organic acid, so it is not readily soluble in water, but it can be removed rapidly with ethylene glycol (antifreeze). Like hydrofluoric acid, phenol not only causes local damage but is also a systemic poison and, as with many chemical burns, the prognosis usually depends more on the systemic effects of absorption than on the surface area of the burn.

White phosphorus

White phosphorus is used in the manufacture of explosives and continues to burn when in contact with air. Particles may become embedded in the skin and have to be covered with water to prevent further combustion. A dilute solution of copper sulphate added to the water will make the phosphorus go black, which makes it easier to identify and remove.

Electrical burns

A clear distinction should be made between flash and contact electrical burns.

Flash electrical burns result in a high dry air temperature for a brief period, which produces a superficial charring of the skin. This charring is almost always less severe than it looks and usually heals without the need for grafting unless there has been associated thermal injury from clothing that has caught fire.

Contact electrical burns are the result of an electric current passing through the tissues and damaging the tissue in its passage.

These burns are almost always worse than they look because much of the damage may be in the deeper tissues in spite of a relatively minor injury visible on the skin.

Contact electrical burns are usually divided into low voltage and high voltage, the dividing point being 1000 volts. In practice, this means the difference between household and industrial currents, and the distinction may help in deciding how severe an injury is likely to be. Lethal injuries do, however, occur at household voltages. Voltage is the only variable that may be gleaned from the history as density of current, resistance and duration of exposure will not be known.

Alternating current (mains) can provoke a tetanic contracture of the muscles that makes it difficult to release the contact. Direct current (lightning) tends to throw the injured person away. In an emergency, NEVER attempt to pull somebody off a current source unless you are CERTAIN that the current has been switched off or the person is pulled off with an insulated agent such as a dry wooden stake.

The passage of an electric current causes damage because of the heat it generates; the amount of heat is related to the density of the current, the resistance of the tissues through which the current passes, and the volume of tissue through which the current passes. Dry skin offers a high resistance and can therefore generate high temperatures, with obvious tissue damage. If the current passes through a large contact area both in and out of the body, there may be no visible skin injury; this is seen when a large contact plate is used in unipolar diathermy. Therefore, although an electrical contact will produce entry and exit points, it differs from a bullet wound in that the visible damage at either site will be related to the contact surface area.

An electrical current will follow the path of least resistance and will travel in the most direct line between the points of contact, of which there must be at least two (source and earth) to form a circuit (Figure 23.8). A current that passes from the palm to the dorsum of the same hand will not deviate to affect the myocardium or brain, but a current that passes from hand to hand or hand to foot will almost certainly affect the myocardium; this may produce arrhythmias that must be carefully monitored and treated if necessary. With high voltages arcing injuries may occur (Figure 23.9), in which the current will jump from forearm to upper arm or upper arm to chest, causing thermal skin injuries at each site.

A current that is forced to travel through tissues of low cross-sectional area or volume (for example, a finger) or through tissues of high resistance (for example, bone) will generate temperatures of up to thousands of degrees Celsius and cause severe tissue damage, even though the overlying skin looks normal. Contact electrical burns should be treated with respect and usually the patient should be admitted to hospital for observation or treatment by appropriate staff. If there is any possibility of myocardial damage, and in all lightning injuries, patients should be monitored with an electrocardiogram because delayed arrhythmias may occur.

Summary

The initial management of severe burns can be intimidating for those who are unfamiliar with them. As with most major trauma,

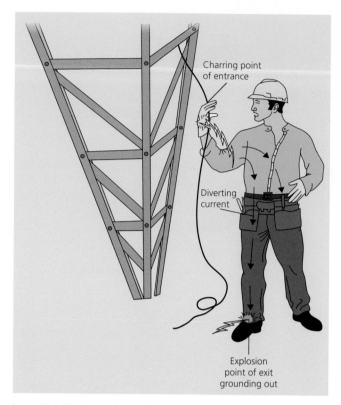

Figure 23.8 Worker receiving a high-voltage electrical injury.

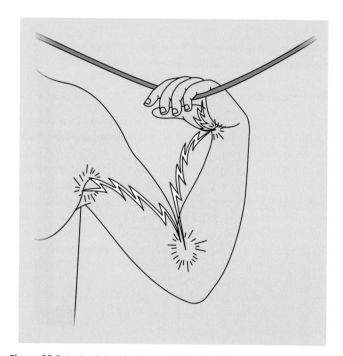

Figure 23.9 Arcing injury, between wrist, cubital fossa and axilla.

however, the management of burns is amenable to logical procedures, following the Advanced Trauma Life Support principles. The history can be as important as the physical examination in determining the likely severity of the burn and early consequences, such as airway impairment, chemical toxicity, electrical myocardial damage, etc.

Common mistakes are failure to:

- keep a patient with a major burn warm after the cause of the burn injury has been established
- assess the size of the burn properly, because of a failure to look at the whole patient
- carry out an early intubation in a patient with significant airway burns, especially if transport over any distance is contemplated.

Emergency intubation in a moving ambulance must be avoided at all costs.

Further reading

Herndon DN. (1996) *Total Burn Care*. Philadelphia: Saunders.
Settle J (ed). (1996) *Principles and Practice of Burns Management*. Edinburgh: Churchill Livingstone.

CHAPTER 24

Chemical Incidents

Virginia Murray

Health Protection Agency, London, UK

OVERVIEW

- Chemical incidents are a risk to both the public and front line rescuers and clinicians.
- The provision of information from statutory bodies can minimise risk and allow casualties to be effectively treated.

Recent experience at the Centre for Radiation, Chemical and Environmental Hazards (CRCE), part of the Health Protection Agency, has given rise to concern about the safety of emergency department staff when they find themselves managing patients contaminated during a chemical incident, and about the viability of emergency departments in the presence of contaminated patients. The objectives of this chapter are to outline chemical incident management for emergency clinicians and details of how to obtain information and help.

Common problems encountered

The CRCE has found that emergency departments have been closed, in part or entirely, as a result of chemical incidents. In the experience of the CRCE, the main causes for such closures appear to be:

- contaminated patients arriving at emergency departments, with or without warning
- spill or chemical release within the department, such as a leaking refrigerator or spillage of a pharmaceutical preparation.

Major chemical accidents cause problems for emergency departments that are different from those recognised in other major incidents – for example, identification of the toxin, safety issues and the risk of chemical cross-contamination of staff, and difficulties in patient management such as the need for specific antidotes. Particular attention should therefore be given to preparation and planning.

What is a chemical incident?

A chemical incident is the accidental or intentional release, or impending release, of a hazardous material (Box 24.1). No definition of chemical incident is ideal but that currently used by the CRCE is 'an acute event in which there is, or could be, exposure of the public to chemical substances which cause, or have the potential to cause ill health' (Centre for Radiation, Chemical and Environmental Hazards 2009). This includes all incidents with an off-site impact, as well as on-site incidents where members of the public are affected. Although this chapter is mainly concerned with the response by emergency departments to large-scale acute chemical incidents, experience at the CRCE has shown that equipment and training in some departments are not complete, therefore making it difficult for them to manage even one or two chemically contaminated patients.

Box 24.1 **Examples of chemical incidents**

- Cases of non-intentional gas poisoning.
- All workplace incidents with an off-site impact, as well as on-site incidents where members of the public are affected.
- Incidents leading to contamination of emergency service personnel and/or hospital staff.
- Spills of chemicals in a school laboratory, resulting in the admission of pupils to hospital or exposure of staff or pupils.
- Potential chemical terrorism events.
- Deliberate contamination of food or water supplies.

How can emergency departments plan for chemical incident response?

Preparation, planning, availability of decontamination facilities and personal protective equipment are essential elements in developing an emergency department response. The NHS emergency planning guidance, 2011, provides detailed advice (Department of Health 2011).

This, with the Civil Contingencies Act (www.cabinetoffice .gov.uk/content/civil-contingencies-act), and accompanying non-legislative measures, delivers a single framework for civil protection

ABC of Major Trauma, Fourth Edition. Edited by David V. Skinner and Peter A. Driscoll.
© 2013 Blackwell Publishing Ltd. Published 2013 by Blackwell Publishing Ltd.

in the United Kingdom capable of meeting the challenges of the 21st century. The Act is separated into two substantive parts: local arrangements for civil protection and emergency powers. Acute trusts are Category 1 responders and, with others, are those organisations at the core of the response to most emergencies (e.g. emergency services, local authorities, NHS bodies). Category 1 responders are subject to the full set of civil protection duties.

Therefore acute hospital trusts must ensure that satisfactory arrangements are in place for the provision of healthcare to casualties following a chemical incident (Box 24.2).

Box 24.2 Requirements for Category 1 responders

- Assess the risk of emergencies occurring and use this to inform contingency planning.
- Put in place emergency plans.
- Put in place business continuity management arrangements.
- Put in place arrangements to make information available to the public about civil protection matters and maintain arrangements to warn, inform and advise the public in the event of an emergency.
- Share information with other local responders to enhance co-ordination.
- Co-operate with other local responders to enhance co-ordination and efficiency.

What are the local chemical hazards?

Under the Civil Contingencies Act 2004, a risk assessment by emergency occurring is necessary under the new guidance. Departments may find it useful to strengthen their links with the local health protection units (www.hpa.org.uk/AboutTheHPA/WhoWeAre /LocalServices/) (the frontline service of the Health Protection Agency), local emergency services, the fire brigade and local or county authorities, including the emergency planning officers, by participating in local and regional resilience forums. Information about such forums and other important emergency planning is available on the UK Resilience website (www.cabinetoffice.gov .uk/ukresilience).

Many of these agencies will have information on methods of assessment, control and mitigation in the event of accidents, much of which concludes with 'seek medical advice'. Few of them have experience in acute medical toxicology, and as a result they rely on advice from emergency departments (Box 24.3).

Box 24.3 What is a large-scale chemical incident?

For the purposes of an emergency department, a large-scale chemical incident is any event where one or both of the following apply.

- The agent involved is present in large quantities or is potentially of high toxicity.
- A large number of people are exposed or at risk of being exposed.

Health effects from chemical incidents

Initial symptoms usually relate to, but are not confined to, the route of exposure; inhalation will cause respiratory effects, but systemic effects may occur where the substance is absorbed. Most effects will appear within a few hours of exposure but some may be delayed. In particular, respiratory symptoms can be delayed for up to 48 h after inhalation. Because effects may be delayed, it is important to identify and document as early as possible all those who were exposed or are suspected of having been exposed. With proper records and contact details, individuals who do not initially require continuing hospital management can, if necessary, be recalled for further assessment.

Susceptible groups that are particularly at risk from a toxic exposure are the young, old, pregnant women and their fetuses, and those who have chronic illnesses. The route of exposure is an important factor in predicting which illnesses will result in increased susceptibility: for example, patients with chronic obstructive pulmonary disorder (COPD) are particularly sensitive to respirable gases.

Multiple hazards such as smoke from a chemical fire may present a complicated picture with both trauma and toxic effects.

What emergency facilities are required?

Facilities for triage (Figure 24.1), resuscitation, decontamination, investigation and treatment, and also short- and long-term follow-up of those exposed should be provided. The facilities for decontamination are available. Other equipment includes personal protective clothing. In addition, adequate training and rehearsals in the use of equipment and facilities are essential. Emergency clinicians should check their own emergency department equipment to make sure that it can:

- manage the incident and prevent staff becoming the next casualties
- manage the patients.

See Box 24.4.

Actions

To allow early assessment of the toxic hazard, the emergency department must obtain as much information as possible about:

- chemical(s) involved
- type of incident
- route(s) of exposure
- type(s) of initial clinical effects.

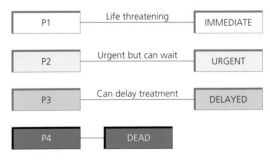

Figure 24.1 Triage categories.

Box 24.4 **Essential actions in developing an emergency department's response to a chemical incident**

• Preparing and maintaining plans.
• Ensuring that staff are prepared and trained, and have access to the advice and expertise needed to provide medical care for the casualties.
• Having carried out a risk assessment, providing the facilities and equipment necessary to provide a safe working environment, including decontamination facilities and personal protective equipment.

It is important to identify and document everybody who has been exposed to chemicals. Some who are initially symptom free may develop symptoms or become concerned about the effects of exposure at a later date.

On-site support

The need for a mobile medical team is likely to arise only where patients who have been exposed to chemicals are also injured or if many, for example school children, have potentially been exposed and it is easier to triage locally rather than transfer to the emergency department for assessments. The following section deals with important factors that should be considered when undertaking on-site support.

At the site of an incident, protection of the mobile medical team is essential, though there is no single set of protective clothing suitable for protection against every hazardous chemical. To minimise the risk of injury, the fire service usually has responsibility for control of the incident, with the site being divided into 'dirty', 'contamination reduction' and 'clean' zones.

The principles of management of walking or stretcher patients include initial rescue, triage and strip to remove contaminated clothing, decontamination and resuscitation and evacuation. The emergency services control centres should advise the mobile aid or triage and should stay in communication. Preferably only decontaminated casualties should be attended (Box 24.5).

Box 24.5 **Management of walking or stretcher patients after a chemical accident**

• Initial rescue.
• Triage.
• Strip to remove contaminated clothing.
• Decontamination and resuscitation.
• Evacuation.

Extensive work has been undertaken to facilitate the ambulance service response in a chemical incident. This includes the provision of personal protective clothing and decontamination facilities. In an extension of this work, the provision of early emergency care in a contaminated zone has been developed via the Hazardous Area Response Teams (HART). HART teams are now operational in each of England's 11 Ambulance Trusts. Scotland has an equivalent Special Operations Response Team (SORT) and Wales has its own Welsh HART team. HART teams are designed to provide triage and treatment of patients inside the contaminated area (hot zone) of a chemical, biological, radiological or nuclear (CBRN) incident. HART teams have a range of customised vehicles and are engaged in an ongoing training programme.

In addition, under the New Dimension programme, decontamination facilities are provided by the fire brigade. The New Dimension programme supplies the fire and rescue service with equipment and procedures to enhance its capability to respond to a range of incidents.

The New Dimension programme has already delivered new equipment and procedures to the fire and rescue service to enable it to decontaminate large numbers of the public at the site of a CBRN incident (Figure 24.2). If a CBRN attack were to occur, it is likely that the fire and rescue service would be among the first to arrive at the site. The service also has the ability to mobilise large numbers of firefighters and equipment rapidly (www.cabinetoffice .gov.uk/ukresilience). For this reason it has, in partnership with the Department of Health, accepted responsibility for the management of public mass decontamination in the event of CBRN attack.

New equipment and procedures enable casualties to be decontaminated immediately on site, reducing the effects on their health. They can then be transported safely to hospitals or shelter for further treatment or support without the risk of contaminating others. Phase 1 of the new dimension involved deployment of mass decontamination/incident response and further phases have added additional fleet and capabilities, e.g. urban search and rescue, high volume pumps.

Mass decontamination units structures can be easily carried and erected on site within minutes and are capable of decontaminating up to 200 people per hour. The tents consist of three sections for disrobe, showering and re-robe and have been designed to

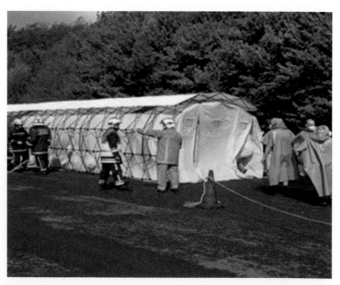

Figure 24.2 Exercising the New Dimensions mass decontamination facilities. (www.nao.org.uk/publications/0708/enhancing_fire_and_rescue.aspx).

ensure comfort and modesty for casualties. Casualties requiring decontamination can remove their clothing underneath special lined and hooded orange cloaks before moving into the heated, warm-water shower units to wash with detergents. They are then provided with re-robe packs containing green jump suits, sanitary products and shoes. Non-ambulant casualties can be decontaminated using a specially designed trolley system that can be set up to convey stretchers through the centre of the tent at the rate of 25 casualties per hour. See Box 24.6.

Box 24.6 Groups particularly at risk from toxic exposure

- Any person directly contaminated by a chemical.
- Susceptible groups – young, old, chronically ill, pregnant.
- First responders – fire, police, ambulance and medical personnel.
- Environmental and other clean-up workers.

The fire and rescue services have gas-tight suits enabling firefighters to rescue in hazardous environments and decontaminate people safely. These suits can be deployed during CBRN incidents as well as for day-to-day operations.

The management of physical injuries follows the routine already described. For the benefit of the casualty and emergency responders, all contaminated clothing should be removed, bagged, labelled and sealed in double clear plastic bags, preferably at the incident site, and stored in a secure area away from staff and patients. Valuables will be stored separately.

Chemical contamination of the skin, eyes and wounds may require prolonged irrigation or even immersion of the affected part.

At the emergency department

The above principles also apply to casualties arriving at the hospital. Early notification of an incident and of any casualties allows final preparation of hospital decontamination facilities and protective clothing by senior staff to minimise any spread of contamination hazard inside the hospital.

Preparation for triage assessment of chemical exposure and toxic risk assessment will probably require support from the local health protection unit who can access additional support from the CRCE. In addition, the medical staff may find it helpful to seek advice from other experts on and off the incident site. A list of such contacts should be held ready for use.

Arrangements should be made as early as possible to obtain antidotes, if appropriate, and to provide facilities for supportive care. Collection of blood, urine, vomit and other relevant biological samples is valuable for confirming exposure and dose received, and should be carried out as soon as possible after an incident in consultation with the local health protection unit and the CRCE.

When discharging patients who have attended the emergency department, it is important not to return any patient to a previously contaminated environment without checking that it is safe to do so.

How to obtain help following a chemical incident

Compared with other trauma emergencies, major chemical incidents which pose a threat to medical responders are relatively rare. When a chemical incident occurs medical responders require information and support. These are available from the following sources.

Health Protection Agency

The Health Protection Agency (HPA) is a government body that protects the health and well-being of the population (www.hpa.org.uk). The Agency plays a critical role in protecting people from infectious diseases and in preventing harm when hazards involving chemicals, poisons or radiation occur. The Agency also prepares for new and emerging threats, such as a bio-terrorist attack or virulent new strain of disease.

Centre for Radiation, Chemical and Environmental Hazards

Centre for Radiation, Chemical and Environmental Hazards (CRCE), part of the Health Protection Agency, provides comprehensive expert advice and support for chemical incidents across England and Wales (www.hpa.org.uk/AboutTheHPA/WhoWeAre /CentreForRadiationChemicalAndEnvironmentalHazards). The centre's strategic goal is to anticipate and prevent the adverse effects of acute and chronic exposure to hazardous chemicals and other poisons.

Every day in Britain, serious chemical incidents occur which threaten people's health. Such potential health threats might involve chemical fires, chemical contamination of the environment or the deliberate release of chemicals and poisons. Exposure to hazardous substances can also occur during accidents at home and work, and as a result of deliberate, malicious releases. The long-term consequences of low-level, chronic exposure to chemicals and poisons are currently not well understood and there is increasing public concern about the possible impact, especially in relation to reproductive health, asthma and cancers. The centre is undertaking intensive research to improve our understanding of these issues.

The Health Protection Agency provides authoritative scientific and medical advice to the NHS and other bodies about the known health effects of chemicals, poisons and other environmental hazards. This advice covers clinical issues such as:

- personal protective equipment
- decontamination and evacuation
- toxicological and epidemiological advice on impact on public health
- clinical advice on antidotes and medical treatment
- the public health impact of industrial sites
- health effects from chemicals in the environment (including water, soil, waste).

The CRCE head office is located in Chilton, Oxfordshire, and there are four specialist centres in Birmingham, Cardiff, London and Nottingham.

Guidance is available round the clock from medical toxicologists, clinical pharmacologists, environmental scientists, epidemiologists and other specialists (Box 24.7). The Centre also advises doctors and nurses on the best way to manage patients who have been poisoned through a contract with the National Poisons Information Service (NPIS).

Box 24.7 **Contact telephone numbers**

- CRCE 0844 982 0555
- NPIS 0844 892 0111

National Poisons Information Service

The NPIS is a clinical toxicology service for healthcare professionals working in the NHS and is a service commissioned by the HPA (www.hpa.org.uk/ProductsServices/ChemicalsPoisons /PoisonsInformationService/). The service consists of a network of units across the UK, providing information and advice on the diagnosis, treatment and management of patients who may have been accidentally or deliberately poisoned. Information on management of poisoning is available on its Internet database TOXBASE (available to registered professionals) or via a 24-h telephone service for more complex cases requiring specialist advice (see Box 24.7). These services are not for members of the public; NPIS supports NHS Direct and NHS 24 in providing advice to members of the public.

There are currently four NPIS units (Birmingham, Cardiff, Edinburgh, Newcastle upon Tyne) providing advice to medical professionals. These units provide a second-tier consultant-led service providing the poisons information necessary for the diagnosis, treatment and management of cases which are clinically more complex.

TOXBASE is the primary clinical toxicology database of the NPIS. All NPIS units contribute to and authenticate the content of TOXBASE and it represents the most authoritative source of information available. It should be used by all medical practitioners and other healthcare professionals working in the NHS as the primary source of poisons information. The TOXBASE database provides information about routine diagnosis, treatment and management of patients suffering from exposure to a wide range of pharmaceuticals, chemicals (agricultural, household and industrial), plants and animals.

Summary

Although the management of injuries sustained in a chemical incident is the same as that of injuries from any other cause, special precautions must be taken by mobile teams attending such an incident and by the receiving emergency department. These should be taken in conjunction with the local health protection unit and the emergency services. Remember that the CRCE with the NPIS can provide invaluable information and advice.

References

Centre for Radiation Chemical and Environmental Hazards. (2009) Chemical Surveillance Report 1st January–31st December 2009. www.hpa.org.uk /Publications/ChemicalsPoisons/ChemicalsSurveillanceReports/

Department of Health, Emergency Preparedness Division. (2011) NHS Emergency planning guidance http://www.dh.gov.uk/en/Publicationsand statistics/Publications/PublicationsPolicyAndGuidance/DH_125840

London Ambulance Service NHS Trust. (2006) Meeting of the Trust Board. Tuesday 28th November 2006. www.londonambulance.nhs.uk/aboutus /trustboard/media/Trust%20Board%20agenda%20-%2028%20November %202006.pdf

CHAPTER 25

Ballistic Injury

Rob Russell,[1] Jon Clasper,[1] Bruce Jenner,[2] Timothy J. Hodgetts[3] and Peter F. Mahoney[1]

[1]Royal Centre for Defence Medicine, Birmingham, UK
[2]Royal Air Force, UK
[3]University of Birmingham, Birmingham, UK

OVERVIEW

- Ballistic weapons can produce very complex injuries.
- Managing a ballistic incident includes managing threats to rescuers as well as managing casualties.
- Weapon design is influenced by international regulations and conventions.
- Surgery for ballistic injury follows principles developed in wartime.

'Ballistics' is the study of thrown objects. Ballistic injury (from *thrown* or *projected* material) may be caused by a number of weapon systems including firearms and explosives.

The damage to tissues caused by projectiles depends on a number of factors.

- The *kinetic energy* of the projectile (influences the amount of energy that the object has available to deliver to tissue). This is given by the equation $KE = \frac{1}{2} \times mass \times velocity \times velocity$.
- The size and shape of the projectile influence how the object behaves in contact with tissue and in turn how much kinetic energy is given up. For example, the energy given up by a bullet will vary if it strikes nose first, side first, 'tumbles' in tissue or breaks into pieces in the tissue.
- The nature of the tissue (how 'elastic' a tissue is influences the amount of energy it can absorb before damage occurs).
- Intervening structures between the tissue and the projectile (such as ballistic protection – 'body armour').

Bullets and firearms

Firearms work by applying an explosive force (e.g. gunpowder ignited in a confined space) to a projectile (e.g. a cannon ball), propelling it down a tube towards a target.

During the 19th century, *cartridges* were developed, packaging the bullet (*boulette* – 'little ball'), propellant and primer within a case. This in turn allowed further development of firearms to include housing a number of rounds within the weapon or within a *magazine* and increasing the rate at which bullets could be fired.

The term 'small arms' generally means weapons that can be carried by an individual. These include *short-barrelled* weapons, e.g. revolvers and pistols, and *long-barrelled* weapons, e.g. rifles, carbines, assault rifles, some machine guns. Modern rifles have a spiral groove in the barrel to spin the bullet and make it more stable in flight.

Machine guns can be fed by magazines or by *belts* of ammunition: a fully automatic weapon will keep firing while the trigger is depressed or until the ammunition runs out.

Light weapons are larger weapons that need a crew of two or more to operate them.

The design of a bullet is influenced by its purpose and legal issues surrounding who is going to be using it and where.

Types of bullets

- *Full metal jacket*: metal casing around a soft core. The round is non-expanding and deep penetrating. Military rounds are generally of this type. The legality of military rounds is governed by the Hague Convention of 1899.
- *Soft point*: the bullet has an exposed lead tip and expands rapidly in tissue. There are many types of expanding rounds (Box 25.1). Rounds used in hunting are often expanding rounds which 'dump' as much energy as possible into the animal to ensure it is killed. Some police and antiterrorist forces use expanding ammunition to ensure their target is rapidly killed or disabled and that the bullets do not go through the target and into someone else.
- *Altered ammunition*: this is altering manufactured ammunition by cutting the jacket or altering the shape of the nose of the bullet or cutting a cross into the nose of the bullet. The intention is to cause the bullet to expand, flatten or fracture, causing increased injury. This type of ammunition is outlawed by the Hague Convention of 1899.

Box 25.1 **Dum-Dum**

A term used to describe altered or expanding ammunition. Dumdum was the site of an arsenal in India which produced soft-nosed bullets for the British Army in the early 1890s.

ABC of Major Trauma, Fourth Edition. Edited by David V. Skinner and Peter A. Driscoll.
© 2013 Blackwell Publishing Ltd. Published 2013 by Blackwell Publishing Ltd.

Velocity and cavitation

High-velocity rounds are generally regarded as those traveling at over 2000 ft/sec. However, the wound caused by such a round soon after it leaves the barrel of a weapon will be much greater than the same round as it is reaching the end of its journey when it will have slowed considerably.

More useful terms are 'high energy transfer' and 'low energy transfer', indicating how much energy the projectile has transferred to tissue.

There are two types of 'cavity' produced by projectiles in tissue.

- The permanent cavity is a localized area of tissue destruction caused by the projectile passing through the tissue.
- The temporary cavity is a transient phenomenon – the displacement of tissue away from the path of the missile after it has passed (Figure 25.1).

High-energy transfer wounds are associated with a large temporary cavity, and this in turn can affect the nature of the exit wound.

Shotguns

Shotguns also use cartridge ammunition. The cartridge contains shot, i.e. metal pellets. These pellets can vary in size from the very small (hundreds of pellets per cartridge) through to those used in 'combat shotgun' cartridges (nine or fewer large balls).

Shotguns have an effective range of 30–50 metres. The injuries produced depend on whether the weapon is fired close to the target (pellets hit close together, creating one large wound) or at a distance (pellets have spread out, creating multiple small wounds).

Explosive injury

Injury produced by an explosive device is the result of complex interactions but for ease of understanding has been broken down into a number of mechanisms. Explosives are categorised as *high order* or *low order* depending on how rapidly they change their state once initiated.

High-order explosives undergo almost instantaneous change from solid to gas, rapidly releasing energy, and are associated with

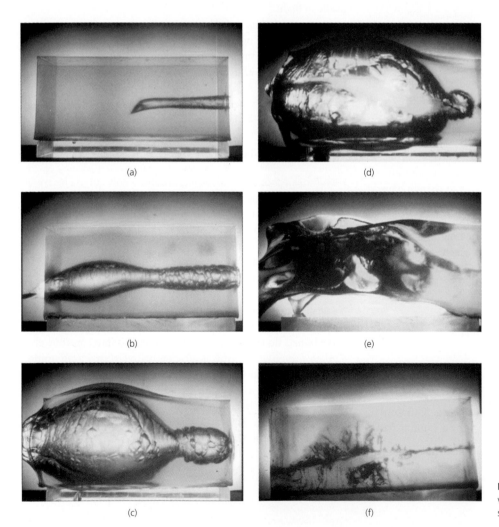

(a)

(b)

(c)

(d)

(e)

(f)

Figure 25.1 (a–f)Progressive track of a high velocity missile (bullet) through gelatin showing cavitation.

sudden increases in pressure and a supersonic shockwave/shock front. Velocity of explosion is 1000–9000 m/sec and a shattering effect is produced.

Low-order explosives change less rapidly (cms/sec to 400 m/sec) and are not associated with the overpressure wave.

Blast injury has been classified as follows.

- *Primary*: due to the actions of the blast (overpressure) wave. This can completely disintegrate a casualty. The blast wave interacts with the body or component tissue, dumping energy into the tissue and producing stress waves (microvascular injury) and shear waves (produce asynchronous tissue movement, causing tearing).
- *Secondary*: due to fragments projected by the energy of the explosion. Fragments can be 'natural' (from the random fragmentation of the bomb's components) or 'preformed' (notched wire, metal balls or squares packed into the bomb). These cause multiple penetrating injuries.
- *Tertiary*: due to the casualty being thrown/displaced by the explosion or injured due to structural collapse. This is generally 'blunt' injury.
- *Quaternary*: this has been used to cover 'all other' effects including fires (from the explosive components or from ignited fuel), toxic effects of fumes, and exacerbation of medical conditions.

There is a question as to whether or not human tissue (from suicide bombers or people disintegrated in bombings in crowded places) that ends up embedded in another victim should be classified as a separate wounding mechanism.

Practically, casualties will often have complex combinations of these types of injury.

- A casualty in a military vehicle blown up by a bomb may be sheltered from the worst of the fragments but injured by the blast wave and fires within the vehicle.
- A soldier injured by a roadside bomb may escape the blast effect but suffer multiple penetrating injury from fragments and be knocked down.

This can lead to conflicting requirements during surgery and anaesthesia.

Improvised explosive devices

The term 'improvised explosive device' (IED) implies an explosive device made by a group or an individual rather than an industrial manufacturing process (Box 25.2). The distinction can be blurred when insurgent groups are supplied with manufactured devices by sympathetic governments or use abandoned military materials in the construction of such devices.

Box 25.2 **Explanation of abbreviations**

IED = improvised explosive device
SBIED = suicide bomber IED
VBIED = vehicle-borne IED
SBVBIED = suicide bomber VBIED

A variant IED is the explosively formed projectile/penetrator (EFP) or 'shaped charge'. This uses a technique first described in mining operations (and adapted by the military) to use explosive to shape and propel a sheet of metal into a very fast-moving 'slug' of molten material. It has been used to attack vehicles.

Managing the ballistic incident

At any incident, whilst care of the injured is of high priority to healthcare workers, failure of scene management will lead to loss of valuable information and may endanger rescuers and casualties.

Scene management

At incidents in which bombs are involved or secondary devices suspected, the '4 Cs' must be adopted (Box 25.3). It is important that healthcare workers have an understanding of the principles used so that they can work with other rescue services. It is important to note that these are not the same 4 Cs that surgeons use when assessing tissue, which are described below.

Box 25.3 **The 4 Cs**

- Confirm
- Clear
- Cordon
- Control

Confirm

Incident commanders must be clear about what is happening and the risk and position of further hazards. Before rushing into action, commanders should take a quick 'time out' to plot their response and communicate their plan. Factors that must be considered are clearance priorities, cordon locations, safe areas, access and egress routes and rendezvous points.

Clear

The scene should be cleared to a safe distance to prevent distraction and preserve forensic evidence. The distance will vary depending on the terrain. The method and urgency of clearance will depend on the incident. Existing casualties and some of the local population may be unable or unwilling to move. A decision must be made as to what provision can be made for these 'stay-behinds' balanced against the risks involved.

Cordon

Cordons establish the area in which the rescue effort is taking place and define safe zones and tiers of command. An outer cordon should be established as a physical barrier preventing accidental or unauthorised access to the site. An inner cordon may be set up around wreckage, especially if hazards still exist. The incident commanders from each service are the Silver Commanders and the Silver area is defined by the outer cordon. Silver Commanders may appoint Bronze Commanders to work within the Bronze area designated by the inner cordon. Gold Commanders co-ordinate the response at regional and national levels.

Control

Once set up, the control of the cordons and scene is maintained by clear rendezvous and access points. The locations of these and access routes to them must be communicated clearly. Personnel should be logged through the cordons. Should a further event occur, commanders will have a record of the staff on site.

Medical management

Once the 4 Cs have been established, medical management and support can begin. This should follow the principles listed in Box 25.4 .

Box 25.4 **Medical management and support principles**

- Command and control.
- Safety.
- Communication.
- Assessment.
- Triage.
- Treatment.
- Transport

Source: Advanced Life Support Group. (2002) *Major Incident Medical Management and Support*, 2nd edn. London: BMJ Books.

Command and control

This is the paramount principle. If good command and control are not established, the initial chaos will continue and the injured will suffer regardless of how well some individual casualties are treated. Command operates vertically within each emergency service. Control operates horizontally across all the services. In the UK, the police have control at the scene – the exception to this is when there are still active hazards and the fire service may take control of the Bronze area. The Silver Commanders for each service must ensure they are easily identifiable and that they communicate with each other. In particular, the ambulance and medical commanders must liaise closely. By using the 4 Cs, many elements of command and control will already have been established. The ambulance and medical commanders should determine where the casualty clearing station, ambulance circuit and other key locations will be as soon as possible. An outline scene is shown in Figure 25.2.

Safety

Healthcare workers must remember that their own safety is paramount and that they must not become casualties themselves. If hazards are present, the fire service will either neutralize them or carry out 'snatch' rescues. In a terrorist incident, secondary devices will often be placed to target the rescue effort and all healthcare workers must remain vigilant for this possibility.

Communication

Every major incident inquiry has identified failings in communications. Without good communication, command and control are impossible. Incident commanders must work closely and hold regular meetings. Communication between the Silver Commanders and receiving hospitals is vital to determine the best use of available resources. Whilst radios are the mainstay of communication, all modalities should be considered. If there is any suspicion of a

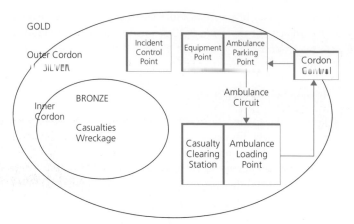

Figure 25.2 Major incident cordons and locations.

secondary device, mobile phones and radios must not be used at the scene until it is declared clear.

Assessment

This is a constant process. The Silver Commanders must always be considering what the current situation is, what extra resources are required and where these can be obtained.

Triage

In any situation when there is more than one casualty, a system of triage must be used. The triage sieve which is the standard UK method for primary triage is shown in Figure 25.3. Triage allots priorities to patients so that the most can be done for the greatest number of patients. The standard triage categories shown in Table 25.1 should be used. Patients must also be labelled with their

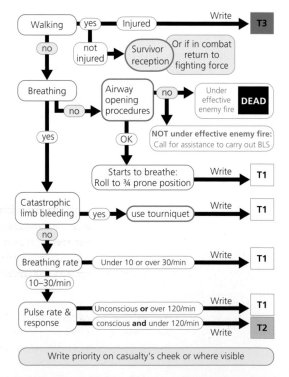

Figure 25.3 Triage sieve (civilian). (Reproduced from Hodgetts T. and Porter C. 2002.)

Table 25.1 Triage categories

Priority	Label colour	Description
T1	Red	Immediate
T2	Yellow	Urgent
T3	Green	Delayed
Dead	White or black	Dead
T4	Blue (not standard)	Expectant – only for mass casualty situation

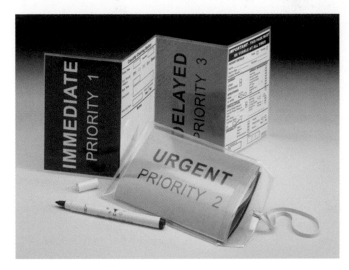

Figure 25.4 Triage cards.

category to avoid duplication of work and allow easy identification of the sickest by the treatment teams. Patients will be triaged many times on their journey to and once at the hospital so the labelling system must be able to cope with patients improving and deteriorating. A typical triage card is shown in Figure 25.4.

Treatment

At the scene of any ballistic incident, treatment teams may be faced with casualties with multiple serious injuries. Figure 25.5 shows the injury map of a casualty injured by an improvised bomb.

Treatment must follow the <C>-ABC paradigm (Box 25.5) but the focus must be to deliver the patient to hospital safely. Any treatment procedure that can safely wait until arrival in the emergency department should be postponed. Box 25.6 outlines particular considerations in the ballistic casualty.

Box 25.5 **<C>-ABC paradigm**

<C>	Control of catastrophic haemorrhage
A	Airway
B	Breathing
C	Circulation

Source: Hodgetts TJ, Mahoney PF, Russell MQ, Byers M. (2006) ABC to <C> ABC: redefining the military trauma paradigm. Emerg Med J 23: 745–6.

Box 25.6 **Clinical considerations in the ballistic casualty**

Ballistic casualties are likely to have a combination of blunt and penetrating injury. Bombing victims may also have burns.

<C> Catastrophic haemorrhage

Penetrating wounds to the groins, axilla and neck. Consider haemostatic agents.

Penetrating wounds to major limb vessels/traumatic amputations. Consider use of tourniquet.

Airway and C-spine

Airway at risk from:

- burn injury
- disruption from fragments
- compression from penetrating vascular injury in the neck.

Consider early anaesthesia and intubation (use of small-diameter endotracheal tubes) or early surgical airway

Cervical collars: these have a limited role in pure penetrating injury and may conceal developing haematoma in the neck. In mixed injury, as occurs in bombings, the use of cervical collars is a balance of risk.

Breathing

Manage sucking chest wounds with adhesive chest seals incorporating a one-way valve and then consider chest drainage.

Circulation

Catastrophic bleeding should have been controlled early. Smaller external bleeds can be managed with simple first aid measures of compression and elevation. Ongoing internal bleeding from penetrating cavity injury needs to be suspected or recognised from history and clinical findings.

UK practice has been hypotensive resuscitation initially until surgical control of bleeding is achieved. Sustained hypotension in blast casualties results in irreversible acidosis. Normotensive resuscitation after the first hour of hypotensive resuscitation is now current UK military practice.

Deficit

The majority of casualties who sustain a high-energy penetrating brain injury do not survive to medical care. Casualties who survive to care from penetrating injury are generally a preselected group and in the absence of obvious devastating injury should be resuscitated as above to minimise secondary injury. There is an obvious conflict between hypotensive resuscitation for cavity bleeding and the need to maintain cerebral perfusion and this becomes a judgement call at the time.

Environment

Hypothermia needs to be managed with warm air blankets and environmental control.

Source: Adapted from Wood PR, Brooks AJ, Mahoney PF. (2005) Resuscitation and anaesthesia for the ballistic casualty. In: *Ballistic Trauma: A Practical Guide*. London: Springer Verlag.

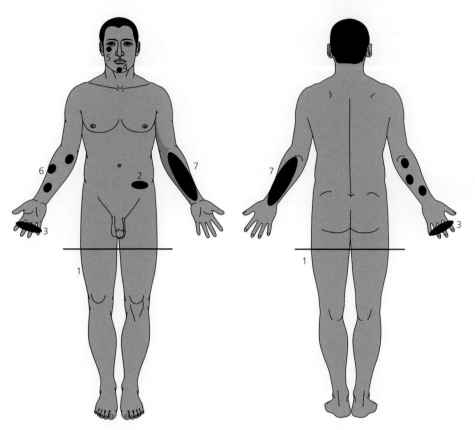

Figure 25.5 Schematic casualty injury map. (1) Bilateral traumatic amputation through femurs; (2) Penetrating abdominal wound; (3) Wounds to fingers; (4) Open jaw; (5) Penetrating eye injury; (6) Multiple wounds to right arm; (7) Burns to skin not covered by clothing.

Transport

The Silver Commanders must ensure optimum use of all transport assets. Not every patient needs to travel in an ambulance, and buses or other multi-passenger vehicles should be used to move the walking wounded. Often these casualties (T3) may be taken to hospital before the more seriously injured as they will require less packaging. Wherever possible, the seriously injured (T1s) should be 'pulsed' to receiving hospitals so that their resuscitation facilities are not overwhelmed. Patients with injuries requiring specialist care (e.g. isolated head injuries, burns) should be considered for transport direct to specialist centres if these centres have the ability to manage the initial reception.

Surgical treatment of ballistic injuries

The most significant problems following ballistic wounds are bleeding, the main cause of death in modern times, and infection, the most common cause of morbidity. In survivors the two principal sites of major blood loss are the abdomen and the limbs, particularly proximal limb injuries. Infection can occur with any penetrating wound but again is most likely to occur with abdominal wounds, due to intestinal perforation, or with limb wounds due to the high-energy nature of these injuries.

Although the principles of surgical control of abdominal haemorrhage or hollow viscus penetration are similar to those of civilian wounds, approximately 20% of casualties will have sustained multivisceral abdominal wounds, will require urgent laparotomy and may be too unstable to tolerate a standard, prolonged operation. In these casualties, damage control techniques can be considered (Box 25.7).

For proximal limb injuries, surgical control of bleeding may be required, but overall few limb wounds are associated with a significant vascular injury. Infection is a major problem with ballistic wounds, and was the main killer before the importance of surgical debridement was recognised.

Due to the nature of ballistic wounds, the surgical control of infection is much more important than with most other wounds. The infection rate from ballistic wounds is far higher than that from civilian-type wounds, particularly from high-energy transfer ballistic wounds, which are often associated with fractures or significant soft tissue wounds. The equivalent civilian wounds are those from agricultural accidents. In addition, military ballistic injuries are often associated with a significant delay in initiating treatment, which effectively means the wounds are infected rather than contaminated. Antibiotics are an adjuvant but are not a substitute for surgery.

Most military ballistic wounds should be explored surgically to determine the extent of the wound and associated contamination. Civilian ballistic wounds can be treated non-operatively providing they are low-energy transfer wounds and regular review is possible. High-energy transfer wounds are associated with large wounds, retained metallic fragments or bony injury, and are usually caused by blast, rifle or close-range shotguns. All high-energy transfer wounds must be explored and debrided, regardless of whether they are civilian or military injuries.

Box 25.7 **Details of damage control laparotomy**

Phase 1

- Rapid (1 h) operation.
- Full-length midline incision.
- Four-quadrant packing of the abdomen .
- Major blood vessel tears are simply tied off or bypassed.
- Bleeding liver lacerations are packed.
- Small bowel penetrations are stapled over.
- Large bowel perforations are tied shut with tape.
- Any spillage of bowel contents is copiously washed out and the abdomen is temporarily closed, often with a sterile plastic sheet .
- Management of hypothermia, coagulation and electrolyte abnormalities in the operating room.

Phase 2

- Ventilated patient is transferred to an ICU for resuscitation.
- Continued reversal of biochemical abnormalities.
- Continued correction of clotting, and further rewarming.

Phase 3

- Definitive repair is undertaken at a planned reoperation when the patient is maximally stabilised.
- Bowel injuries are repaired.
- Vessels are repaired.
- Feeding tubes placed.
- Missed injuries looked for.
- The patient returns to ICU.

Source: Bowley DMG, Barker P, Boffard KD. (2000) Damage control surgery – concepts and practice. J RAMC 146: 176–82.

The principles of surgery are as follows.

- Skin edges should be excised together with any necrotic or degloved skin, and the wounds extended to allow full visualisation of the wound track (Figure 25.6).
- Deep fascia should be incised longitudinally along the full length of the wound.
- Fasciotomies (full-length division of the fascia) should be considered for all high-energy transfer wounds, or those associated with vascular or bony injury. This is carried out to prevent the expected soft tissue swelling producing further ischaemia and necrosis.
- All devitalised or necrotic muscle must be excised, and all foreign accessible foreign material should be removed. Non-viable muscle will be associated with the 'Surgical 4 Cs': pallor (**C**olour) and lack of **C**apillary bleeding, although this may be due to hypovolaemia rather than local injury. In addition, lack of **C**ontractility and abnormal **C**onsistency are present, although this will take several hours to develop (these are obviously different to the 4Cs of incident control!) (Figure 25.7).

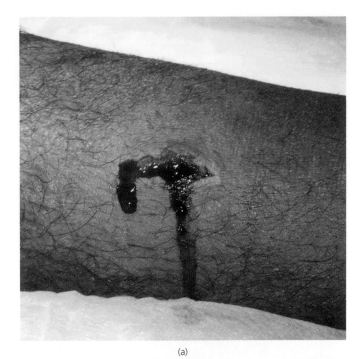

(a)

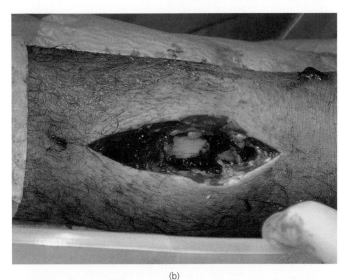

(b)

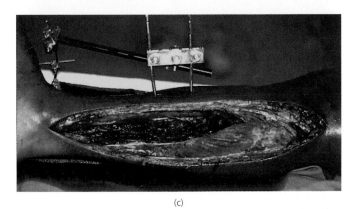

(c)

Figure 25.6 (a–c)Excision, exploration and debridement of bullet wound/track.

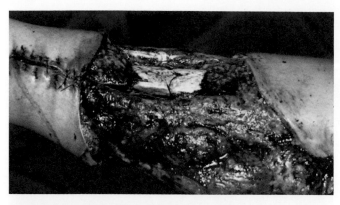

Figure 25.7 Subsequent overt necrosis of de-vitalised tissue.

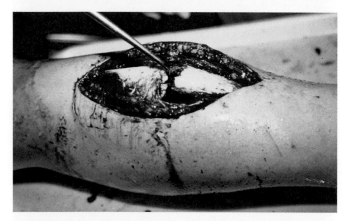

Figure 25.8 Delivering the bone ends into the wound.

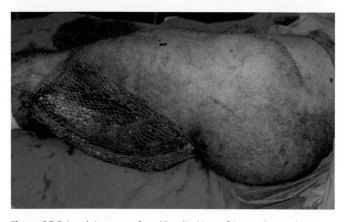

Figure 25.9 Local tissue transfer with split skin grafting to the resulting defect.

- Bone ends should be debrided and must be adequately visualised, if necessary delivering the bone ends into the wound (Figure 25.8). All loose bony fragments with no soft tissue attachment should be removed.
- All wounds should be thoroughly irrigated with 6–9 L of isotonic fluid.
- Following debridement, the wounds should be dressed with, but not packed with, gauze.
- All bony and extensive soft tissue wounds should be immobilised to minimise further tissue trauma. This can be with plaster of Paris or by external fixation (see Figure 25.6C).

With very few exceptions, ballistic wounds should never be closed primarily. This will lead to swelling of subcutaneous tissue and further ischaemia, resulting in a very high infection rate. Ignorance of this has unfortunately has led to complications in virtually all military conflicts, including recent wars.

Delayed primary closure can be carried out after 2–5 days. With high-energy transfer wounds, plastic surgical techniques are frequently required (Figure 25.9).

Summary

Management of the ballistic casualty is a combination of :

- understanding ballistic mechanisms
- managing the scene of the incident
- understanding clinical priorities and the particular problems posed by ballistic injury.

This chapter has given an introduction to these issues and guidance on further reading is provided below.

Online resources

There are many good online resources about ballistics and ballistic injury. Resources the authors found particularly useful are as follows.

Ross AH. Gunshot wounds: a summary. www.soton.ac.uk/~jb3/bullet/gsw.html.

http://en.wikipedia.org. Articles on history and development of firearms and ammunition. Good material on different types of expanding ammunition.

www.brooksidepress.org/Products/OperationalMedicine/DATA/operationalmed/Manuals/FMSS/INJURYMECHANISMSFROM CONVENTIONALWEAPONSFMST0424.html. Good basic descriptions of wounding mechanisms.

Further reading

Immediate management of ballistic casualties

Coupland R, Molde A, Navein J. (2001) *Care in the Field for Victims of Weapons of War*. Geneva: ICRC. www.icrc.org.

Hodgetts TJ, Mahoney PF, Evans G, Brooks A (eds). (2006) Battlefield Advanced Trauma Life Support, Parts 1 to 3. J RAMC 152 (suppl). This is the revised 3rd edition of the BATLS manual.

Hodgetts T, Porter C. (2002) *Major Incident Management System*. London: BMJ Publishing.

Husum H, Gilbert M, Wisborg T. (2000) *Save Lives, Save Limbs: Life Support for Victims of Mines, Wars and Accidents*. Penang, Malaysia: Third World Network.

ICRC. (2006) *First Aid in Armed Conflict and Other Situations of Violence*. Geneva: ICRC. www.icrc.org.

War surgery

Borden Institute. (2004) *Emergency War Surgery, Third United States Revision*. Washington, DC: Borden Institute.

Coupland RM. (2000) *War Wounds of Limbs: Surgical Management*. Oxford: Butterworth Heinemann.

Dufour D, Kromann Jensen S, *et al.* (1998) *Surgery for Victims of War*, 3rd edn. Geneva: ICRC.

Giannou C, Baldan M. *War Surgery* (2009). Geneva, ICRC.

Husum H, Ang SC, Fosse E. (1995) *War Surgery Field Manual*. Penang, Malaysia: Third World Network.

Roberts P (ed). (2004) The British Military Surgery Pocket Book. AC No 12552. British Army Publication. Crown Copyright.

Ballistics: history, mechanisms, ballistic protection and casualty management

Brooks AJ, Clasper J, Midwinter M, Hodgetts TJ, Mahoney PF. (2011) *Ryan's Ballistic Trauma – a practical guide*. London: Springer-Verlag.

Ryan J, Rich N, Morgans B, Dale R, Cooper G. (1997) *Ballistic Trauma: Clinical Relevance in Peace and War*. London: Hodder Arnold.

CHAPTER 26

Trauma in Hostile Environments

Mark Byers,[1] Peter R. Davis,[2] Timothy J. Hodgetts[3] and Peter F. Mahoney[4]

[1]Ministry of Defence, London, UK
[2]Southern General Hospital, Glasgow, UK
[3]University of Birmingham, Birmingham, UK
[4]Royal Centre for Defence Medicine, Birmingham, UK

OVERVIEW

- Hostile can mean many things, from direct threat to isolation.
- Care has to be adjusted according to the prevailing circumstances.
- Always assess the emergency medical system backing you up in remote areas, and know how to access it.

The term 'hostile' can mean many things, from a threat directed at an individual (intent to kill or injure), through isolation in a remote location to an adverse external environment (extremes of temperature and altitude, or contamination). Working in a conflict zone can encompass all of these.

Threat and levels of care

The experience of military medical services has been that, during fighting, individuals who leave cover to attempt to help casualties frequently become casualties themselves. This led Butler *et al.* (1996) to describe three stages of combat casualty care, where the treatment given is modified by the level of threat. These stages included *Care Under Fire* (a fire-fight is ongoing) and *Tactical Field Care* (the fight is over but resources are limited).

The UK Defence Medical Services have adopted and enhanced this approach within the multidisciplinary Battlefield Advanced Trauma Life Support (BATLS) programme (Table 26.1). Field resuscitation represents team-based resuscitation by a doctor and military medics far forward of the deployed hospital. Advanced resuscitation is led by consultants and involves a higher level of treatment and diagnostic equipment, experience and judgement.

Central to this approach to combat casualty care is the modified paradigm of <C>-ABC, where <C> is the control of catastrophic haemorrhage. This has developed from evidence of the different injury patterns seen in military trauma (blast and ballistics) compared to civilian trauma (largely blunt injury); this is expanded upon in Chapter 25.

The main initial effort is to eliminate the threat or to move the casualty away from the threat. As the threat reduces, the level of care can increase. A tourniquet placed during *Care Under Fire* should be reviewed in *Tactical Field Care* and other methods of haemorrhage control attempted; a needle decompression performed in *Tactical Field Care* should be reviewed in *Field Resuscitation* for the need to place a chest drain before onward evacuation to hospital.

Although the example used is that of military conflict, the principles equally apply to other hostile situations. A casualty trapped in a burning vehicle or a building in danger of collapse needs rapid removal and delay for spinal immobilisation is unjustified because of the threat to the casualty and the rescuers.

Table 26.1 Actions within the four stages of BATLS

Stage of care	Actions taken
Care Under Fire	Win the fire-fight. Rescue the casualty from danger. Apply tourniquet for catastrophic limb bleeding <C>. Roll face down, head to one side, for postural airway drainage <A>.
Tactical Field Care	Perform a tactical rapid primary survey (TRaPS). Use external haemostatic agents (e.g. *Celox Gauze*) to control <C> in areas where a tourniquet is impractical. Use suction and simple adjuncts to maintain the airway. Immobilise the C-spine for blunt injury (but not penetrating trauma without signs). Treat open pneumothorax with (1) vented chest type dressing and (2) monitor respiratory rate. Decompress tension pneumothorax. Dress wounds; splint fractures; give analgesia.
Field Resuscitation	This environment offers (limited) environmental control and a horizontal approach to trauma resuscitation. Additional interventions will be possible that include surgical airway, chest drain, intraosseous access and fluids, additional analgesia options, and antibiotics.
Advanced Resuscitation	This environment offers robust environmental control and a consultant-based team, together with blood and blood products, plain X-ray, FAST ultrasound, laboratory support, CT imaging and experienced trauma surgery.

CT, computed tomography; FAST, focused assessment with sonography in trauma. (Extracted from BATLS Manual 2008, reproduced from J R Army Medical Corps with permission.)

The ballistic environment: key points

- Ballistic individual protective equipment (IPE) both protects and hinders casualty and rescuer.
- Special cutting tools may be required to remove ballistic protection ('body armour') from victims in order to expose the patient for the primary and secondary survey.
- The wearing of cumbersome ballistic protection may make it difficult for rescuers to perform basic or advanced life support techniques.
- A risk/benefit evaluation will have to be made as to just how much IPE to remove from either victim or rescuer at the point of injury in order to facilitate initial resuscitation.
- Wearing night vision goggles has been shown to prolong the time taken to perform advanced life support techniques in the field. There is poor depth perception that makes it difficult to manipulate instruments and equipment, although it is not impossible to do so.

Isolation

In simplistic terms, isolation may be due to the following.

- *Geography*: medical treatment facility located miles from a centre of population and/or relying on aircraft or airdrops for supplies. Examples are a remote area expedition or a military camp.
- *Human activity*: a hospital or community where access to supplies or free movement of people is being deliberately prevented.
- *Damaged infrastructure*: access to supplies or people is disrupted, for example following a natural disaster.

There is a paradox: a well-supplied and supported geographically isolated facility (Figure 26.1) still may provide an excellent standard of care, including safe cavity surgery and postoperative intensive care with ventilation. This is what the military do particularly well.

Conversely, a large hospital (Figure 26.2) previously used to delivering a high standard of care may be unable to do so due

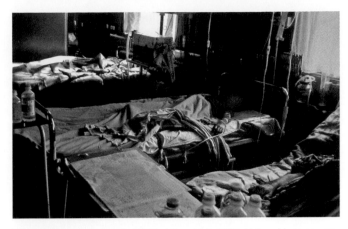

Figure 26.2 Pristina Hospital Critical Care Unit, 1999. Vulnerable to power cuts and supply shortages.

to supply chain interruption for consumables (drugs, dressings, sutures), inadequate power or inadequate removal of hospital waste (including cadavers). This will frequently be seen in conflict and postconflict settings.

Current UK thinking involves triaging patients into priorities according to urgency of clinical need based on physiological parameters and anatomical injury. In resource-limited areas, triage will necessarily select those casualties who need the least resources; for example, the surgeon may select those who do not need postoperative ventilation, and who do not need cavity surgery. Now read the vignette in Box 26.1

Based on the experience of the ICRC surgeon working in a resource-limited hospital, three lessons were identified.

- Intravenous fluids and antibiotics buy time for most patients.
- Patients with severe life-threatening injuries die despite treatment unless the equipment resources, the number of nursing staff and the organisation of the hospital infrastructure are adequate.
- When the hospital infrastructure is disrupted, surgical resources are easily wasted by operating on patients whose prognosis is hopeless (underlining the importance of realistic triage for treatment) and the death rate is unacceptably high among those who should survive.

When making a medical assessment in an isolated environment, it is worth considering the emergency medical system and the pathway a casualty will follow systematically

- *Call*: how is help summoned following an incident? By radio signal, mobile phone or satellite phone or by sending a second vehicle to get help?
- *Response*: what help is likely to come? What are their skills? How far away is trained medical aid? Must you rely on self-aid at the scene?
- *Topography*: what is the terrain? Are there access issues in reaching the casualty? What vehicle will be needed? Does a ground vehicle need to be armoured? Can a helicopter landing site be secured? How will the incident site be marked (smoke/flare/fluorescent clothing) and is this safe?

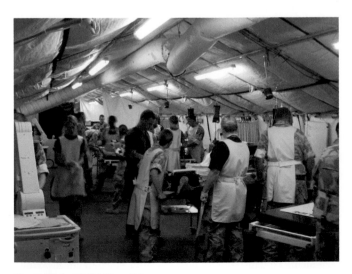

Figure 26.1 UK field hospital.

- *Destination*: where will the casualties be taken (local civilian hospital, NGO hospital, private hospital, military facility)? Do you have right of access to this facility? Is it safe for these casualties?

Box 26.1 Trauma in a hostile environment: a vignette

I was a team surgeon in one of four teams with the International Committee of the Red Cross in Kabul in 1992 when we received roughly 600 new casualties over a period of six days. Most were civilians from the vicinity of the hospital. About 250 with small soft tissue wounds were sent home with antibiotic tablets after having tetanus prophylaxis. They had instructions to return if they developed problems: few did. This is in keeping with a non-operative policy for small soft tissue wounds, but the extreme circumstances did not allow the patients to remain in hospital for observation. We were able to admit all patients with large wounds to dress the wound and give fluids intravenously, benzyl penicillin, tetanus prophylaxis and analgesia. Owing to fatigue and the proximity of the battle, we were able to operate only for some hours each day and those with abdominal wounds had priority. The perioperative mortality was high. Those who were rushed into the operating theatre because of the severity of their wounds usually died during or soon after surgery because the admission procedure had become so disrupted that many arrived on the operating table having received insufficient intravenous fluid replacement. After surgery more died through lack of postoperative supervision. Much valuable surgical time and energy was wasted. The patients with abdominal wounds who survived were those who required laparotomy for perforation and not for bleeding. The few patients admitted with thoracic wounds whose condition was not stabilized by fluid resuscitation and chest drainage died before they could reach the operating theatre. Most patients with severe wounds of the limbs that required amputation or wound excision had to wait three or four days for their surgery, but those with massive multiple wounds died in the meantime.

Source: Coupland RM. (1994) Epidemiological approach to surgical management of the casualties of war. BMJ 308: 1693–7.

External environment

Broadly speaking there are four extremes of environment in which humans regularly live, work or survive, these being at altitude and depth, and at extremes of cold and heat.

Trauma at altitude

High altitude is considered to be heights above 2500 m, with very high altitude being above 3500 m and extreme altitude greater than 5800 m. At Everest base camp (5400 m), the atmospheric pressure is about half that at sea level; at the summit (8848 m) it is around one-third.

Arterial oxygen saturations remain above 90% up to 2500 m, but fall progressively after this height. Altitude illness is common above 3500 m and no further acclimatisation occurs above 5800 m.

Trauma at high altitude raises issues that are both clinical and ethical.

- Will the summit attempt continue and the casualty be collected on the return leg or will the attempt be aborted?
- Do resources need to be brought to rescue the casualty (and what are the risks to the rescuers) or must the retrieval take place only with existing resources?

Rapid ascent above 2500 m, especially when accompanied by high levels of physical exertion, predisposes to acute mountain sickness (AMS). High-altitude cerebral oedema (HACE) is considered an extension of AMS whilst high-altitude pulmonary oedema (HAPE) can develop *de novo*.

Oxygenation at altitude

Maintaining oxygenation will be challenging. Where only bottled oxygen is available, conservation of gas becomes an imperative. At base locations, oxygen concentrators may be available and should be utilised. Oxygen may be titrated to maintain an optimum peripheral oxygen saturation by way of a finger probe pulse oximeter.

A lower threshold is required for intervention in thoracic trauma at altitude. The subject will already be hypoxic. Injury will further reduce functional residual capacity (FRC) and the victim becomes more vulnerable to hypoxia. In the clinical presence of any or all of the following features, tube thoracostomy should be considered for intrapleural drainage:

- multiple rib fractures
- surgical emphysema
- decreased thoracic excursion and worsening hypoxia.

Analgesia and anaesthesia at altitude

At altitude, opiate analgesia is hazardous because respiratory drive, hypoxic ventilatory response (HVR) and hypercapnic ventilatory response (HCVR) are all depressed. In reducing a fracture or fracture dislocation, the combination of opiate and benzodiazepine commonly used for procedural sedation in a lowland emergency department (ED) would be ill advised at altitude. Although midazolam itself does not reduce HVR, the combination of drugs would reduce both HVR and HCVR. The adverse pharmacological effects coupled with lack of monitoring and resuscitation facilities militate against this therapy at high altitude.

Inhalation anaesthesia at altitude is logistically problematic and will exacerbate hypoxia. An inspired oxygen concentration of 72% is required to maintain a normal PaO_2 at 4000 m and this would be difficult to achieve with scant resources in the wilderness. For this reason, general anaesthesia at very high altitude must be avoided unless absolutely necessary. Intravenous ketamine is the most suitable agent when general anaesthesia is a necessity. The Indian Army Medical Services have recorded its successful use at very high altitude in trauma laparotomy.

- Controlling pain or agitation will decrease oxygen demand. Remember that simply splinting a broken limb effectively, and reducing a fracture or fracture dislocation will dramatically reduce pain.

- Regional anaesthetic blocks are an invaluable adjunct to managing extremity injury. Conisder the addition of one of the many superb pocket handbooks on regional anaesthesia to your medical kit.
- For strong oral analgesia, oral or buccal tramadol is recommended by the International Committee for Alpine Rescue. HVR is maintained during administration of tramadol. For intravenous analgesia or procedural sedation, ketamine is the drug of choice. HVR is maintained and HCVR is increased with ketamine.
- Above 2000 m, oxygen/nitrous oxide gas mixtures (Entonox) are contraindicated as inspired oxygen concentrations greater than 54% are required to maintain a normal SpO_2. The concentration of nitrous oxide required to achieve adequate analgesia or anaesthesia would critically decrease the amount of available oxygen for a patient and so would worsen hypoxia.

Spinal immobilisation at altitude

Formal cervical spine and vertebral column immobilisation is usually advisable in urban situations in blunt polytrauma victims. At altitude or in hostile environments, the ability to move a victim even a short distance may mean the difference between successful rescue and death. Maintaining correct spinal immobilisation may be impossible due to lack of resources, or may be so logistically cumbersome that both rescuers and victim may be placed at unacceptable further danger.

Therefore a pragmatic approach must be taken: where possible, spinal injury must be excluded on clinical grounds and the need for formal immobilisation ignored. The NEXUS criteria have been proposed for use in the wilderness medical setting to clinically exclude spinal injury.

Trauma at depth

Trauma occurring at depth may result in the casualty rising to the surface with excessive haste. This will predispose to decompression illness and barotrauma.

Decompression illness is due to bubbles of inert gas (usually nitrogen) forming in the tissues and circulation. The amount of nitrogen taken up by the tissues is a function of the depth and duration of the dive. The longer spent at depth, the more gas needs to be excreted on ascent. If decompression is too rapid then bubbles form and disrupt tissues and the microcirculation. Gas bubbles can also produce an arterial gas embolism. Barotrauma can affect all gas-filled structures, but most commonly the lungs, ears and sinuses.

On rescue from the water, casualties should be kept horizontal to prevent reflex hypotension. Hypothermia is likely to be a concomitant problem. Symptoms of decompression illness may be delayed and the injured diver's buddy must also be considered to be at risk.

- This environment will be particularly challenging for the rescuer. For the patient, remember that oxygen demands will be increased through pain and the need to maintain perfusion of injured tissues.
- Analgesia should be intravenous where possible, again considering the use of intravenous ketamine both for analgesia and for dissociative anaesthesia where painful procedures may have

to be performed. There are many reports of the successful use of ketamine anaesthesia on board submerged submarines, where clearly inhalational anaesthesia is contraindicated. It could equally be used in a hyperbaric chamber.

- When a patient has been exposed to an underwater explosion, be very suspicious of occult injury to the lungs. In particular, blast lung and arterial gas embolism may occur, the latter often presenting with bizarre neurological signs.

Trauma in cold environments

Hypothermia is a common factor associated with major trauma even in the UK temperate environment. Hypothermia is defined as a core temperature below 35°C: it is considered severe when <32°C.

A simple practical tip is that patients who are cold but not shivering will have severe hypothermia: a patient with a cold axilla is also likely to have severe hypothermia.

The 'lethal triad' of hypothermia, acidosis and coagulopathy has been identified as a major cause of morbidity and mortality in the critically injured patient. Studies from urban trauma centres have shown that more than 50% of patients with penetrating injury are hypothermic upon admission to the ED. This is predominantly due to the initial hypovolaemia associated with penetrating injury, or the major visceral injury caused by blast or by blunt trauma. Mortality has been shown to increase by as much as 50% in case-matched trauma studies where patients are hypothermic compared to normothermic upon arrival.

The wilderness environment will produce conditions conducive to hypothermia, and this will complicate the management of trauma in such settings. Those most at risk in the wilderness are the young and old and patients with extremity, head, spinal or burns injury. Patient transport in a helicopter with open cabin doors in a combat zone, for example, will induce hypothermia even in hot climates, due to the flow of cool air over exposed skin. Prevention through a high index of suspicion is better than treatment.

Sheltering the patient, preventing further heat loss and instituting rewarming are the key steps in managing hypothermia. Any wet clothing should be removed and the casualty insulated from conductive, convective and evaporative heat loss (i.e. insulate from ground and from cool air flow over the patient). The patient should be managed in dry underwear, or else naked, in a sleeping bag, preferably within a shelter such as a bivouac sac or a thermally insulated casualty or survival bag, e.g. Blizzard Sac. Commercially available heat packs should be applied to the body at the root of the neck, axillae, abdomen and groin areas to warm the large vessels and so conduct heat back to the core. Heat packs can be improvised with hot water in drinks flasks, but be careful not to burn the patient by applying a hot metal flask directly to the skin.

Passive rewarming is achieved by insulating the patient and allowing him or her to produce heat endogenously through shivering. The patient must be effectively insulated within a sleeping bag, one that is both wind and waterproof, or a commercial survival device such as a Blizzard Sac. The use of metallic foil blankets can no longer be recommended; indeed, more heat may be lost through conduction than is retained through reflection of body heat. Warming the patient's immediate environment (vehicle, room) will also contribute to passive heat transfer.

Passive rewarming is only practicable where the patient can shiver and produce heat endogenously. When the core temperature has dropped so far that shivering has ceased, then heat will continue to be lost through conduction, evaporation and the 'after drop' phenomenon, and the patient will become more hypothermic irrespective of the quality of the insulating equipment around him or her.

Active rewarming is mandatory for the non-shivering patient or the asystolic patient, and this is a hospital level intervention. The non-shivering patient with vital signs and a detectable cardiac output can be warmed with a convective heating blanket system such as a Bair Hugger. The asystolic patient will be most effectively warmed through extracorporeal circulation (ECC) such as extracorporeal membranous oxygenation (ECMO) or cardiopulmonary bypass (CPB).

In the case of the profoundly hypothermic victim in whom vital signs are still detected, circum-rescue haemodynamic collapse with ventricular fibrillation is likely to occur with rough handling and rapid changes in body orientation. In the cold patient, the complex cardiovascular reflex mechanisms are ineffective at adapting to fluid shifts. As an example, rapid venous pooling occurs in the lower limbs when a patient moves from supine orientation to vertical orientation, as in a hauling or vertical winch rescue. Due to depression of the cardiovascular reflexes, heart rate and cardiac output cannot be raised, venous return to the heart decreases critically and syncope ensues, with the risk of ventricular fibrillation. This can be mitigated by maintaining the patient supine throughout the rescue when this is logistically possible. When circum-rescue collapse does occur, cardiopulmonary resuscitation must commence, but only if it can be maintained through to definitive care.

Drugs, fluids and medical equipment should be stored so as to prevent degradation through freezing.

Trauma in hot environments

Dealing with trauma in a hot environment is uncharacteristic in the UK. However, military experience in conflicts in the Middle East has presented trauma casualties with concomitant heat injury which may have been emerging before the physical injury was inflicted or has arisen due to continued exposure following the physical injury.

Heat illness is a spectrum with lethargy, nausea, headaches and cramps at the minor end of the spectrum progressing in severe cases to produce hypoglycaemia, cardiac dysrhythmias, rhabdomyolysis (and renal failure), muscle compartment syndromes, convulsions, coma and death.

Prevention of heat illness is clearly the best practice (protect any injured casualty from the sun where possible). Once established, heat illness is best treated by active external cooling (strip-spray-fan) and the use of cool intravenous fluids.

A key aspect to managing trauma in hot climes is to appreciate that victims may be several litres depleted in terms of body fluids through poor intake and insensible losses. Make adjustments and allow for this during resuscitation and during induction of anaesthesia, when peripheral vascular resistance may drop precipitously. Paradoxically, hypothermia may still supervene in the exposed, multiply injured patient so do not discount this.

Drugs, fluids and medical equipment must be stored so as to prevent them degrading through exposure to very high ambient temperatures.

Trauma in a chemical environment

The outcome for wounds contaminated by chemical agents is worse than the conventional injury alone. The priority for an injured casualty in a contaminated environment is to remove them from the hazard and decontaminate, then treat their conventional and chemical injuries in parallel according to their relative need: is the patient's immediate problem life-threatening external bleeding or is it symptoms from a chemical agent for which there is an available antidote? Traditional linear systems teaching for trauma resuscitation may poorly link trauma, medical toxicological and environmental problems. The UK military has devised a single gateway to all clinical emergencies (Clinical Guidelines for Operations) to ensure these issues are assessed, diagnosed and treated concomitantly.

Clinical interventions in the 'hot zone' are realistically limited and can be equated to the level of care available during *Care Under Fire* or at best to *Tactical Field Care* (see Table 26.1). Rescuers will have their stamina and dexterity degraded by the necessary personal protective equipment and skilled technical interventions will often be impractical.

Clinical interventions in the 'hot zone' should include control of catastrophic haemorrhage and simple airway management, coupled with an appropriate life-saving antidote if available (<C>, A), whereas care in the 'warm zone' includes the full <C>-ABC care with antidotes and decontamination prior to handing over a clean casualty to the 'cold zone' into the field resuscitation phase of care.

- Individual protective equipment will limit the scope of interventions available to the rescuer due to manipulation constraints, etc.
- The key is to limit interventions and to extract and decontaminate the casualty as quickly as possible.
- Triage must be rapid and effective.
- Rescuers must not expose themselves to further risk through remaining 'on scene' any longer than absolutely necessary in order to provide basic life support and to establish the priority for evacuation of casualties.

Further reading

Butler FK, Hagmann J, Butler EG. (1996) Tactical combat casualty care in special operations. Military Med 161(suppl 1): 3–16.

Coupland RM. (1994) Epidemiological approach to surgical management of the casualties of war. BMJ 308: 1693–7.

Hodgetts T, Mahoney P, Evans G, Brooks A (eds). (2006) *Battlefield Advanced Trauma Life Support*, 3rd edn. Joint Service Publication 570.

Hodgetts TJ, Mahoney PF, Russell MQ, Byers M. (2006) ABC to <C>ABC: redefining the military trauma paradigm. Emerg Med J 23: 745–6.

Hoperus Buma APCC, Burris DG, Hawley A, Ryan JM, Mahoney PF (eds). (2009) *Conflict and Catatrophe Medicine: a practical guide*, 2nd edn. London: Springer Verlag.

Kuehl A. (1994) *Prehospital Systems and Medical Oversight*, 2nd edn. St Louis, MO: Mosby Year Book.

Macnab C, Mahoney PF. (2002) Pre-hospital planning. In: Ryan J, Mahoney P, Greaves I, Bowyer G (eds). *Conflict and Catastrophe Medicine: A Practical Guide*. Heidelberg: Springer.

Redmond A, Mahoney P, Ryan J, Macnab C. (2006) *ABC of Conflict and Disaster*. London: BMJ Books.

CHAPTER 27

Psychological Trauma

Martin P. Deahl

South Staffordshire and Shropshire Healthcare NHS Foundation Trust, Stafford, UK

OVERVIEW

- The psychological consequences of trauma may be delayed in onset and easily overlooked in a patient with extensive physical injuries.

- It is easy to be complacent and fail to treat psychological abnormalities simply because they seem reactive and appropriate to the circumstances. Just because psychological symptoms are understandable doesn't make them any less treatable.

- Depression and other anxiety disorders are more common than post-traumatic stress disorder following trauma.

- Although there is no evidence that early intervention reduces the likelihood of long-term psychological abnormalities following trauma, patients should be monitored and reviewed as the earlier abnormalities are detected, the more responsive they are likely to be to treatment.

- Trauma staff are emotionally vulnerable and robust systems of staff support should be in place to allow staff access to confidential help without fear of stigma or humiliation.

More than 60% of us suffer potentially traumatising events at some point in our lives. For those who go on to suffer long-term psychological sequelae, the aftermath is often undetected, untreated and yet may be more disabling than any physical injury. This is particularly the case when there are concomitant physical injuries; these may mask psychological symptoms, yet paradoxically increase the likelihood of long-term psychological disorder. Although post-traumatic stress disorder (PTSD) is the most widely known reaction (indeed, after road traffic crashes, for example, more than 20% of patients attending the emergency department go on to suffer PTSD), depression and other anxiety disorders are also common and no less a cause of enduring social handicap than PTSD (Box 27.1).

A variety of disorders often occur after traumatic incidents whether or not physical injuries are present (Box 27.2). Clinicians involved in trauma care should be able to identify and manage common psychological reactions following trauma, and know when to refer for a specialist psychiatric opinion.

ABC of Major Trauma, Fourth Edition. Edited by David V. Skinner and Peter A. Driscoll.
© 2013 Blackwell Publishing Ltd. Published 2013 by Blackwell Publishing Ltd.

Box 27.1 Psychological sequelae of road traffic crashes

After road traffic crashes more than 20% of patients attending the emergency department go on to suffer PTSD. Driving phobias and major depressive disorders are also seen in 10–20% of survivors. These may be a social handicap and persist for years, despite the patient having made a satisfactory physical recovery.

Box 27.2 Psychological responses to trauma

- Immediate emotional reactions to trauma.
- Adjustment disorders.
- Acute stress disorder (ASD).
- Post-traumatic stress disorder.

Psychological responses to trauma

Immediate emotional reactions to trauma

A wide range of emotional reactions is seen after physical or psychological trauma. Many individuals show little or no immediate emotion. However, an absence of emotional distress does not mean that an individual is immune to subsequent disorder. Emotional reactions may be delayed or precipitated by secondary events such as media coverage, inquests and police investigations. Intense fear, anxiety and distress are generally short-lived and respond well to reassurance, empathic concern and practical support. However, brief courses of hypnotic and anxiolytic drugs may be needed for more severe reactions.

Adjustment disorders

Several patients experiencing stress or significant life change (for example, as a result of illness or disability following trauma) develop psychiatric symptoms which, although a handicap, are insufficient to meet diagnostic criteria for any other specific psychiatric disorder. These adjustment disorders generally develop within a month or so after significant life change and generally resolve within 6 months. Various clinical features are recognised but most patients typically manifest depressive or anxiety symptoms.

These disorders may respond to simple reassurance and supportive specific counselling, but symptom-targeted treatment with psychotropic drugs or cognitive-behavioural psychotherapy may be indicated in more severe cases.

Acute stress disorder

Acute stress disorders (ASD) are defined in the *Diagnostic and Statistical Manual of Mental Disorders* (DSM-IV) as occurring within 4 weeks of a life-threatening traumatic event, lasting for at least 2 days and resolving within that 4-week period. Symptoms include intrusive phenomena (nightmares, flashbacks, etc.), avoidance of reminders of the trauma, hyperarousal, and dissociative symptoms such as emotional numbing and depersonalisation (Box 27.3).

Box 27.3 Symptoms of ASD

- Intrusive phenomena (nightmares, flashhacks, etc.).
- Avoidance of reminders of the trauma.
- Dissociative symptoms such as emotional numbing and depersonalisation.

It is important to distinguish ASD from normal 'understandable' distress. Although the condition often resolves spontaneously, it identifies a group of patients at high risk of going on to develop long-term disorders and requiring careful follow-up. As many as 75% of patients suffering ASD after traumatic events will suffer from clinically significant PTSD 2 years later. There is now clear evidence that trauma-focused cognitive-behavioural therapy (CBT) is not only an effective treatment for ASD but also reduces the likelihood of subsequent PTSD.

Post-traumatic stress disorder

Post-traumatic stress disorder is a common and potentially disabling condition affecting all age groups; it may, if untreated, run a life-long relapsing course. Diagnostic criteria for PTSD are operationally defined (Box 27.4), although many individuals experience symptoms of PTSD that themselves are insufficient to meet the full diagnostic criteria: so-called 'partial PTSD'. Intrusive symptoms such as flashbacks and avoidance symptoms are a normal part of the stress response after trauma and are considered pathological only when they become excessive in frequency, duration or intensity.

The point prevalence of PTSD in the population is at least 1–2% and lifetime prevalence figures for the full-blown PTSD syndrome may exceed 10%. Between 30% and 50% of survivors of combat, man-made and natural disasters (including rescue workers), as well as personal tragedy such as torture, accidents, abuse and rape will go on to suffer from PTSD. Compared to the rest of the population, individuals with PTSD are much more likely to make negative life course decisions. Teenagers with PTSD are less likely to succeed academically or complete secondary or higher education. The unemployed are less likely to obtain stable employment and those in work are more likely to become unemployed. Single people with PTSD are less likely to marry, and those in stable relationships are more likely to divorce. The indirect socioeconomic costs of PTSD are therefore incalculable.

Box 27.4 'Core' diagnostic criteria for post-traumatic stress disorder

- A life-threatening event outside normal human experience.
- Re-experiencing the trauma:
  - intrusive memories
  - dreams/nightmares
  - flashbacks: a sense of reliving the event, distress at exposure to events resembling trauma.
- Avoidance of stimuli associated with the trauma.
- Evidence of increased arousal:
  - sleep disturbance
  - irritability
  - hypervigilance
  - exaggerated startle response.
- Duration beyond 1 month.

Vulnerability to post-traumatic stress disorder

Whether an individual develops PTSD or other psychiatric disorders after traumatic events depends upon an amalgam of the event itself, its context and the emotional significance attributed to it by an individual. In addition, several predisposing factors have been identified. These include the emergence of an ASD after the trauma, a past history of psychiatric disorder, a 'neurotic' anxiety-prone personality, exposure to previous traumatic experiences, including childhood abuse, and perceived threat to life and personal safety at the time of a traumatic event. Important gender differences have been noted; for example, women are more likely than men to develop PTSD after interpersonal, and especially sexual, violence. The presence of premorbid vulnerability factors also increases the likelihood of persisting, long-term PTSD and the development of co-morbid psychopathology, particularly affective disorder and substance misuse (Boxes 27.5 and 27.6).

Box 27.5 Post-traumatic stress disorder: important facts

- Post-traumatic stress disorder may present with dysfunctional social behaviour such as the breakdown of previously stable relationships and antisocial behaviour.
- Other psychiatric disorders such as depression, alcohol and drug misuse are often associated with PTSD.
- No single intervention effectively treats PTSD, and combinations of treatment are usually necessary.
- Families may suffer as much as the patient and should always be involved in treatment.

> **Box 27.6 Factors predisposing to the development of post-traumatic stress disorder**
>
> - Emergence of an ASD after the trauma.
> - Past history of psychiatric disorder.
> - 'Neurotic' anxiety-prone personality.
> - Exposure to previous traumatic experiences, including childhood abuse.
> - Perceived threat to life and personal safety at the time of a traumatic event.

Co-morbid disorders and behavioural sequelae of post-traumatic stress disorder

A 'pure' PTSD syndrome is unusual, and the condition is often complicated by concurrent affective disorder, particularly major depression, generalised anxiety and panic disorder, alcohol and drug misuse. The presence of co-morbidity not only makes treatment more difficult, but is an important risk factor for subsequent suicide.

Pre-existing psychiatric disorders may also be significantly exacerbated following psychological trauma. Dysfunctional behaviour often co-exists and may be the only presenting feature of an underlying PTSD. Occupational instability, antisocial behaviour and the breakown of previously stable relationships occur frequently and should raise the possibility of PTSD in any individual following traumatic events.

The biology of post-traumatic stress disorder

Several enduring biological abnormalities have been identified in individuals with PTSD. Abnormalities of the hypothalamo-pituitary-adrenal (HPA) axis include hypocortisolaemia and enhanced adrenocorticoid sensitivity to the effects of dexametasone suppression ('supersuppression'), which is proportional to the clinical severity of PTSD. It has been suggested that central glucocorticoid receptor hypersensitivity occurs in PTSD. Other neurochemical findings include evidence of increased central catecholamine activity, particularly noradrenaline and 5-hydroxytryptamine (HT), both neurotransmitters that play a part in the encoding and retrieval of memory. Anatomical changes, particularly hippocampal volume, have also been demonstrated in PTSD.

Management of psychological responses to trauma

Primary prevention (prophylaxis)

True prevention means reducing trauma by measures such as improving safety in the workplace, on the roads and in the home, crime prevention and preventing war. Specific measures include the preparation of emergency service workers, soldiers and others routinely exposed to traumatic events, to help them cope with anticipated trauma. Thorough recruit selection to 'screen out' vulnerable individuals, realistic training and establishing 'tightly knit' cohesive teams can all mitigate the effects of trauma. 'Stress inoculation' programmes are increasingly used in training; these programmes include the exposure of prospective body-handlers to human remains and postmortem examinations, and educational briefings before combat that explain the likely effects of trauma to service personnel.

Secondary prevention

After traumatic events, a variety of general and specific measures is used to reduce immediate emotional distress and help reduce the incidence of post-traumatic illness such as PTSD. General measures ('tea and sympathy') may seem intuitively obvious but can be easily overlooked in a busy department, particularly after major incidents when staff are preoccupied with major trauma rather than the minor physical injuries. Paradoxically, in the immediate post-trauma period, the psychological needs of the patient are inversely proportional to the extent of any physical injury; consequently, those with minor injuries often require proportionately more psychological support.

The patient should be made as physically comfortable as possible as quickly as possible, for example, by expediting physical and forensic examinations, and allowing the patient privacy and the opportunity to remove wet or soiled clothing and wash themselves. Allocating a specific staff member to supervise the patient facilitates a therapeutic relationship and provides an opportunity for the patient to discuss their experience and feelings should they wish to do so. Simple support is not only a matter of kindness but also allows staff to make a brief mental state assessment. After major incidents, telephones should be made available for patients to contact friends and family, to let them know they are safe and make arrangements to be collected. Neither distressed patients nor those with marked emotional numbing or other dissociative symptoms should be allowed to leave the department unescorted. Chaplains and agencies such as the Salvation Army should be enlisted to provide comfort and immediate psychological support following major incidents with multiple casualties. In the immediate aftermath of trauma the patient needs a sympathetic ear and practical advice from someone who has time to listen. Mental health workers are neither necessary nor desirable.

The role of psychiatric services in the aftermath of trauma is controversial. The main purpose of early intervention by mental health workers is to assess mental state and identify psychiatric disorder as, without doubt, the earlier a specific disorder is identified and treated, the better the long-term outcome. However, trauma staff are sometimes understandably reluctant to involve mental health workers because of stigma and the fear that focusing on emotional reactions may create or exacerbate psychological problems. In an ideal service, an integrated approach to management using appropriately trained staff within the trauma team, attuned to the physical health needs of the patient, may be best placed to assess mental state.

Specific measures designed to reduce long-term psychiatric morbidity after trauma include various forms of acute intervention, such as brief CBT for acute stress disorders. There is little evidence to suggest that any other interventions are effective. Critical incident stress debriefing (CISD) or psychological debriefing (PD) have been widely practised, but numerous studies have now clearly demonstrated that the technique is ineffective and may even be harmful.

Some elements of debriefing (such as psycho-education) may be helpful and seem intuitively appropriate but further research is needed to demonstrate effectiveness.

The best long-term psychological outcome is likely to be achieved when any early intervention is used as one element of an integrated 'stress management' package which includes immediate support, practical help and adequate follow-up to identify those who go on to develop long-term disorders. A number of initiatives embracing these principles are currently undergoing evaluation, such as trauma incident management (TRIM) developed and used by the armed forces.

Treatment of established post-traumatic stress disorder

A variety of psychological interventions and drug treatments has been shown to relieve at least some PTSD symptoms. The diversity of available treatments is an indication that none in isolation is particularly effective and an eclectic approach combining psychotherapy, drug treatments and social support is most likely to succeed. PTSD victims can be difficult to engage and are often reluctant to discuss symptoms or seek help. Time should be taken to establish a good therapeutic relationship with the patient before embarking on specific therapies (Box 27.7). The therapist should also be prepared to be proactive and include facilities for community outreach. PTSD creates secondary victims among families and it is important to involve significant others wherever possible in any treatment programme.

Box 27.7 **Early intervention: factors to consider**

- Establishing rapport and a therapeutic relationship.
- Continuity and consistency of approach.
- Don't look for problems where they don't exist.
- Sensitive review of emotional symptoms and signs to identify ASD.
- Where present consider referral for CBT.
- Education including description of normal trauma response, coping strategies and where, when and how to obtain help and support if symptoms fail to improve.
- 'Joined-up' care liaising with trauma team and A&E staff.
- Arrange review to assess coping and adjustment and to detect emerging PTSD and other disorders.

Psychological therapies

A variety of psychological treatments have been advocated in the treatment of PTSD. Group-based therapies may be particularly useful when dealing with the victims of a shared trauma such as combat or in disaster rescue workers. Cognitive techniques and exposure-based behavioural interventions are popular and have proven efficacy. Anxiety management programmes used alone are probably less effective. Audiotape desensitisation is an effective and commonly used technique based on the principle of 'imaginal' exposure. The patient writes a detailed script, describing not only events but also the feelings, sights, sounds and smells of the trauma. These are then recorded onto audiotape. Repeated exposure to the audiotape using a personal stereo often reduces symptoms of hyperarousal to tolerable levels within 2–3 weeks. Eye movement desensitisation and reprocessing (EMDR) is a popular but controversial technique which is nevertheless supported by a firm evidence base. The patient relives traumatic memories while the therapist induces saccadic eye movements, which is claimed to produce rapid symptom relief in PTSD. Its mechanism of action is uncertain but is almost certainly due in part to exposure.

Drug treatment

Although drugs alleviate some of the symptoms of PTSD, they are not generally as effective as psychological treatments and should always be combined with psychotherapy. Drug treatments tend to be most effective following acute PTSD and are of particular benefit in reducing 'positive' symptoms such as nightmares and intrusive thoughts. Co-morbid depression and other psychiatric disorders are also indications for drug treatment.

Drugs acting on central serotonergic transmission appear to have the most beneficial effects on the symptoms of PTSD. These include selective serotonin reuptake inhibitors (SSRIs) such as fluoxetine. Doses considerably in excess of those used to treat depression are commonly required and treatment maintained for 2 months or more before the full therapeutic effect is observed. Although benzodiazepines are occasionally useful in reducing symptoms of hyperarousal, they should generally be avoided, particularly if there are concurrent problems with alcohol and other substance misuse.

A variety of other drugs have been used to some effect, including more sedative antidepressants acting primarily on 5-HT systems such as nefazadone, tricyclic antidepressants, monoamine oxidase inhibitors (MAOIs) and non-psychotropic drugs such as clonidine that act by reducing central noradrenergic activity. The 5-HT antagonist cyproheptadine is occasionally useful in preventing nightmares.

Summary

Psychological trauma is common and disabling. Stigma, shame and the avoidance symptoms associated with PTSD mean that patients all too often suffer in silence or present with dysfunctional social lives and a variety of diverse and seemingly unrelated difficulties. Many cases go undetected and a high incidence of clinical suspicion is required, particularly in high-risk groups such as emergency service workers, participants in combat and rape and accident victims, to enable them to have access to treatment and therapeutic facilities. Health professionals are not immune to the psychological effects of trauma. They are also more likely to deal with their difficulties by self-medicating with drugs and alcohol than face the stigma and professional opprobrium associated with seeking help.

Public attitudes towards psychological trauma are ambivalent and at times downright hostile ('after all, they're lucky to be alive', 'they're malingerers only after compensation'). Contrary to popular opinion, when litigation follows trauma a successful resolution for the plaintiff seldom brings about any significant clinical improvement. In the aftermath of traumatising events, psychological symptoms are easily disregarded.

There can be no room for complacency and symptoms should not be dismissed merely because they are understandable in the context of trauma. Any patient with significant psychological distress more than 6 months after a traumatic event, or whose symptoms are socially handicapping, should be referred for a psychiatric assessment. The earlier the treatment of psychological trauma, the more effective it is and trauma victims should not have to wait for a crisis before receiving help. Follow-up should be offered to all trauma victims seen in the emergency department.

Major incident planning must include provision to inform the general practitioner (GP) of all patients involved in an incident, including those sustaining only minor injuries (Box 27.8). The report should include brief details of the incident, information about the possible sequelae of psychological trauma, and how and where the GP can obtain specialist advice. Most importantly, the GP should review the patient 6 months to 1 year after the incident, to assess the patient's mental state and lifestyle before and after the incident.

Box 27.8 **Information for the GP**

- Brief details of the incident.
- Possible sequelae of psychological trauma.
- How and where the GP can obtain specialist advice.

A significant change in personality, deterioration in relationships and social or occupational functioning, excessive alcohol or substance misuse, in addition to obvious signs of psychological disorder should alert the GP to the possibility of an underlying post-traumatic illness (Box 27.9). This should trigger a more detailed examination and specialist referral if necessary.

Box 27.9 **Signs of post-traumatic illness**

- Significant change in personality.
- Deterioration in relationships and social or occupational functioning.
- Excessive alcohol or substance misuse.
- Obvious signs of psychological disorder.

Further reading

Black D, Newman M, Mezey G, Hendriks JH (eds). (1997) *Psychological Trauma: A Developmental Approach.* London: Gaskell Press. A small but comprehensive work covering all aspects of traumatic stress throughout the life-cycle. The first book on PTSD to be written from a British perspective.

Deahl MP, Wessely S. (2003). In debate: psychological debriefing is a waste of time. Br J Psychiatry 183: 12–14. A brief but informative debate demonstrating the politicisation and controversies surrounding early intervention.

Foa EB, Keane TM, Friedman MJ, Cohen JA (eds). (2009) *Effective Treatments for PTSD.* London: Piatkus Books. A comprehensive textbook on PTSD and one of the best up-to-date reference sources available.

CHAPTER 28

Major Incidents

Lizle Blom[1] and John J. M. Black[2]

[1] Royal Berkshire Hospital, Reading, UK
[2] John Radcliffe Hospital, Oxford, UK

OVERVIEW

- Definition.
- Initial response.
- Phases of a major incident:
  - preparation
  - response
  - recovery.

The Department of Health's Strategic National Guidance to the NHS for Major Incident Emergency Planning (2005) defines a major incident as any occurrence that presents a serious threat to the health of the community, disruption to the service or causes such numbers or types of casualties as to require special arrangements to be implemented by hospitals, ambulance trusts or primary care organisations (Box 28.1). Varying types of casualties and medical incidents fall into this category. The type of incident will indicate the resources required. Every hospital should therefore have a major incident plan to use when normal resources are unable to cope. Whereas natural disasters account for most deaths worldwide, accidents (Figure 28.1) or terrorist incidents involving the transport system, such as the London bombings in 2005 (Figure 28.2), remain a significant risk in the United Kingdom.

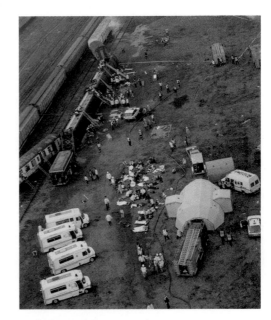

Figure 28.1 Clapham rail disaster, London.

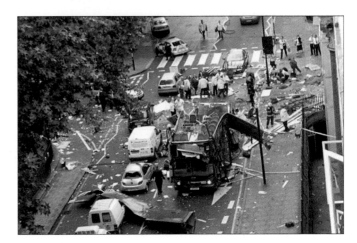

Figure 28.2 London bombing incident.

Box 28.1 **Major incident definition**

Major incidents can be:

- Simple or compound
- Compensated or uncompensated
- Natural or man-made.

Most incidents are:

- Simple (environment intact)
- Compensated (patient load less than capacity available)
- Man-made.

Major incidents can arise in a variety of ways.

- Big bang: a serious transport accident, explosion or series of smaller incidents.

ABC of Major Trauma, Fourth Edition. Edited by David V. Skinner and Peter A. Driscoll.
© 2013 Blackwell Publishing Ltd. Published 2013 by Blackwell Publishing Ltd.

- Rising tide: infectious disease epidemic or a capacity/staffing crisis.
- Cloud on the horizon: a serious threat such as a major chemical or nuclear release developing elsewhere and needing preparatory action.
- Headline news: public or media alarm about a personal threat.
- Deliberate release of chemical, biological, radiological or nuclear materials (CBRN incident).
- Preplanned major events that require planning: demonstrations, sports events, air shows.

The initial response

The hospital is usually alerted to a major incident by ambulance control, who may alert the switchboard or speak directly to the emergency department (ED) as determined by local protocol. Standard phrases are used to avoid confusion. 'Major Incident Standby' is used to warn of a potential incident, for example a multiple vehicle crash on a motorway or a commercial airliner that has declared an inflight emergency. Generally speaking, only a limited number of key staff are alerted: duty ED consultant and ED nurse co-ordinators, duty surgeons, intensivists, operating theatres, blood bank, operations manger and hospital matron.

When a major incident has been confirmed, a full hospital response is initiated by the phrase 'Major Incident Declared – Activate Plan'. The response can be terminated at any stage by 'Major Incident – Cancelled'. Ambulance control will inform receiving hospitals when the scene is clear of live casualties.

Hospitals may also need to activate their own major incident plans either as a consequence of an internal incident on the hospital site (e.g. a fire requiring staff and patient evacuation) or when significant numbers of patients self-present necessitating extraordinary measures to be implemented to manage the surge in demand at the hospital. It is very important that the Ambulance Service is informed of a major incident declaration by the hospital.

When a 'Major Incident Declared' message is received (Box 28.2), the following information should be established from ambulance control.

- Time that major incident occurred.
- Exact location of incident (grid reference, nearest road junction, etc.).
- Type of incident has occurred (road/rail/terrorism)?
- Hazards (present and potential)
- Approximate numbers and severity of the casualties?
- Clinical personnel (if any) required at the scene? (Medical incident commander /medical emergency response incident teams)

If a medical incident commander (MIC) or medical emergency response incident team (MERIT) is required at the scene (see below), the ambulance service will endeavour to avoid dispatching hospital based clinical teams from the nearest receiving hospitals that are most likely to receive significant numbers of casualties.

Box 28.2 **Standard major incident phrases**

'Major Incident – Stand By.' A major incident is imminent. Warn key staff and assemble the hospital co-ordination team.
'Major Incident Declared – Activate Plan.' The incident has occurred. A full response is required.
'Major Incident – Cancelled.' There is no longer the threat of a major incident.
'Major Incident – Stand Down.' The last live casualties have left the major incident scene.

Preparation for major incidents

The phases of major incidents are shown in Box 28.3.

Box 28.3 **Phases of major incidents**

1 Preparation.
2 Response.
3 Recovery.

Planning

Major incident plans should include on-call lists for available staff, action cards readily available at all times, standard alerting messages, co-ordination between police, ambulance service and hospitals, good use of security to control traffic flow and to lock down the emergency department and hospital site, updated equipment and infrastructure. This plan should be revised regularly and major incident practice sessions held at appropriate intervals (see below).

An all-hazard approach should be followed where one plan should be able to deal with any type of major incident. Mass casualty incidents will require modifications to the standard major incident plan: for example industrial accidents, sports stadium events, terrorist attacks using chemical and biological materials, chemical spillage, radiation incidents, large numbers of children and natural disasters. The hospital's intranet is a valuable resource for storing and accessing major incident plans and action cards in the event of an emergency.

Equipment

Protective clothing for major incident clinical responders (MIC/MERIT) responders should meet British standards and the current recommendations of the ambulance and police advisory groups (Box 28.4). For example, the helmet should be made of kevlar composite, green with white lettering, with a visor and chin strap; jackets must be high visibility and should be clearly labelled in green 'DOCTOR' or 'NURSE' (Figure 28.3). Incident commanders (including the medical incident commander) will wear checkered tabards to facilitate identification at the scene (Figure 28.4). National standardisation of clothing and clinical equipment will help recognition at the scene and facilitate control and emergency clinical care, especially when mutual aid arrangements are activated across neighbouring ambulance services in large-scale incidents.

Box 28.4 **Protective clothing for field responders**

Personal protective clothing for staff on site at a major incident

- Warm underclothing.
- Fire-retardant suit.
- High-visibility jacket marked 'DOCTOR' or 'NURSE'.
- Hard hat with visor.
- Gloves (robust and latex pairs).
- Ear defenders.

Additional essential equipment

Everybody

- Personal identification and money.
- Notebook (ideally plasticised with water-resistant pen).
- Action card.

Medical incident commander

- Radio and spare battery.
- Optional:
  - action cards
  - camera
  - dictaphone
  - mobile phone/ tetra radio handset.

Medical supplies are best carried in rucksacks with partitions clearly dividing them into functional equipment modules: 'airway', 'breathing' and 'circulation', etc. Checklists on the wall of the major incident room can be useful to remind teams deploying from hospitals not to forget important analgesic or anaesthetic drugs from the controlled drugs cupboard if such items are to be taken to the scene.

Following the July 7th bombings in London in 2005, emergency dressing packs have now been pre-positioned on major transport hubs at over 200 locations in England which are suitable for use by bystanders with first aid skills and first responding ambulance personnel, the major focus being to control significant external haemorrhage (Box 28.5). These dressings packs are stored at marked rail staff manager's offices for immediate deployment.

Since 2008, all ambulance service trusts in England have been issued with sufficient emergency medical equipment and drugs to treat up to 100 trauma P1 and P2 priority casualties (100 modular

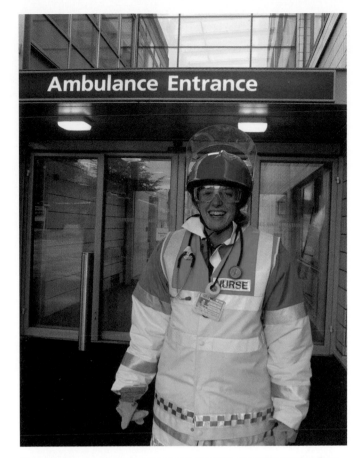

Figure 28.3 A member of an Emergency Department MERIT Nursing Team appropriately dressed and protected to support clinical care at a major incident.

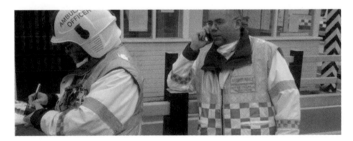

Figure 28.4 Ambulance Incident commanders wear distinctive green and white checkered tabards at major incidents over protective clothing (PPE) to facilitate identification and complex scenes.

trauma packs in 80:20 adult-to-paediatric ratio) (Box 28.6), and up to 250 P3 (for ambulant casualties) (Box 28.7; Figure 28.6) in the event of a major incident as part of the Ambulance Service National Capabilities Programme co-ordinated through the Emergency Preparedness Division, Department of Health. In addition, multiple oxygen delivery systems suitable for delivering oxygen to up to 50 casualties simultaneously have been supplied (Figure 28.7).

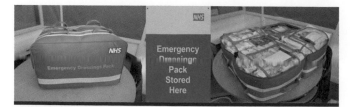

Figure 28.5 NHS emergency dressings packs for use by first responders for control of significant external haemorrhage.

Box 28.5 Contents of NHS emergency dressing packs (Figure 28.5)

- Elasticated compression dressings (20).
- Extensive wound dressings (25).
- Extra large sterile dressings (96).
- Large, medium and small sterile dressings (96 of each).
- Boxes of large and extra-large gloves sterile gloves (1 of each).
- Paramedic shears (5).
- Cling film (1 roll).

Box 28.6 Contents of Priority 1 and 2 trauma packs stored in Ambulance Mass Casualty Equipment Vehicles

- Scene assessment, triage/documentation equipment.
- Basic and advanced airway management and breathing equipment.
- Haemorrhage control: elasticated compression dressings, amputation and burns dressings, arterial and venous tourniquets, celox haemostatic dressings.
- Vascular access (peripheral IV cannulation and intraosseous needles).
- Drug administration accessories.
- Splintage (femoral traction and pelvic) and survival blanket.
- Amputation sets.
- P1 and P2 drugs (100 trauma packs per pod):
    - chemical countermeasures
    - rapid-sequence induction and procedural sedation drugs.

Box 28.7 Ambulant Casualty (P3) Equipment stored on ambulance mass casualty vehicles (250 casualties)

- Triage labels.
- Triangular bandages.
- Emergency dressings.
- Extremity splints.
- Eye casualty irrigation equipment and dressings.
- Sterile gloves/sheers.
- Intravenous cannulae.
- G-proxymetacaine and chloramphenicol eye drops.
- Morphine.
- Ibuprofen/paracetamol.

Training

Acute hospitals should ensure adequate training, exercising and testing of its major incident plans (Box 28.8). The Department of Health recommends a minimum of one 'live' exercise every 3 years, a 'table-top' exercise every year and a test of communications cascades every 6 months. The Prehospital Emergency Care Certificate and the Diploma in Immediate Medical Care prepare clinicians to the proper standards but doctors should also take courses in medical management of a major incident (MIMMS) if they are likely to undertake medical incident command roles or to be a member of MERIT delivering

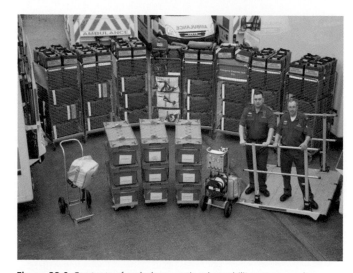

Figure 28.6 Contents of ambulance national capability mass casualty equipment vehicles containing trauma packs for 100 P1 and P2 trauma packs for adults and children, and equipment and drugs for up to 250 ambulant (P3) casualties.

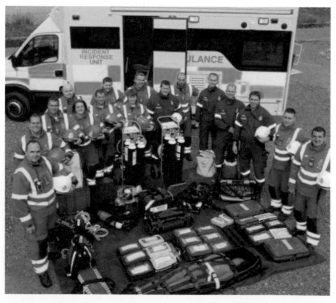

Figure 28.7 Hazardous Area Response Teams (HART) Emergency Clinical Equipment which also includes mass oxygen delivery systems.

medical care at the casualty clearing station at the major incident scene. MERIT team members should have also undertaken appropriate trauma and resuscitation training, for example Advanced Trauma Life Support (ATLS) and Advanced Paediatric Life Support (APLS) training. Hospital-based clinical and management teams responding to a major incident may also benefit from table-top exercises (EMERGO training) and hospital major incident medical management and support (HIMMS) courses.

Box 28.8 **Suggested staff training requirements**

Medical incident officer

- Diploma in Immediate Medical Care (Royal College of Surgeons of Edinburgh) or Prehospital Emergency Care Certificate

  and

- Major Incident Medical Management and Support (MIMMS) course (3 days) (other major incident training courses available)

  and

- Advanced life support instruction (Advanced Trauma Life Support/Prehospital Trauma Life Support)

Member of mobile medical care team

- Prehospital Emergency Care course

  and

- Major Incident Medical Management and Support (MIMMS) course (first 2 days only)

  and

- Advanced life support instruction (Advanced Trauma Life Support/Prehospital Trauma Life Support)

Incident scene organisation

Figure 28.8 illustrates the organisation of the incident scene.

Command

Overall control of the scene is the responsibility of the police, who will place a secure outer cordon around it. A second inner cordon may be established around the immediate incident scene if it is necessary to control the movement of emergency service personnel into a potentially hazardous area.

Each emergency service will appoint a commander who is usually a senior officer; this role will be initially undertaken by the first emergency service personnel from all three services at the scene. Incident commanders will usually be located closely to their emergency command vehicles that are normally co-located to facilitate interagency communication. These vehicles should be the only vehicles not to switch off their coloured beacons. Incident commanders at the scene will form Silver (tactical) level command

whereas their chief officers will meet remotely at an agreed location to form Gold level command for strategic level planning. Forward incident commanders (Bronze) will be appointed to co-ordinate rescue efforts.

Since 2007, newly formed ambulance service hazardous area response teams (HART) have been trained to deliver emergency clinical care in hazardous and semi-permissive environments inside the inner cordon of a major incident in order to save the lives of salvageable patients who may not reach casualty clearing stations (CCS) alive without prior clinical intervention (Figure 28.9).

If the incident is spread over a large area it will be broken into smaller (Bronze) sectors to facilitate effective scene management, each with its own forward Bronze commanders.

The police

In addition to securing the incident scene and saving life, the police will establish clear routes into and out of the incident, and control the public and bystanders, liaise with the media, activate the voluntary aid societies (at the request of the ambulance service) and local authorities. They will set up a casualty bureau to collate information regarding survivors and the dead, identify the dead and organise their removal from the scene in conjunction with the local coroner. They have responsibility for ensuring preservation of forensic evidence and prosecuting any criminal activity that may have contributed to the incident occurrence.

The fire service

If there is fire, chemical or any other significant environmental hazard within the inner cordon, the senior fire officer will assume primacy for management within the inner cordon and will be responsible for the rescue of casualties. The fire service has access to specialist cutting and rescue equipment, and has specialist resources for undertaking urban search and rescue.

The ambulance service

The ambulance service is responsible for assessment and treatment of all casualties and for their onward transport to hospital. The ambulance service provides an essential link between the NHS and other services involved in a major incident and it is therefore imperative that ambulance service personnel rapidly identify and declare the potential for a major incident. The first responders at the scene will use a structured universal report system to ensure quality of initial information and to guide an appropriate response from the emergency services and the NHS. The following mnemonic is widely adopted to ensure that key information is relayed early to ambulance control and onto receiving hospitals (Box 28.9).

Principles of management and medical support

All members of the health services should use a structured response, both prehospital and within the hospital. This encapsulates major

Scene Organisation

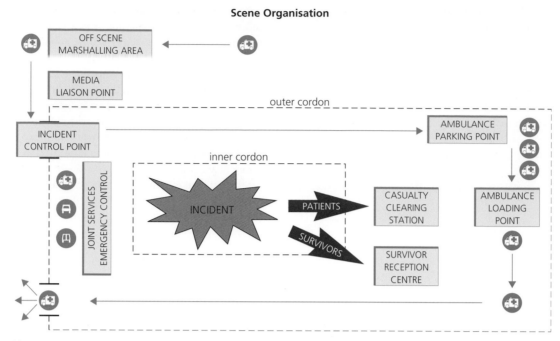

Figure 28.8 Incident scene organisation.

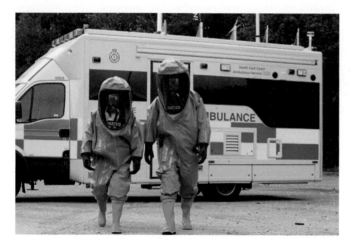

Figure 28.9 Ambulance HART teams can now safely deploy alongside fire and rescue teams in semi-permissive hazardous environments to save life (e.g. following a chemical/radiological incident). See Chapter 21.

Box 28.9 **'METHANE' – initial situation report**

M   Major incident declared or hospitals on standby
E   Exact location
T   Type of incident
H   Hazards, present and potential
A   Access to site
N   Numbers and types of casualties
E   Emergency services present and required

---

incident medical management where 'CSCA' represents the incident management aspects of the response and 'TTT' represents the clinical support that is provided (Box 28.10).

Box 28.10 **Principles of management and medical support at major incident scene**

C   Command
S   Safety
C   Communications
A   Assessment

T   Triage
T   Treatment
T   Transport

C – COMMAND

In addition to specialist paramedical clinical skills, ambulance officers have a number of other key roles to establish at the scene of a major incident. These include a loading officer (to record hospital destination of individual casualties), a primary and secondary triage officer to prioritise casualties for rescue, treatment and transport to hospital (see below), a casualty clearing station officer (to locate a suitable area and set up the CCS), a safety officer (to identify hazards and supervise personal protective equipment and staff) and a communications officer. It is the ambulance incident commander's (AIC) responsibility to nominate receiving hospitals and to arrange the provision of a medical incident commander (MIC) and medical emergency response incident teams (MERIT) teams to support the incident if necessary.

Medical incident commanders are responsible for all medical resources at the scene, including their tasking and safety (see Box 28.10). It is essential they liaise closely with, and remain in close proximity to, the AIC who has primacy in terms of overall command. As MERIT personnel arrive at the scene, they may be appointed to a number of different roles by the MIC but their main effort is likely to be delivering emergency clinical treatment at the CCS. Suitably trained clinicians may also be deployed to forward areas to support and co-ordinate triage and emergency treatment.

The composition of NHS MERIT teams is currently under review but it is likely that in the future they will be drawn from both acute hospitals (e.g. emergency physicians, emergency nurses and operating department assistants) as well as BASICS immediate medical care schemes, dependent on local circumstances and available resources. Responsibility for the equipping, deployment, training of these teams now rests with the ambulance service.

S – SAFETY

Staff, and their safety, take priority over the incident scene and survivor management. Appropriate personal safety equipment is essential. Highly visible jackets with tabards specific for role, warm and waterproof underclothing, hard hats, goggles, gloves, both heavy duty and latex, steel capped boots, and chemical resistant personal protective clothing if required, should always be worn (see Figure 28.3). Always remember safety protocol: Self, Scene, Survivors.

C – COMMUNICATION

Communications are frequently problematic at major incidents because of the challenges and constraints of the environment. Training should be provided in radio use, as knowledge of radio voice procedure will be assumed. Spare batteries must always be readily available. Alternative methods of communication should be considered and planned. Don't forget the value of a runner, especially when all radios are busy. Make sure to use written messages to avoid confusion. All the incident commanders must liaise regularly, but the ambulance and medical incident commanders should be almost inseparable.

A – ASSESSMENT

The first on scene should estimate the magnitude and severity of the incident, including estimating the numbers of live casualties as soon as possible. This information will determine the response needed. Information should then be upgraded regularly in order to provide the necessary resources. The scene should also be assessed for potential hazards to the teams and appropriate precautions instigated.

T – TRIAGE

Triage is the sorting of casualties into priorities for emergency treatment and/or for evacuation to higher echelons of care (e.g. to the casualty collection point within the inner cordon, casualty clearing station or onto hospital). There are three treatment priority groups: those needing immediate emergency treatment to sustain life (e.g. airway support or decompression of tension pneumothorax), those requiring urgent treatment (e.g. placement of traction splint for a fractured femur), and those who priority for treatment can be delayed (e.g. a simple superficial wound).

Initial primary triage takes place at the location where casualties are found and will usually be performed by ambulance personnel. Secondary triage takes place at the casualty clearing station and will usually be performed by ambulance personnel supported by MERIT/enhanced care medical teams.

Triage is a dynamic process and must be regularly repeated as patients may deteriorate whilst awaiting treatment. Ordinarily the sickest patients are the highest priority not only for emergency treatment but also for rescue/evacuation to hospital unless the incident is truly overwhelming and there are not adequate resources to undertake this. The underlining principle when dealing with large numbers of casualties with finite resources is to 'do the most for the most'.

The most widely used systems to undertake initial triage by the ambulance service uses a simple system that makes an assessment of the physiological well-being of the patient. The most widely used system currently is the Triage Sieve (Figure 28.10). Ambulant patients (classified as P3) are unlikely to have an immediately life threatening injury but will require further careful clinical assessment when circumstances permit. All non-ambulant patients are either priority P1 (with evidence of respiratory distress or shock), P2 (no evidence of respiratory distress or signs of shock), or dead if they show no signs of life on opening the airway. As soon as a P1 criterion is established the triage process is completed, i.e., there is no need to establish the presence of shock in a patient with a persistently abnormal (fast or slow) respiratory rate. The limitation of the triage sieve is that it takes time to complete (at least 1 minute to identify a P2 casualty), and the triage process itself if done in isolation does not in itself benefit the casualty in need of immediate life saving treatment (e.g. catastrophic external haemorrhage control using a tourniquet), and it does not take into account specific anatomical patterns of injury. This limitation was highlighted by the London Coroner Lady Justice Hallett following her investigation of the London in 2005, published in 2011, which resulted in a Rule 43 ruling being issued, requiring the ambulance services to review their casualty triage systems.

Ambulance triage systems are in the process of being further refined on the basis of recent military operational experience in Iraq and Afghanistan. The military triage sieve has recently been modified for use on the battlefield that links the initial

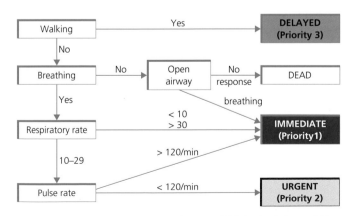

Figure 28.10 Triage sieve. Capillary refill is unreliable in the dark or cold but can be used instead of pulse rate. CRT >2 indicates Priority 1.

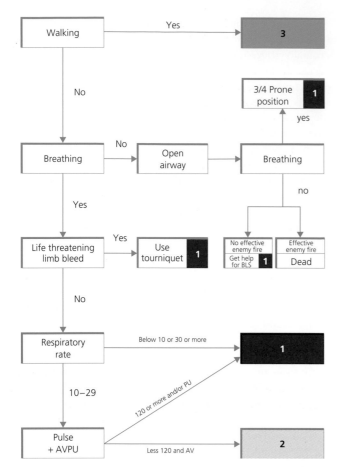

Figure 28.11 Military triage sieve. It will rarely be appropriate to undertake BLS in a mass casualty incident.

In truly hazardous environments, there are two purposes for triage: to prioritise patients for rescue and for treatment. In semi-permissive environments with limited resources for extrication and rescue it may be more appropriate to undertake 'reverse' triage, i.e., to rescue those with less severe injury in the first instance in order to potentially save the most lives with the finite available resources for rescue.

In some challenging environments with limited patient access, it may not be straight forward in rapidly confirming that death has occurred, especially should it prove necessary to wear to wear high levels of protective clothing/chemical suits. Simple detection systems for detecting expired carbon dioxide (e.g. face mask with Easycap calorimetric CO_2 detector attached) may provide more rapid confirmation – if in doubt it may be appropriate to initially triage as P1 as this will trigger repeat clinical assessment as circumstances permit.

Labelling of patients should ideally be visible and firmly secured. Labels must clearly show standard triage category, injuries noted, treatments provided and drugs administered. They should also allow for the priorities of the patient to be changed. Specifically designed triage cards (Figure 28.12) and simple snapper systems have been designed for this purpose, but in their absence casualties can be marked using indelible pens on the face or exposed chest. The 'SMART' label system is increasingly being used by ambulance services/MOD in the UK for this purpose and includes a simple system for keeping a running tally of triage category numbers that greatly facilitates the triage process.

Ambulance triage systems are continuing to evolve and it is now recognized, following the London Bombings in July 2005, and recent operational military experience in Iraq and Afghanistan, that there is merit in combining primary triage with undertaking a quick, but immediately life saving intervention, by two-person clinical triage teams (e.g. application of tourniquet and placing

casualty prioritization process with quickly administered effective therapeutic intervention (application of a tourniquet, the placement of unconscious patients semi or fully prone position (Figure 20.11). This can be readily implemented by two- person 'therapeutic triage' team as outlined below. As soon as it has been established that a patient is P1 the triage assessment process is complete. This system also appropriately accommodates a sub-group of ambulant patients being appropriately prioritized as P1 if a tourniquet has been applied to control catastrophic haemorrhage following severe upper limb amputation/injury. The assessment of conscious level (AVPU), which can be very quickly established even in high levels of PPE, is also incorporated into this system and removes the requirement to assess respiratory rate and heart rate in unconscious patients (as determined by inability to obey commands or an AVPU score of P or less). It will rarely be appropriate to undertake cardio-pulmonary resuscitation in a mass casualty incident.

Secondary triage at the casualty collection point or casualty clearing stations can be more sophisticated and may also factor in specific anatomical patterns of injury, if there is an experienced clinician to undertake this. When prioritizing patients for onward transport to hospital, further refinement of P1 casualties can be undertaken by subdividing them into P1 airway, P1 breathing, P1 shock , P1 haemorrage control, etc.

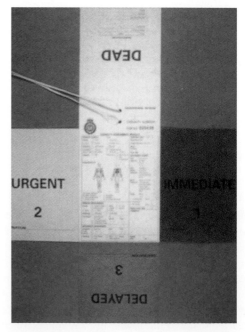

Figure 28.12 Triage label.

unconscious patients in the recovery position for airway maintenance. It is likely that the UK military approach for combat casualty triage will be adopted by UK Civilian Ambulance Services for use in major incidents caused by blast and ballistic injury (see Figure 28.11).

T – TREATMENT

Initial treatment will often be bystander first aid. The ambulance service is thereafter responsible for the subsequent and overall treatment of patients. They may be supported by doctors and nurses from immediate medical schemes or from hospital-based medical emergency response incident teams (MERIT), formerly known as mobile medical teams (Box 28.11).

Box 28.11 **MERIT functions at major incident**

- Experienced clinicians to perform secondary triage at CCS.
- Additional clinical personnel to perform life-saving haemorrhage control, airway, breathing and circulation interventions.
- Administration of analgesia.
- Delivery of critical care (including rapid-sequence induction/procedural sedation)) as required.
- Emergency surgical procedures to facilitate extrication (rarely required).
- Communication with MIC re. appropriate disposal and distribution of patients.
- Treatment and appropriate discharge of patients at the scene with minor injury and illness.

Once the hierarchy is in place, treatment is predominantly delivered at the CCS (Figure 28.13). The principal aim of treatment is to deliver life-saving care to enable patients to reach hospital alive. Priority1 patients may require the equivalent of ED resuscitation room interventions and the procurement of mass-casualty equipment vehicles should greatly facilitate the provision of such care should this be required in a large scale incident. Treatment is therefore mostly confined to external compressible haemorrhage control, airway maintenance, ventilatory support, pelvic and long bone splintage, spinal packaging, and analgesia. A proportion of these patients may require procedural sedation to facilitate these interventions, and unconscious patients with airway and or respiratory compromise may need to undergo rapid sequence induction of anaesthesia for stabilization and safe onward transport to hospital, either by road or by helicopter, if there are the resources and personnel available to undertake this. The recent procurement of mass casualty equipment vehicles should greatly facilitate the delivery of such care. Although P3 (ambulant) casualties may be moved to hospital immediately with minimal treatment on scene treatment using public transport assets (e.g. by minibus/coach), with appropriate prehospital emergency medicine/nursing secondary care support (MERIT) many such patients could potentially be assessed, treated and discharged from scene. In structural building collapse, such as occurred on 9/11 in New York, in addition to trapped patients with crush injuries, there may be significant numbers of ambulant patients with concrete dust-related eye injury in need of prompt eye irrigation/treatment. England's ambulance services now hold the necessary equipment and drugs to potentially undertake this at the scene.

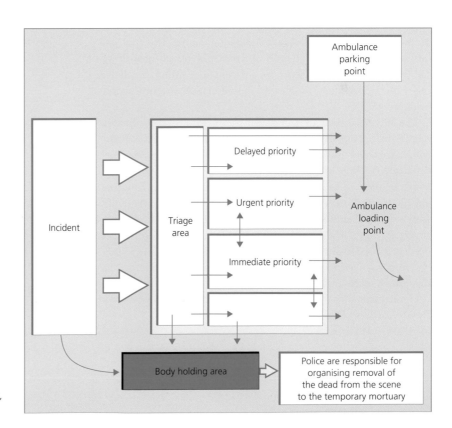

Figure 28.13 Organisation at the site of a major incident, including layout of the casualty clearing station.

T – Transport

The ambulance service is responsible for transporting injured patients to hospital. To decide the most appropriate transport, the ambulance incident commanders should consider its capacity, availability and suitability, such as access to difficult terrain. Before the patient is loaded into the ambulance, it should also have been decided which hospital is most appropriate under the circumstances, what observations and treatment will be needed on the way, and if the patient should be escorted.

In addition to these seven areas of responsibility, the MIC will monitor the medical response to ensure that it is adequate and that there is a continuing supply of equipment. He will observe the team members for signs of fatigue, and organise relief staff – usually every 4 hours. A debrief of all medical personnel involved at the scene should be held within 24 hours.

Hospital response

The key to successful hospital management of a major incident is, once again, command and control. This depends on early establishment of an effective hospital co-ordination team (HCT) staffed by senior hospital medical, nursing, administration and support staff. The principles for managing the hospital's response are similar to the procedures that are used to manage the incident scene. Its role is to effectively lead and co-ordinate the wider hospital's response to support the incident (Box 28.12). All should be as senior and experienced as possible – the hospital's medical director, director of nursing/matron and chief executive/director of operations, or their nominated deputies, should be well placed to take on this role. They must be familiar with the hospital's major incident plan and effectively function at the Silver (tactical) level of hospital command, and will be based at the hospital's Silver control suite/operation centre. The strategic health authority will take on the health the Gold role, co-ordinating the wider NHS's response to the incident if required and liaising with Department of Health should national coordination be required.

The duty ED consultant will take on the ED medical co-ordinator role providing operational level (Bronze) command of the ED and will lead, oversee and co-ordinate patient care within the emergency department. Other clinical and support personnel should also be aware of their roles in the response to a major incident, but to anticipate a lack of familiarity and to assist junior staff, everybody with a key role should be issued with an 'action card' when they report for duty. These cards are distributed according to clinical need and not personal choice.

Ordinarily a MERIT team response would not be requested from the nearest receiving hospital following a major incident.

Upon receipt of 'Major Incident Declared' by the hospital's switchboard or ED, a series of events should follow.

- Hospital areas cleared and readied.
- Off-duty staff call-in list activated using cascade systems.
- Set-up of communication systems.
- Command and control implemented (see Boxes 28.12, 28.13 and 28.14).

Box 28.12 Hospital response to an incident

Actions on receiving 'Major Incident – Stand By'

Medical, nursing and administrative co-ordinators meet and establish the control centre. They then:

- liaise with the ambulance service about the details and status of the incident
- start to prepare the emergency department for the reception of casualties
- warn theatres, the intensive care unit and outpatients department about the possible disruption of activities
- establish an accurate bed state.

Actions on receiving 'Major Incident Declared – Activate Plan'

If no prior warning, co-ordinators meet and establish the control centre. They then:

- establish whether MERITs are required; collect the teams, ensure the members are properly clothed and equipped, and dispatch them to the scene
- establish a triage point
- clear the emergency department of existing casualties and prepare for the reception of casualties
- inform theatres and outpatients department that normal activities must be suspended; ask the intensive care unit to clear beds if possible
- designate a ward for the reception of admitted casualties and start emptying it of existing patients
- organise staff as they arrive
- arrange facilities for the police, relatives and the media.

Box 28.13 Control centre equipment

- Stationery including triage labels and pre-issued patients' notes, labels and ID bracelets.
- Staff control board, with a list of staff roles and allocations.
- Patient control board, with the names of casualties, their triage priority and disposal details.
- Telephones for internal hospital use, plus a line to the press room and police documentation team.
- Signs to direct staff, relatives and the press.

Hospital staff should deploy initially to their usual work areas at predetermined locations, in or adjacent to the ED, as per their hospital's major incident plan

The HCT immediate priorities are to ensure that the ED is promptly cleared of patients and that steps are to taken to create inpatient capacity. Early decisions will need to be made about what other scheduled care (outpatients/elective operations, etc.), if any, will take place during the incident, and which additional clinical and administrative personnel should be deployed to support patient care in the ED.

Ambulance control, in liaison with the HCT, will constantly review the requirement as to whether or not non-major incident emergency patients are admitted to the EDs of receiving hospitals supporting the major incident or whether they are diverted to other hospitals further afield.

The ED medical co-ordinator (ED consultant) is in charge of co-ordination of clinical care in the ED receiving patients and will appoint an experienced clinician (triage officer) to assess patients on arrival at the ED and determine which clinical area of the ED will be used for their care. Additional ED co-ordinators (medical and nursing) will oversee clinical care in all key areas of the ED and ensure the appropriate composition of resuscitation teams, their resupply and rotation. Other key co-ordination roles within the ED include surgical, radiological and critical care prioritising patients for imaging, and damage control surgery, and critical care. A blood transfusion liaison officer will have a key role ensuring that sufficient blood and blood products are available for use in the ED/operating theatres and to oversee the early implementation of mass transfusion protocols if appropriate.

One of the key roles for the hospital's medical co-ordinator and the ED medical co-ordinator will be to ensure that the surge capacity of the ED is maintained throughout the duration of the incident. Central to this is ensuring that only absolutely essential investigations are undertaken in the ED and that early decisions are made by experienced surgeons regarding the requirement for emergency damage control surgery. Those not requiring immediate surgery should be transferred to appropriate wards/ITU at the earliest opportunity. In an overwhelming incident it may be necessary to secondarily transfer existing inpatients to other hospitals to ensure adequate ward capacity. Patients requiring complex multidisciplinary trauma care may also require secondary transfer to regional major trauma centres. Every effort will be made by the ambulance service to transfer such patients directly from the scene to tertiary hospitals, if there are the resources to do so.

The use of tabards in the ED, just as at the major incident scene, can greatly facilitate the ready identification of key ED staff, clinical co-ordinators and management personnel, and can contribute to the smooth running of the department throughout the incident.

Preparation usually depends on how much warning is received. Staff should report to pre-assigned designated areas and are allocated roles according to action cards. The reporting area should be outside the main ED to avoid congestion.

Special arrangements for other vital infrastructures such as portering, security, pharmacy, CSSD, facilities, clinical equipment and drug resupply will also need to be anticipated and actively managed by the HCT.

Patient identification and tracking are essential and appropriate documentation is vital if acceptable standards of clinical care and risk are to be maintained throughout a major incident. Pre-issued case notes and labels, bar-coded patient identity bracelets using standard hospital numbering systems, should be used for laboratory and imaging requests, and labelling patient property/clothing.

Close liaison with the police-run Casualty Bureau will be essential to ensure effective handling of enquiries from the public attempting to establish the whereabouts and well-being of family members caught up in the incident.

Equipment should be frequently checked and stored in a major incident room. Single-use emergency medical equipment should be stored in such a way to facilitate timely resupply of clinical areas. The use of white boards and information boards, communication/radios/runners/cellular phones, and special equipment such as showers, personal protective equipment suits, antidotes/vaccines and mobile surgical equipment may also be required. Equipment should be easily transportable and disposable items should be easily replaceable.

Recovery phase

When the medical or ambulance incident officer reports that the last casualty has left the site, and when all patients have been admitted to, or discharged from, the ED, the medical co-ordinator will declare a 'stand-down' of the major incident at the scene.

After such a major event, each service has a duty to restock and make itself operational again. There is also an important duty to staff for proper debriefing. It is an essential process to learn valuable lessons, both positive and negative, make recommendations for change and adapt service protocols if needed. Inevitably important lessons will be learned and acted upon; existing major incident plans should be reviewed and refined on the basis of such experience. It is also important to recognise that all hospital staff exposed to such incidents are vulnerable to psychological trauma and should be provided with appropriate information, support and follow-up as required.

Further reading

Advanced Life Support Group. (2011) *Major Incident Medical Management and Support. The Practical Approach at the Scene*, 3rd edn. Oxford: Wiley-Blackwell.

Department of Health. (2006) *NHS Emergency Planning Guidance 2005: Mass Casualties*. London: Department of Health.

Department of Health. (2007) *NHS Emergency Planning Guidance 2005: Underpinning Materials*. London: Department of Health.

Hodgetts TJ. (2002) EU Triage Position Statement: http://ec.europa.eu/echo/civil_protection/civil/prote/pdfdocs/disaster_med_final_2002/d6.pdf

Hodgetts TJ, Porter C. (2002) *Major Incident Management System*. Oxford: Wiley-Blackwell.

Major Incident Medical Management and Support: Hospital. http://www.alsg.org/uk/HIMMS

UK Department of Health Mass Casualty Clinical Equipment Vehicles: Background, Rationale & Contents (video) www.vimeo.com/6099244

CHAPTER 29

Trauma Systems in Developing Countries

Douglas Wilkinson

Oxford University Hospitals NHS Trust, Oxford, UK

OVERVIEW

- Trauma kills, prevention is best.
- A systematic approach to treating trauma victims saves lives.
- Any trauma system has been shown to be better than no system.
- The system should be appropriate, adaptable and affordable.
- A multidisciplinary doctor/nurse training programme is desirable to promote best practice in the treating trauma teams.

Trauma statistics in developing countries are notoriously difficult to assess accurately. In 1998 developing countries accounted for more than 85% of all deaths due to road traffic crashes globally, and for 96% of all children killed. Well over two-thirds of trauma worldwide occurs outside developed countries and over 50% of the trauma in developing countries occurs outside urban areas. Trauma is the second most common cause of death in 15–44 year olds. The Gross Domestic Product (GDP) of any country is dependent on this age group as its working populace and it is therefore vital that trauma management and the need for injury prevention are highlighted worldwide. In addition to road deaths and injury, developing countries also have a high incidence of other forms of injury including violent crime, civil and military unrest, landmine injuries, etc.

The need for a worldwide response to injury prevention and reducing the incidence of trauma has been highlighted for many years. However, the problems of trauma management in developing countries are legion.

Low economic countries often differ in social infrastructure, expenditure on health, political persuasion and educational levels of healthcare, making the use of a single uniform trauma training template to meet all needs very difficult.

Any trauma system in such countries needs to be:

- appropriate
- affordable
- adaptable
- sustainable.

ABC of Major Trauma, Fourth Edition. Edited by David V. Skinner and Peter A. Driscoll.
© 2013 Blackwell Publishing Ltd. Published 2013 by Blackwell Publishing Ltd.

Appropriate

Developing countries by definition have a differential between rich and poor, educated and uneducated and often huge geographical expanses make integration and corporate growth difficult. Different trauma systems will be briefly reviewed below but the challenge for a trauma system to be appropriate to that country or that region remains paramount.

Affordable

With the GDP of several countries being less than 20 US dollars per person per annum, affordable healthcare is essential. Issues relating to HIV prevention and maternal mortality take up much of a health budget alongside issues pertaining to immunisation, sanitation, etc. The indirect effect from trauma deaths has therefore not been included by healthcare budget planners in many countries both developed and developing. Many trauma systems are simply too expensive to be used in many developing countries.

Adaptable

In many developing countries teaching hospitals strive for western standards in education and in trauma training, which is questionable, whereas district hospital and clinics in the remoter areas often have very little appropriate trauma training, if any. 'One system to treat all' is a very tricky concept in a developing country as it is often necessary to vary the level of trauma training from a teaching hospital to a district hospital as in many areas doctors are simply not available. A trauma system therefore needs to be able to train up the healthcare professionals who are actually doing the work in their remote areas rather than solely relying on training doctors and senior clinicians in the centres.

Sustainable

The trauma system managed by a country's own Department of Health free of external donations, aid organisations and external interference may be seen as utopia. There is little doubt that financial sustainability in a developing country is a regular cause for failure of any trauma training scheme because trauma does not attract a high national and international profile, and local and national trauma prevention strategies and management schemes are often low down the list in a national healthcare budget. In addition to financial sustainability difficulties, quality assurance, levels of training and indeed audit of existing trauma systems in remote areas of countries which are financially challenged are difficult to set up and maintain. If a trauma system is going to be sustainable, it needs to have the support of the country's Ministry of Health, full support of the local medical societies and colleges and enjoy the benefits of World Health Organization (WHO) and other non-governmental organisation support.

The scale of the problem

Over the last 15 years the WHO and other organisations have begun to stress the importance of injury prevention and effective trauma care across the globe. It would appear that mortality resulting from trauma occurs in three time scales.

The **first peak** of death occurs immediately on impact due to internal injuries such as irruption of major vessels, acute injury, asphyxiation and massive internal organ disruption. No matter how advanced a nation's trauma system is, the only way to reduce the mortality in this initial stage is to prevent the injury happening in the first place. **Prevention** of injury is by far the most cost-effective and life-saving strategy that a country can embark on. The WHO's Department of Injuries and Violence Prevention in Geneva is working with governments throughout the world to look at strategies for reducing the incidence of trauma through education and legislation.

The **second peak** of death following an injury would be in the first hours after the injury where patients have survived the initial impact but could die from potentially survivable injuries such as lung damage, pneumothorax, haemothorax, slow internal bleeding and unstabilised limb fractures. Early diagnosis and a systematic approach of assessing a patient in these early hours would seem to reduce the mortality. It is not so much the 'golden hour' but the 'silver day' or the 'bronze week' that is realistic in remote areas.

It is encouraging to see that several developing countries are now working on improving prehospital training and first responders in their urban areas.

The **third peak** of deaths occurring several days to weeks after a traumatic event result from infection, sepsis and the delay in treating a patient earlier. Intensive care units are very expensive and therefore relatively rare in developing countries.

It is the prevention and early management of a severely traumatised patient that is cost effective in reducing mortality. The question therefore arises: what trauma systems are available to the developing countries and do they fulfil the above criteria?

Guidelines for Trauma Essential Care is a WHO publication which endeavours to identify and promote inexpensive ways of reinforcing trauma treatment worldwide. It is a laudable handbook seeking to accomplish this goal by better defining what essential trauma treatment services should realistically be made available to almost every injured person worldwide. It lists but does not quantify different trauma systems worldwide. Due to limited space, we will review Advanced Trauma Life Support and Primary Trauma Care systems in the context of this review.

Advanced Trauma Life Support

The American College of Surgeons started the very successful trauma system Advanced Trauma Life Support (ATLS) over 25 years ago which was designed for training doctors in America in the management of severely injured patients. It is a very comprehensive course, which is reviewed regularly. It is centrally controlled with a consistent quality assurance level for both the provider and the instructor course candidates. Many industrialised countries have adopted it with good effect.

Pertaining to the review of trauma systems in developing countries, the question is whether ATLS is an appropriate, affordable, adaptable and sustainable programme that can be used in such countries.

As mentioned above, a single system appropriate for teaching hospitals and smaller rural areas is unusual. ATLS is often restricted to large teaching institutions as it is expensive, and only a few chosen clinicians have access to this facility. The two-look concept of primary and secondary survey has been shown to be valuable in treating patients and is appropriate to all levels of care. The start-up and course costs for ATLS are expensive, and in order to maintain quality and training consistency, local adaptation is not possible. There has been some recent review of the ATLS system in the journals, considering its position and progress as well as questioning the validity of not having a national trauma scheme, as compared to paying another country to use their trauma scheme.

Primary Trauma Care

The Primary Trauma Care (PTC) management system is a robust, flexible cascade training model organised by the Primary Trauma Care Foundation and is designed to train doctors and nurses in developing countries in the management of the severely traumatised patient. It has been running since 1997 and is now available in 34 countries worldwide. The PTC manual (Figure 29.1) can be found free on the internet and is translated into 11 languages. The manual is also published by the WHO as an annexe to the *Surgical Care at the District Hospital* publication.

The PTC manual is intended to be used in conjunction with the two-day PTC course which trains people to review trauma prevention strategies and to manage the severely traumatised patient in a systematic protocolised way.

These PTC courses are designed to be run by local healthcare professionals, thereby providing trauma training at the local level.

This trauma system is designed to empower local educational and medical facilities to use the course material and trains doctors and nurses with equipment they have to treat the patients effectively. The initial courses run though the Primary Trauma Care Foundation are offered to a country free and once the manual and slides have been adapted and translated to the local country, they are offered to the medical organisations or Ministry of Health to adapt as a basis for a national trauma scheme. The PTC programme is therefore appropriate and affordable and encourages adaptation to the local environment. In order to be financially sustainable any revenue raised by the organisers is used to offset local and basic costs. Quality assurance and regular audit are essential to ascertain levels

Primary Trauma Care

Introduction

Trauma transcends all national boundaries. Many less affluent countries have a significant proportion of road and industrial trauma in a generally young population. Morbidity and mortality associated with such trauma can be reduced by early and effective medical intervention.

This Primary Trauma Care course is intended to provide basic knowledge and skills necessary to identify and treat those traumatised patients who require rapid assessment, resuscitation and stabilisation of their injuries. This course will particularly highlight the need for early recognition and timely intervention in specific life-threatening conditions.

This course is intended to provide material by lectures and practical skill stations that represents an acceptable method of management for trauma. It provides a very basic foundation on which doctors and health workers can build the necessary knowledge and skills for trauma management with minimal equipment and without sophisticated technological requirements.

There are several very successful and well organised trauma courses and manuals available, including the American College of Surgeons ATLS™ course and the EMST Australian course. These courses are directed to medical personnel in well equipped hospitals with oxygen, communication and transport etc. and offer a comprehensive syllabus. The Primary Trauma Care is not a substitute for these courses, but uses similar basic principles and emphasises basic trauma care with minimal resources.

The Objectives

At the completion of this course you should:

1. Understand the priorities of trauma management
2. Be able to rapidly and accurately assess trauma patients needs
3. Be able to resuscitate and stabilise trauma patients
4. Know how to organise basic trauma care in your hospital.

Primary Trauma Care

Trauma in Perspective

Most countries of the world are experiencing an epidemic of trauma, but the most spectacular increase has been in the developing countries. Proliferation of roads and use of vehicles has led to a rapid increase in injuries and deaths and many peripheral medical facilities find themselves faced with multiple casualties from bus crashes or other disasters. Severe burns are also common in both urban and rural areas.

A number of important differences between high and low-income countries make development of a specifically designed Primary Trauma Care Course beneficial. They include:

- the great distances over which casualties may have to be transported to reach a medical facility
- the time taken for patients to reach medical care
- the absence of high-tech equipment and supplies
- the absence of skilled people to operate and service it.

PREVENTION of trauma is by far the cheapest and safest mode to manage trauma. This depends on the location's resources and factors such as:

- culture
- manpower
- politics
- health budget
- training.

Every effort should be made by the medical trauma teams to address the above factors in the prevention of trauma. Much of this lies beyond the scope of this manual, but time will be spent on the course looking at local circumstances and prevention possibilities.

Figure 29.1 An extract from the PTC manual. (Extracted from the Primary Trauma Care Manual with permission from the Primary Trauma Care Foundation.)

Primary Trauma Care

ABCDE of Trauma

The management of severe multiple injury requires clear recognition of management priorities and the goal is to determine in the initial assessment those injuries that threaten the patient's life. This first survey, the 'primary' survey, if done correctly should identify such life-threatening injuries such as:

- airway obstruction
- chest injuries with breathing difficulties
- severe external or internal haemorrhage
- abdominal injuries.

If there is more than one injured patient then treat patients in order of priority (Triage). This depends on experience and resources (Discussed in the practical sessions).

The ABCDE survey (Airway, Breathing, Circulation, Disability and Exposure) is undertaken. This primary survey must be performed in no more than 2–5 minutes. Simultaneous treatment of injuries can occur when more than one life-threatening state exists. It includes:

• Airway

Assess the airway. Can patient talk and breathe freely? If obstructed, the steps to be considered are:

- chin lift/jaw thrust (tongue is attached to the jaw)
- suction (if available)
- guedel airway/nasopharyngeal airway
- intubation. NB keep the neck immobilised in neutral position.

• Breathing

Breathing is assessed as airway patency and breathing adequacy are re-checked. If inadequate, the steps to be considered are:

- decompression and drainage of tension pneumothorax/haemothorax
- closure of open chest injury
- artificial ventilation.

Give oxygen if available.

Primary Trauma Care

• Circulation

Assess circulation, as oxygen supply, airway patency and breathing adequacy are re-checked. If inadequate, the steps to be considered are:

- stop external haemorrhage
- establish 2 large-bore IV lines (14 or 16 G) if possible
- administer fluid if available.

• Disability

Rapid neurological assessment (is patient awake, vocally responsive to pain or unconscious). There is no time to do the Glasgow Coma Scale so a

- awake   A
- verbal response   V
- painful response   P
- unresponsive   U

system at this stage is clear and quick.

• Exposure

Undress patient and look for injury. If the patient is suspected of having a neck or spinal injury, in-line immobilization is important. This will be discussed in the practical sessions.

NOTES….✎

Reassessment of ABC's must be undertaken if patient is unstable

Figure 29.1 (Continued)

of teaching in this cascade model, as without local national levels of competence, consistent trauma training could vary widely.

The PTC manual and more information on the Primary Trauma Care Foundation can be found at www.primarytraumacare.org.

Further reading

Ali J, Adam R, Butler A, *et al.* (1993) Trauma outcome improves following the advanced trauma life support programme in a developing country. J Trauma 34: 890–8.

Carmont M. (2005) The origins, development and success of the ATLS course. Postgrad Med J 81(952): 87–91.

Davis M. (2005) Should there be a UK based advanced trauma course? Emerg Med J 22(1): 5–6.

Driscoll P, Wardrope J. (2005) ATLS: past, present and future. Emerg Med J 22(1): 2–3.

Krantz BE. (1999) The international ATLS programme. Trauma Quart 14: 323–8.

Krug E. (2004) *Road Traffic Injuries.* Geneva: World Health Organization.

Nantulya N, Reich M. (2002) The neglected epidemic of road traffic injuries in developing countries. BMJ 324: 1139–41.

Nolan J. (2005) ATLS in the UK: time to move on. Emerg Med J 22(1): 3–4.

Wilkinson D, Skinner M. (2000) *Primary Trauma Care Manual.* Oxford: Primary Trauma Care Foundation.

World Health Organization. (2003) *Surgical Care at the District Hospital.* Geneva: World Health Organization.

World Health Organization. (2004) *Guidelines for Essential Trauma Care.* Geneva: World Health Organization.

Zwi A, Forjuoh S, Muruqusampillay S, Odero W, Watts C. (1996) Injuries in developing countries – policy response needed now. Trans Roy Soc Trop Med Hyg 90: 593–5.

Index

Note: Page numbers in *italics* refer to Figures; those in **bold** refer to Tables and Boxes

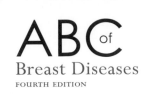

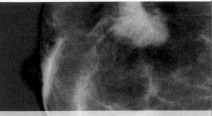

ABC of Breast Diseases

4TH EDITION

J. Michael Dixon
Western General Hospital, Edinburgh, UK

Breast diseases are common and often encountered by health professionals in primary care. While the incidence of breast cancer is increasing, earlier detection and improved treatments are helping to reduce breast cancer mortality. The *ABC of Breast Diseases, 4th Edition*:

- Provides comprehensive guidance to the assessment of symptoms, how to manage common breast conditions and guidelines on referral
- Covers congenital problems, breast infection and mastalgia, before addressing the epidemiology, prevention, screening and diagnosis of breast cancer and outlines the treatment and management options for breast cancer within different groups
- Includes new chapters on the genetics, prevention, management of high risk women and the psychological aspects of breast diseases
- Is ideal for GPs, family physicians, practice nurses and breast care nurses as well as for surgeons and oncologists both in training and recently qualified as well as medical students

AUGUST 2012 | 9781444337969 | 168 PAGES | £27.99/US$46.95/€35.90/AU$52.95

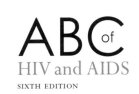

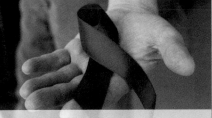

ABC of HIV and AIDS

6TH EDITION

Michael W. Adler, Simon G. Edwards, Robert F. Miller, Gulshan Sethi & Ian Williams
University College London Medical School; Mortimer Market Centre, London; University College London; St Thomas' Hospital, London Medical School; University College London Medical School

Since the previous edition, big advances have been made in treatment, knowledge of the disease and epidemiology. The problem of AIDS in developing countries has become a major political and humanitarian issue.

- Edited by the Director of the Department for Sexually Transmitted Diseases, *ABC of HIV and AIDS, 6th Edition* is an authoritative guide to the epidemiology, incidence, and most up to date management of HIV and AIDS
- Reflects the constantly changing knowledge of the disease and its manifestations, new developments in drug and non-drug management, sociological and political issues
- Includes 6 new chapters on conditions associated with AIDS and further concentration on the community effects of the disease, and the situation of women with AIDS
- Ideal for all levels of health care workers caring for HIV and AIDS patients

JUNE 2012 | 9781405157001 | 144 PAGES | £24.99/US$49.95/€32.90/AU$47.95